Occupational Medicine

Diagnostic Testing

Guest Editor:

Michael H. LeWitt, MD, MPH
Medical Director
Occupational Medicine
Great Valley Health
Paoli Memorial Hospital
Jefferson Health System
Paoli, Pennsylvania

Publisher: HANLEY & BELFUS, INC.
210 South 13th Street
Philadelphia, PA 19107
(215) 546-4995
Fax (215) 790-9330
Web site: http://www.hanleyandbelfus.com

OCCUPATIONAL MEDICINE: State of the Art Reviews is included in *Index Medicus, MEDLINE, BioSciences Information Service, Current Contents* and *ISI/BIOMED.*

Authorization to photocopy items for internal or personal use, or the internal or personal use of specific clients, is granted by Hanley & Belfus, Inc. for libraries and other users registered with the Copyright Clearance Center (CCC) Transaction Reporting Service, provided that the base fee of $1.00 per copy plus $0.25 per page is paid directly to the CCC, 21 Congress St., Salem, MA 01970. Identify this publication by including with your payment the fee code, 0885-114X/96 $1.00 + .25.

OCCUPATIONAL MEDICINE: State of the Art Reviews	(ISSN 0885-114X)
July-September 1997 Volume 12, Number 3	(ISBN 1-56053-244-0)

© 1997 by Hanley & Belfus, Inc. under the International Copyright Union. All rights reserved. No part of this book may be reproduced, reused, republished, transmitted in any form or by any means, or stored in a data base or retrieval system without written permission of the publisher. An exception is chapters written by employees of U.S. government agencies; these chapters are public domain.

OCCUPATIONAL MEDICINE: State of the Art Reviews is published quarterly by Hanley & Belfus, Inc., 210 South 13th Street, Philadelphia, Pennsylvania 19107. Periodical postage paid at Philadelphia, PA, and at additional mailing offices.

POSTMASTER: Send address changes to OCCUPATIONAL MEDICINE: State of the Art Reviews, Hanley & Belfus, Inc., 210 South 13th Street, Philadelphia, PA 19107.

The 1997 subscription price is $88.00 per year U.S., $98.00 outside U.S. (add $40.00 for air mail).

Occupational Medicine: State of the Art Reviews
Vol. 12, No. 3, July–September 1997

DIAGNOSTIC TESTING
Michael H. LeWitt, MD, MPH, Editor

CONTENTS

Preface xi
Michael H. LeWitt

Neuropsychological Evaluation 413
James D. Seward

> The neuropsychological evaluation is differentiated from psychiatric, psychological, and neurological evaluations, with attention to the neuropsychologist's function and accreditation. Common neuropsychologic tests, such as those used to measure memory, intelligence, visual perception, emotional functioning, and language, are described.

Audiologic Testing: An Overview for Occupational Physicians 433
Robert T. Sataloff and Joseph Sataloff

> This chapter summarizes the audiologic tests likely to be encountered by occupational physicians caring for workers with hearing loss complaints. These include audiometric tests, electrocochleography, evoked-response audiometry, and tests designed to examine for central nervous system damage.

Testing the Afferent Visual System 449
Lawrence G. Gray

> Dr. Gray details a variety of tests that can help to determine the source of reduced acuity and describes how patients prone to malingering or symptom magnification can be revealed through specific challenges.

Clinical Disorders of Smell and Taste 465
Beverly J. Cowart, I.M. Young, Roy S. Feldman, and Louis D. Lowry

> Renewed attention to chemosensory dysfunction has revealed that a substantial portion of the population are affected during their lives, many simply as a result of aging. The authors discuss terminology, assessment, etiology, and prognosis and compare current understanding with that presented by Mackenzie in 1884.

**Occupational Respiratory Function Testing—
An Algorithmic Approach** 485
Philip Harber and David Discher

> The authors stress the importance of matching tests to the functions under examination and offer a systematic approach to selection, performance, and interpretation of tests in occupational medicine practices.

Diagnostic Testing of Cardiac Function 513
Timothy A. Shapiro and Paul M. Coady

> The electrocardiogram's value in detecting atrial abnormalities, ventricular hypertrophy, and myocardial injury is described, with attention to ambulatory monitoring and exercise stress testing. Perfusion imaging, assessment of resting cardiac function with echocardiography, and other techniques also are addressed.

The Independent Medical Examination and the Functional Capacity Evaluation 525
John Kraus

> Independent medical examinations (IMEs) are requested most commonly for conditions related to musculoskeletal problems. This chapter thoroughly delineates the IME process, illustrating points with universal applicability, but focusing on assessment of musculoskeletal disease. The functional capacity evaluation, for determination of task performance ability, also is addressed.

The Role of the Clinical Laboratory in Occupational Medicine 557
Jack W. Snyder

> The pre-analytic, analytic, and post-analytic stages of laboratory testing present challenges to the attainment of accurate and timely information. These include sampling errors, quality control, and interpretation of results. Learning about the benefits and limitations of specific tests allows the physician to use the laboratory more productively and cost-effectively.

Epidemiology and Biostatistics 587
Michael H. LeWitt

> Dr. LeWitt presents an introduction to epidemiology and biostatistics, with a review of commonly used terms and concepts.

Index 601

PUBLISHED ISSUES
(available from the publisher)

January 1989	**The Management Perspective**	
	L. Fleming Fallon, Jr., O.B. Dickerson, and Paul W. Brandt-Rauf, Editors	
April 1989	**Alcoholism and Chemical Dependency**	
	Curtis Wright, Editor	
October 1989	**Problem Buildings**	
	James E. Cone and Michael Hodgson, Editors	
January 1990	**Hazardous Waste Workers**	
	Michael Gochfeld and Elissa Ann Favata, Editors	
April 1990	**Shiftwork**	
	Allene J. Scott, Editor	
July 1990	**Medical Surveillance in the Workplace**	
	David Rempel, Editor	
October 1990	**Worksite Health Promotion**	
	Michael E. Scofield, Editor	
January 1991	**Prevention of Pulmonary Disease in the Workplace**	
	Philip Harber and John R. Balmes, Editors	
April 1991	**The Biotechnology Industry**	
	Alan M. Ducatman and Daniel F. Liberman, Editors	
July 1991	**Health Hazards of Farming**	
	D. H. Cordes and Dorothy Foster Rea, Editors	
October 1991	**The Nuclear Energy Industry**	
	Gregg S. Wilkinson, Editor	
January 1992	**Back School Programs**	
	Lynne A. White, Editor	
April 1992	**Occupational Lung Disease**	
	William S. Beckett and Rebecca Bascom, Editors	
July 1992	**Unusual Occupational Diseases**	
	Dennis J. Shusterman and Paul D. Blanc, Editors	
October 1992	**Ergonomics**	
	J. Steven Moore and Arun Garg, Editors	
January 1993	**The Mining Industry**	
	Daniel E. Banks, Editor	
April 1993	**Spirometry**	
	Ellen A. Eisen, Editor	
July 1993	**De Novo Toxicants**	
	Dennis J. Shusterman and Jack E. Peterson, Editors	
October 1993	**Women Workers**	
	Dana M. Headapohl, Editor	
January 1994	**Occupational Skin Disease**	
	James R. Nethercott, Editor	
April 1994	**Safety and Health Training**	
	Michael J. Colligan, Editor	
July 1994	**Reproductive Hazards**	
	Ellen B. Gold, B. L. Lasley, and Marc B. Schenker, Editors	
October 1994	**Tuberculosis in the Workplace**	
	Steven Markowitz, Editor	

1997 ISSUES

The Pharmaceutical Industry
Edited by Gregg M. Stave, MD, JD, MPH
Occupational Health Services
Glaxo Wellcome Inc.
Research Triangle Park, North Carolina
and Ron Joines, MD, MPH
SmithKline Beecham
Philadelphia, Pennsylvania

Human Health Effects of Pesticides
Edited by Matthew C. Keifer, MD, MPH
Harborview Medical Center
Seattle Washington

Diagnostic Testing
Edited by Michael H. LeWitt, MD
Great Velley Health
Paoli, Pennsylvania

Health Care Hazards
Edited by Melissa A. McDiarmid, MD, MPH
U.S. Department of Labor/OSHA
Washington, DC
and Ellen Kessler, MD, MPH
Fairfax Hospital
Falls Church, Virginia

1996 ISSUES

Law and the Workplace
Edited by Jack W. Snyder, MD, JD, PhD
Thomas Jefferson University Hospital
Philadelphia, Pennsylvania
and Julia E. Klees, MD, MPH
BASF Corporation
Mount Olive, New Jersey

Violence in the Workplace
Edited by Robert Harrison, MD, MPH
California Department of Health Services
Berkeley, California

Occupational Epidemiology
Edited by Ki Moon Bang, PhD, MPH
National Institute for Occupational Safety
  and Health
Morgantown, West Virginia

**Psychosocial and Corporate Issues
in Occupational Dysfunction**
Edited by Ibrahim Farid, MD, PhD
United States Postal Service
South San Francisco, California
and Carroll Brodsky, MD, PhD
University of California School of Medicine
San Francisco, California

Ordering Information:
Subscriptions for full year and single issues are available from the publishers—
Hanley & Belfus, Inc., 210 South 13th Street, Philadelphia, PA 19107
Telephone (215) 546-7293; (800) 962-1892. Fax (215) 790-9330.

1995 ISSUES

Effects of the Indoor Environment on Health
Edited by James M. Seltzer, MD
University of California School of Medicine
San Diego, California

Construction Safety and Health
Edited by Knut Ringen, DrPH,
Laura Welch, MD, James L. Weeks, ScD, CIH,
and Jane L. Seegal, MS
Washington, DC
and Anders Englund, MD
Solna, Sweden

Occupational Hearing Loss
Edited by Thais C. Morata, PhD,
and Derek E. Dunn, PhD
National Institute for Occupational Safety
and Health
Cincinnati, Ohio

Firefighters' Safety and Health
Edited by Peter Orris, MD
Cook County Hospital
Chicago, Illinois
and Richard M. Duffy, MSc
International Association of Fire Fighters
Washington, DC
and James Melius, MD, DrPH
Center to Protect Workers' Rights
Washington, DC

Ordering Information:
Subscriptions for full year and single issues are available from the publishers—
Hanley & Belfus, Inc., 210 South 13th Street, Philadelphia, PA 19107
Telephone (215) 546-7293; (800) 962-1892. Fax (215) 790-9330.

CONTRIBUTORS

Paul M. Coady, MD
Clinical Assistant Professor of Medicine, Department of Medicine, Thomas Jefferson University, Philadelphia; Lankenau Hospital, Wynnewood, Pennsylvania

Beverly J. Cowart, PhD
Member, Monell Chemical Senses Center, Philadelphia; Adjunct Assistant Professor (Research), Department of Otolaryngology–Head and Neck Surgery, Thomas Jefferson University, Philadelphia, Pennsylvania

David P. Discher, MD
Private Consultant, Occupational and Environmental Medicine, Sunnyvale, California

Roy S. Feldman, DDS, DMSc
Chief, Dental Service, Veterans Affairs Medical Center, Philadelphia, Pennsylvania

Lawrence G. Gray, OD
Clinical Assistant Professor of Neurology and Ophthalmology, Allegheny University of the Health Sciences; Chief, Neuro-ophthalmic Disease Service, The Eye Institute of the Pennsylvania College of Optometry; Adjunct Assistant Professor of Neurology, Hospital of the University of Pennsylvania, Philadelphia, Pennsylvania

Philip Harber, MD, MPH
Professor of Medicine, University of California, Los Angeles, California

John Kraus, MD, MMM
Chief Medical Officer, Bryn Mawr Rehabilitation Hospital, Malvern; Instructor, Department of Rehabilitation Medicine, Jefferson Medical College, Philadelphia, Pennsylvania

Michael H. LeWitt, MD
Medical Director, Occupational Medicine, Great Valley Health, Paoli Memorial Hospital, Jefferson Health System, Paoli, Pennsylvania

Louis D. Lowry, MD
Professor and Vice Chairman, Department of Otolaryngology–Head and Neck Surgery, Thomas Jefferson University, Philadelphia, Pennsylvania

Robert Thayer Sataloff, MD, DMA
Professor, Department of Otolaryngology, Jefferson Medical College; Chairman, Department of Otolaryngology–Head and Neck Surgery, The Graduate Hospital, Philadelphia, Pennsylvania

Joseph Sataloff, MD, DSc
Professor, Department of Otolaryngology–Head and Neck Surgery, Jefferson Medical College, Philadelphia, Pennsylvania

James D. Seward, PhD
Neuropsychologist, Department of Psychology, Bryn Mawr Rehabilitation Hospital, Malvern, Pennsylvania

Timothy A. Shapiro, MD
Clinical Associate of Medicine, Department of Medicine, Hospital of the University of Pennsylvania, Philadelphia; Lankenau Hospital, Wynnewood, Pennsylvania

Jack Snyder, MD, JD, MPH, PhD
Associate Professor, Departments of Emergency Medicine and Laboratory Medicine, Thomas Jefferson University, Philadelphia, Pennsylvania

In Min Young, MD
Professor, Department of Otolaryngology–Head and Neck Surgery, Thomas Jefferson University, Philadelphia, Pennsylvania

PREFACE

This issue of *Occupational Medicine: State of the Art Reviews* on diagnostic testing is targeted for the occupational and environmental physician, but also has applicability for the physician in any setting where diagnostic testing is used. The text provides a variety of information about the wide range of tests that are relevant in the practice of occupational and environmental medicine. It also presents, where appropriate, alternative methods for gaining knowledge about potential and actual clinical conditions, whether as a result of exposure, or relating to health in general.

This book arose out of a need for concise yet thorough discussions of testing resources, compiled in one source. The authors and editor hope that the information presented meets the needs of the practicing clinician.

There are other aspects of testing that may be helpful for physicians, but due to space limitations these could not be included. Neurology as it pertains to neuromuscular testing is nicely covered in Occupational Medicine 7(4):765–783, 1992; dermatology is discussed in 7(3):385–401, 1992 and 9(1):1–9, 37–44, and 45–52, 1994; and evaluation of reproductive hazards is presented in 9(3): 387–404 and 423–433, 1994.

I would like to thank all of the authors for their work in preparing the chapters. I also thank my prior teachers for their guidance and encouragement. Additionally, I would like to thank my family from whom I took the time to write and edit.

Michael H. LeWitt, MD, MPH
GUEST EDITOR

JAMES D. SEWARD, PhD

NEUROPSYCHOLOGICAL EVALUATION

From the Bryn Mawr Rehabilitation Hospital
Malvern, Pennsylvania

Reprint requests to:
James D. Seward, PhD
Bryn Mawr Rehabilitation Hospital
414 Paoli Pike
Malvern, PA 19355

A neuropsychological evaluation is an in-depth and comprehensive examination of a patient's mental functioning. Areas assessed include attention and concentration, memory, problem solving, speech and language, intellectual level, motor abilities, sensory and perceptual abilities, academic achievement, and emotional condition.

The purpose of the neuropsychological evaluation is to determine the patient's pattern of mental strengths and weaknesses, with emphasis on how this pattern will affect the patient's ability to perform myriad day-to-day social and vocational tasks. In addition, a neuropsychological evaluation can be an invaluable tool in the process of diagnosing and following conditions such as dementia, brain injury, neurotoxic exposure, and various neurologic conditions. For example, patients who have sustained a traumatic brain injury, stroke, or have some other neurologic condition may be referred to ascertain their level of cognitive functioning and to make recommendations for treatment. Serial evaluations are especially helpful to document the course of recovery. Referrals also may be made to diagnose elderly persons with suspected or possible dementia or to detect brain dysfunction in injured workers with mild traumatic brain injury or exposure to neurotoxins.

The top five referral sources for neuropsychologists, listed in order, are neurologists, psychiatrists, rehabilitation specialists, attorneys, and neurosurgeons.[55]

Due to its comprehensive nature, a neuropsychological evaluation is a long process. The average evaluation, including report writing, takes approximately 9 hours.[55]

Confusion exists as to the difference between a psychiatric, psychological, or neurologic evaluation and a neuropsychological evaluation.[49] A neuropsychological evaluation examines the previously mentioned areas of mental functioning via the use of a clinical interview, observations of the patient, review of collateral information, and the administration of neuropsychological and psychological tests. A psychological evaluation may incorporate portions of these sources of data, but the focus is typically more limited, being restricted to the patient's emotional condition or level of intellectual function. A psychiatric evaluation is usually conducted to establish a diagnosis according to *DSM-IV*[2] and possibly to recommend appropriate treatment, which often involves psychotropic medications. The process consists of a clinical interview and, when appropriate, a review of collateral information. Psychiatrists may administer a standardized mental status examination, such as the Mini Mental State,[16] or a self-report rating scale, such as the Beck Depression Inventory.[6] However, they do not administer comprehensive psychological or neuropsychological tests; in many states, nonpsychologists are prevented by law from administering psychological tests and procedures. Finally, an examination by a neurologist is focused on signs and symptoms of neurologic dysfunction. The neurologist will examine the patient's entire nervous system, including peripheral and spinal nerves. The neurologist also may order studies such as electroencephalogram, magnetic resonance, computed tomography, positron emission tomography, or single photon emission computed tomography.

In the United States, the title "neuropsychologist" is only legally protected in Louisiana. In the other states and territories, any licensed or certified psychologist can call himself or herself a neuropsychologist and can provide neuropsychology services. This results in a wide variation in the quality of these services.

In an attempt to rectify this, Division 40 of the American Psychological Association proposed a definition of neuropsychologist in 1988[12] (Table 1). However, this definition has no legal power.

TABLE 1. Definition of a Clinical Neuropsychologist

THE FOLLOWING STATEMENT WAS ADOPTED BY THE EXECUTIVE COMMITTEE OF DIVISION 40 AT THE AMERICAN PSYCHOLOGICAL ASSOCIATION MEETING ON AUGUST 12, 1988
A Clinical Neuropsychologist is a professional psychologist who applies principles of assessment and intervention based upon the scientific study of human behavior as it relates to normal and abnormal functioning of the central nervous system. The Clinical Neuropsychologist is a doctoral-level provider of diagnostic and intervention services who has demonstrated competence in the application of such principles for human welfare following:
A. Successful completion of systematic didactic and experiential training in neuropsychology and neuroscience at a regionally accredited university;
B. Two or more years of appropriate supervised training applying neuropsychological services in a clinical setting;
C. Licensing and certification to provide psychological services to the public by the laws of the state or province in which he or she practices;
D. Review by one's peers as a test of these competencies.
Attainment of the ABCN/ABPP Diploma in Clinical Neuropsychology is the clearest evidence of competence as a Clinical Neuropsychologist, assuring that all of these criteria have been met.

American Psychological Association
From Division 40, American Psychological Association: Definition of a clinical neuropsychologist. Clin Neuropsychol 3:22, 1989; with permission.

Currently, neuropsychologists are certified largely by two boards: the American Board of Clinical Neuropsychology and the American Board of Professional Neuropsychology. Both organizations will provide a list of diplomates upon request. In addition, several professional organizations are dedicated to neuropsychology: the National Academy of Neuropsychology, the International Neuropsychological Society, and Division 40 of the American Psychological Association. The membership requirements for these organizations are not as stringent as are those for board certification; however, membership in one or more of these societies indicates that a neuropsychologist has access to the recent literature (in the form of the organization's journal) and is a member of the scientific community. There are a number of other organizations that a provider of neuropsychology services may join to bill himself or herself as "board certified"; however, the requirements for many of these boards are minimal, and membership does not necessarily indicate any special competence. When in doubt as to the significance of board certification, the referring physician should ask for specifics about the certifying process and requirements.

Neuropsychologists will sometimes make use of "technicians" to perform some or all of the testing.[10,55] Division 40 of the American Psychological Association provides guidelines for the use of these personnel.[13] The author believes that technicians should be used with caution, in that much information can be obtained by a professional observing the patient engage in a variety of tasks over an extended time. Regardless of whether technicians are used, the neuropsychologist maintains complete responsibility for the evaluation.

THE NEUROPSYCHOLOGICAL EVALUATION

The scope and comprehensiveness of a neuropsychological evaluation are determined by the characteristics of the patient and the referral question. In an inpatient setting, the referral question may be specific (e.g., "Will the patient's memory deficits affect his ability to benefit from physical therapy?") or the patient may be elderly or ill. In these cases, a comprehensive evaluation may not be conducted, and the patient may be seen only for an hour-long consult; implied here is the importance of the referral source providing a specific referral question. However, in outpatient referrals, especially in workers' compensation cases or other situations with legal implications, a comprehensive evaluation is warranted.

The Triad Model of Evaluation

When training students and fellows, the analogy of a three-legged stool helps to illustrate the importance of using different sources of information in a comprehensive neuropsychological evaluation. Each leg represents a general category of information that should be incorporated into the evaluation. In this author's opinion, the integration of diverse sources of information is the difference between neuropsychological testing—that is, administration of a group of standardized tests—and neuropsychological evaluation.

When performing a comprehensive neuropsychological evaluation, the neuropsychologist should not depend solely on the results of testing but should integrate data from a variety of sources, including the patient's records, information from significant others, and observations and interview of the patient during the testing itself and during breaks and other "down time" (Table 2). Some sources of information are discussed below.

TABLE 2. Factors Used in Clinical Assessment in a Neuropsychological Evaluation

Patient's complaints
Observations of significant others
History of Problem
Background history
Childhood/Development
Educational/Achievement
Health/Medical
Occupational/Recreational
Family/Marital
Psychiatric/Neurologic
Criminal/Legal
Drugs/Substance Abuse
Behavioral observations
Review of records
Educational
Medical/Psychiatric
Vocational/Employment
Psychological/Neuropsychological Testing
Quantitative scores
Qualitative analysis

From Purisch AD, Sbordone RJ: Forensic Neuropsychology: Going Beyond the Test Data. Irvine, CA, Neuropsychological Associates of California, undated; with permission.

Background Information

Record Review

The referral source should make as much information available as possible to ensure the comprehensiveness of the report. Valuable sources of information are academic records, including the results of standardized testing; military records; and, in cases of traumatic injury, records from the emergency personnel and the hospital.

Occupational medicine physicians are often in a good position to do this in that they may have access to the patient's employment records. It is especially helpful to examine documents that the employee may have completed premorbidly in his or her own hand, such as requests for time off. This can often help to estimate the employee's premorbid level of functioning.

Reports from Significant Others

An interview with family members or caregivers of the patient is a valuable source of information about the patient's functioning. Rating scales and questionnaires can be completed by significant others to supplement the interviews with these sources. The Cognitive Behavior Ratings Scales[64] (CBRS) is an example of the former. It consists of 116 items that a family member or other reliable observer completes in regard to the patient's day-to-day behavior. The items fall into nine scales: language deficit, agitation, need for routine, depression, higher cognitive deficits, memory disorder, dementia, apraxia, and disorientation. Another example is the Katz Adjustment Scale–Relative's Form[31] (KAS–R). The KAS–R consists of 127 items for which the person filling out the form is instructed to rate the patient's behavior over the preceding few weeks. Factor analysis of these scores produced 13 factors: belligerence, verbal expansiveness, negativism, helplessness, suspiciousness, anxiety, withdrawal, psychopathology, nervousness, confusion, bizarreness, hyperactivity, and stability. The Significant Others Questionnaire[44] provides a more subjective, qualitative approach to information gathering. It consists of a number of short essay-type questions that allow a family member or caregiver to provide information on the patient's deficits with emphasis on how these deficits have affected his or her ability to function at home, at work, in school, socially, and within the family.

Observations and Interview of the Patient

Examples of potential valuable observations of the patient include reports of waiting room behaviors such as informal interactions with other staff and patients and the use of magazines and books. When working in a hospital, it is helpful to note whether the patient can find his or her way back from the restroom during breaks—a task that can be difficult for patients with impaired spatial skills.

The clinical interview with the patient can be supplemented with a questionnaire such as the Neuropsychological Symptom Checklist (NSC), which is part of the Neuropsychological Status Examination.[50] This form lists common symptoms associated with neurologic disease and injury. It is sometimes helpful to give a copy of this form to a family member to complete in regard to the patient. Comparison of the two forms can be diagnostic. A patient with a severe brain injury will often deny or minimize any symptoms, but family members are likely to report a number of difficulties.[49] However, some researchers caution that a checklist such as the NSC may have a "leading nature," thus informing malingering subjects about potential symptoms.[35]

Integration of information from different sources is especially important because a number of factors can influence test results (Table 3). It is only through such knowledge that the applicability of these factors to the evaluation can be determined.

Of particular importance given the multicultural workforce is a knowledge of the possible effects of the patient's linguistic and cultural background on the results of the evaluation. For example, in one study the race of the examiner and the level of mistrust of whites significantly affected the IQ test performance of black students.[57] The American Psychological Association has formulated guidelines for assessing

TABLE 3. Issues that Confound Test Interpretation

Patient failed to understand instructions	Antagonism toward examiner
Sensory difficulties	Time of day
Peripheral neurological difficulties	Low blood sugar level
Poor motivation	Previous assessment history
Fatigue	Pain
Anxiety	Age of patient
Depression	Ethnic background of patient
Psychotic thinking	Cultural background of patient
Medications	Premorbid intelligence level
Medical diseases	History of premorbid learning disability
Malingering	Attentional difficulties
Hysteria	Motor difficulties
Litigation	Familarity with tests
Alcoholism	Background and experience of examiner
Substance abuse	Recent emotional stresses

From Purisch AD, Sbordone RJ: Forensic Neuropsychology: Going Beyond the Test Data. Irvine, CA, Neuropsychological Associates of California, undated; with permission.

members of diverse populations, of which neuropsychologists and psychologists should be aware.[3]

Malingering

The triad approach to evaluation presented in this chapter can be helpful to rule out malingering. The neuropsychologist should look for inconsistencies between the patient's performance on the tests, informal observations of his or her behavior, background information, and the reports of significant others. Other specific ways of ruling out malingering are detailed by Lezak.[37]

SPECIFIC TESTS

This chapter does not present a comprehensive description of various neuropsychological and psychological tests; readers are referred to Lezak's encyclopedic text on neuropsychological assessment.[37] The aim is to provide an introduction to frequently used tests. Only tests designed primarily for use with working-age adults are described.

Although a goal of this chapter is to be descriptive rather than critical, all of the tests discussed, with the exception of "projective" personality tests, have been shown to have some utility in neuropsychological assessment. The neuropsychologist should be aware of the specific psychometric strengths and weaknesses of each procedure.

There are three primary "philosophical" approaches to test selection: the flexible approach, the flexible battery approach, and the standardized battery approach[55] (Table 4). More than half of the clinical neuropsychologists who responded to a recent survey use a flexible battery approach, about a quarter use a flexible approach, and the rest use a standardized battery.[55]

Test Batteries

Test batteries are groups of individual tests assembled with the primary goal of providing a standard data collection procedure by assessing a broad sample of behavior.[37] There are two frequently used batteries: the Luria-Nebraska Neuropsychological Battery and the Halstead-Reitan Neuropsychological Battery.

THE LURIA-NEBRASKA NEUROPSYCHOLOGICAL BATTERY

The Luria-Nebraska Neuropsychological Battery (LNNB) attempts to standardize the assessment procedures of A.R. Luria, a Russian physician and neuropsychologist.[18]

Two forms are available. Form I consists of 269 items, and Form II, which is described as "largely a parallel form," has 279 items.[18] Form I can be scored by hand or computer, and Form II must be scored by computer. The LNNB is divided into 13 clinical scales, or subtests. Form II contains an additional scale that measures delayed recall of some of the memory items (Table 5).

TABLE 4. Approaches to Neuropsychological Test Selection

Flexible	Not uniform, but based upon the needs of the individual patient.
Flexible Battery	Variable but routine groupings of tests for different diagnostic groups, such as head injury, neurotoxin exposure, etc.
Standardized Battery	Routine use of the Halstead-Reitan, Luria-Nebraska, or other grouping of tests that is administered to all patients.

Adapted from Sweet JJ, Moberg PJ, Westergaard CK: Five-year follow-up of practices and beliefs of clinical neuropsychologists. Clin Neuropsychol 10:202–221, 1996.

TABLE 5. Scales of the Luria-Nebraska Neuropsychological Battery

C1	Motor functions	C8	Reading
C2	Rhythm	C9	Arithmetic
C3	Tactile functions	C10	Memory
C4	Visual functions	C11	Intellectual processes
C5	Receptive speech	C12	Intermediate memory (Form II only)
C6	Expressive speech	01	Spelling (optional)
C7	Writing	02	Motor writing (optional)

Scores on the various items are combined to produce three types of additional scales: (1) summary scales, which indicate laterality, severity, and whether brain injury is present; (2) localization scales, which attempt to locate focal deficits; and (3) factor scales, which assess specific neuropsychological functions. "Critical levels" are computed using corrections for patient age and education. Guidelines for qualitative scoring are also presented.

The LNNB is flexible and need not be administered in one setting. The administration time for the whole battery is about 2½ hours. The equipment demands are minimal, and the entire LNNB can be carried in a small briefcase.

HALSTEAD-REITAN NEUROPSYCHOLOGICAL BATTERY

The Halstead-Reitan Neuropsychological Battery[45] (HRNB) is the most frequently used fixed battery.[20] It consists of 10 tests, but neuropsychologists frequently administer only part of it[20] (Table 6). The HRNB is usually given with a version of the Wechsler Intelligence Scales and one or more tests of personality, often the Minnesota Multiphasic Personality Inventory.

The HRNB provides two main summary scores: the Impairment Index and the Neuropsychological Deficit Scale (NDS). The Impairment Index is the proportion of seven test scores derived from five tests in the HRNB that fall below a cutoff assumed to be characteristic of brain-damaged patients. It is therefore considered to be a measure of the consistency of impairment. The NDS is based on 42 scores generated by the HRNB and is considered to be a measure of the severity of impairment.

TABLE 6. Tests Included in the Halstead-Reitan Neuropsychological Battery

Test	Description
Category Test*	Deducing underlying themes in series of designs
Tactual Performance Test*	Putting shapes into a formboard while blindfolded
Seashore Rhythm Test*	Differentiating between pairs of rhythmic beats
Speech Sounds Perception Test*	Discerning nonsense syllables played on a tape
Trail Making Test	Connecting a series of circles on paper as quickly as possible in sequence
Grip Strength	Measures right and left hand grip strength in kilograms
Finger Tapping Test*	Counts number of taps made with counter using right and left index finger in 10 seconds
Aphasia Screening Test	Surveys aphasia and related deficits
Sensory-Perceptual Examination	Examines ability to perceive tactile, auditory, and visual stimuli
Lateral Dominance Examination	Determines hand and foot preference

* Scores from these tests contribute to the Impairment Index

The HRNB has the advantage of the availability of normative data that provide corrections for three variables that have been demonstrated to be related to performance on these tests: age, gender, and education.[26] Computer software is available for scoring the HRNB.[27]

A complete HRNB will take most of a day to administer, especially if intellectual, personality, and additional memory testing is included. (In the author's opinion, the HRNB does not adequately assess memory, necessitating the addition of one or more tests of memory to the HRNB.) Severely disabled or easily fatigued patients lack the stamina to tolerate this lengthy procedure. The HRNB also requires bulky equipment, making it difficult to administer in off-site situations, such as a work location.

The LNNB and the HRNB are comparable in their ability to identify the presence or absence of *generalized* brain damage.[29] Which of these batteries the neuropsychologist may use is a function of the characteristics of the patient, the training and experience of the neuropsychologist, and the circumstances of the case.

Although the HRNB and LNNB are equally sensitive to the presence of brain damage, they vary as to the functional areas assessed. Factor analytic techniques indicate that the LNNB appears to have more of a language loading and thus would presumably be more sensitive to dominant hemisphere dysfunction, and the HRNB has more of a nonverbal emphasis and thus would be better at detecting nonverbal deficits.[51] Therefore, the reason for referral and suspected pathology influence battery selection.

Using a particular group of tests such as a battery is in some ways similar to the process of learning a foreign language. Over time, administering the same group of tests to a variety of patients, observing their behavior, and obtaining corroborating information, the neuropsychologist explicitly or implicitly builds a personal database, becoming sensitive to nuances in the patients' performance. Although some neuropsychologists have extensive experience with two or more batteries, most seasoned clinicians find it most efficient to focus on a core group of tests.[55] The results of standardized testing, while important, are just one source of information.

Circumstances also play a part in the choice of a test battery. For example, the LNNB is easily transported and is thus better suited for on-site evaluations. On the other hand, the HRNB can be administered by properly trained technicians (although interpretation must be done by a neuropsychologist) and would thus be more appropriate than the LNNB in situations where a number of patients are to be tested, such as in an industrial toxic exposure.

The referring physician should inquire as to the test battery being used and the neuropsychologist's justification for the choice.

Other Commonly Used Tests

Other frequently used tests are described below with examples of measures of intelligence, memory, academic abilities, language, problem solving, visual perception, sensory and motor abilities, attention and concentration, and emotional functioning.

THE WECHSLER INTELLIGENCE SCALES

The Wechsler Adult Intelligence Scale–Revised (WAIS–R) is one of the Wechsler Intelligence Scales (WIS) and is the most commonly used test of overall intellectual functioning.[59,60] It consists of 11 subtests (Table 7) and is thus actually a test battery.[37] Six of the subtests require a spoken response, and they make up the

TABLE 7. Subtests of the Wechsler Adult Intelligence Scale–Revised

Test	Description
Verbal Tests	
Information	Questions that tap fund of general knowledge
Digit span	Repeating digits forward and backward
Vocabulary	Defining words
Arithmetic	Solving word problems without use of paper and pencil
Comprehension	Answering questions that require common sense and social judgment
Similarities	Describing how two words are similar
Performance Tests	
Picture completion	Identifying the missing details in a series of pictures
Picture arrangement	Putting comic strip-type panels in proper sequential order
Block design	Reproducing abstract designs using blocks
Object assembly	Putting together puzzle-like objects
Digit symbol	Coding task requiring replacing numbers with symbols

verbal scale. The remaining five subtests make up the performance scale, which consists primarily of visual/perceptual tasks, all of which must be completed within a specified time. Each subtest produces a raw score, which is translated into a scaled score, which has a mean of 10 and a standard deviation of 3. The scaled scores for both the verbal scale and the performance scale are added and, through the use of the appropriate age-adjusted table, converted into a verbal IQ, performance IQ, and full scale IQ. The WAIS–R produces a "deviation IQ" with a mean of 100 and a standard deviation of 15.

Many psychologists calculate three factor scores for the WAIS–R:[48] verbal comprehension, which measures verbal knowledge and understanding; perceptual organization, which reflects the ability to use and manipulate information perceived visually; and freedom from distractibility, which indicates the ability to concentrate and attend.

Some psychologists continue to use the original WAIS.[59] The tests are similar, although the mean WAIS verbal, performance, and full scale IQs are about 7, 8, and 8 points higher than corresponding IQs on the WAIS–R.[60]

A full WAIS–R usually can be administered in 1½ hours, depending on the characteristics of the patient. Numerous short forms of this test are available.[48]

The manual for the test contains normative data for patients 16–74 years old. Heaton published age, education, and gender corrections for the WAIS–R using data from the original standardization sample.[24]

The WAIS and WAIS–R are sensitive to the effects of generalized brain impairment in that, compared to normal controls, patients will tend to have significantly lower verbal IQ, performance IQ, and full scale IQ scores; however, even though the scores tend to be lower, they may be within normal limits.[29] This is especially true in the case of a focal brain injury, which may spare IQ but cause other functional deficits. Therefore, it is important to examine the pattern of subtest scores rather than relying on the IQs, which are averages and thus may obscure relevant patterns of strengths and weaknesses. This pattern analysis can reveal lateralization of brain injury, concrete thinking, difficulties with attention and concentration, and dementia.[37] In addition, untimed verbal scale subtests such as information and vocabulary tap overlearned knowledge generally acquired throughout a lifetime and are thus relatively resistant to the deleterious effects of brain injury in nonaphasic patients. Therefore, performance on these subtests can sometimes be used to estimate premorbid intelligence, though the use of a demographic formula such as the Barona Index also can be helpful.[5] The literature contains much data on WAIS–R findings for various diagnostic groups.[37]

For these reasons, the WAIS–R or one of the other of the Wechsler Intelligence Scales often constitutes the core of a neuropsychological evaluation. Lezak writes: "Excepting very severely impaired adults, a WIS battery typically constitutes a substantial portion of the test framework of the neuropsychological evaluation for persons 16 and older."[37]

MEMORY

Wechsler Memory Scale–Revised. The Wechsler Memory Scale–Revised (WMS–R) is one of the most commonly used measures of overall memory function.[61] It consists of 13 subtests (Table 8) and, like the WIS, is actually a test battery.

The information and orientation subtest contains mental status-type questions and is primarily used for screening. The scores from the other 12 subtests are used to compute five composite indices: verbal memory index, visual memory index, general memory index, attention/concentration index, and delayed recall index. Like the WAIS–R scores, these scores are normally distributed with a mean of 100 and a standard deviation of 15.

The verbal memory, visual memory, and general memory indices primarily measure immediate memory and learning. The delayed recall index, which assesses a person's ability to retain and recall information after a delay, is perhaps most relevant to a person's ability to function in day-to-day life. The manual presents normative data for ages 16–74.

The WMS–R manual also cites studies that indicate the presence of three factors among the subtests:
I. Logical memory, visual reproduction, associate learning
II. Mental control, digit span
III. Personal and current information, orientation

TABLE 8. Subtests of the Wechsler Memory Scale–Revised in Order of Administration

Subtest	Description
Information and orientation	Mental status-type orientation questions
Mental control	Counting backward, saying the alphabet, adding serially
Figural memory	Identifying briefly seen designs from among an array of similar designs
Logical memory I	Repeating spoken passages
Visual paired associates I	Learning a series of color-design combinations
Verbal paired associates I	Learning a series of word pairs
Visual reproduction I	Reproducing briefly seen geometric designs
Digit span	Repeating strings of digits forward and backward
Visual memory span	Repeating series of movements forward and backward
Logical memory II	Delayed recall of spoken passages
Visual paired associates II	Delayed recall of color-design combinations
Verbal paired associates II	Delayed recall of word pairs
Visual reproduction II	Delayed reproduction of geometric designs

The WMS–R takes 45–60 minutes to administer. A brief version of the scale that omits the four delayed recall subtests can be administered, but this results in the loss of important information about the patient's ability to retain what he or she has learned. Many psychologists administer portions of the WMS–R, usually logical memory I and II and visual reproduction I and II; however, this practice should be discouraged because it violates the standardization procedure and therefore limits the applicability of the normative data presented in the manual.

The Wechsler Memory Scale,[58] the original version of this instrument, is still in use by some psychologists. However, it is not as comprehensive, and some of the material has little relevance for patients.

The manual cites studies that indicate that the WMS–R is sensitive to a number of clinical conditions, including psychiatric disorders, alcoholism, dementia, Huntington's disease, Korsakoff's syndrome, closed head injury, stroke, brain cancer, seizure disorder, multiple sclerosis, and worksite neurotoxins.

This author recommends use of the WMS–R in the assessment of older adolescents and young and middle-aged adults. It is not recommended for patients who are severely impaired and older adults, for whom the WMS–R is often too demanding, and patients with sensory or motor deficits that would prevent them from being able to respond to the various subtests. The WMS–R does not adequately assess nonverbal memory; many patients spontaneously adopt a labeling strategy for the "visual" items. Therefore, the WMS–R can be supplemented with a task such as the delayed recall of the Rey-Osterrieth Complex Figure, which seems less amenable to verbal labeling.

The California Verbal Learning Test. The California Verbal Learning Test (CVLT) is a test of auditory-verbal learning and memory.[9] The patient is read a list of 16 words from a "shopping list" five times. The list consists of four items in each of four categories: fruit, spices and herbs, clothing, and tools. After each presentation, the patient is asked to recall the items. After five presentations and recalls, an interference list of 16 different items is presented for one trial. The patient is asked to recall the second list. Immediately following this recall, free recall of the first list is administered, followed by a cued recall, in which the administrator would ask the patient, for instance, to name the items that are clothing. The free and cued recall of the first list is repeated after a 20-minute delay. Finally, a recognition test for the first list is presented.

Scoring of the CVLT quantifies a number of scores, including levels of recall, learning strategies, serial position effects, learning curve, consistency of recall, proactive and retroactive interference, retention over delays, enhancement of recall by cueing and recognition, perseverations and intrusions, and false positives. Software is available to calculate these indices.[17] Norms are provided for ages 17–80.

The CVLT is sensitive to memory impairment in general, and performance patterns can differentiate between various patient groups. The manual presents "score patterns" for chronic alcoholism, Parkinson's disease, multiple sclerosis, Huntington's disease, and Alzheimer's disease.

The Auditory-Verbal Learning Test (AVLT) is a similar, but less comprehensive measure, that uses a list of 15 words.[56]

The CVLT and similar tasks provide an indication of how a person learns. This information is helpful in guiding rehabilitation efforts, especially in patients who will be attending school or participating in some other training program. A particular advantage of the CVLT and similar tasks is that they make no visual-sensory or motor demands. As with the WMS–R, the CVLT and AVLT may be too demanding and disheartening for severely impaired patients.

ACADEMIC ABILITIES

Tests of academic achievement are often incorporated into a neuropsychological evaluation. Although most such tests were originally developed with school uses in mind, they are helpful in an adult neuropsychological evaluation for several reasons. Tests of language-based academic abilities can be useful to establish premorbid level of functioning: abilities such as word recognition tend to be relatively resistant to the effects of brain injury. Conversely, brain-injured patients often do poorly on tests of arithmetic and math. Finally, an awareness of a patient's functional academic abilities is often helpful in making vocational recommendations, especially if the recommendations involve school or other training programs.

The Wide Range Achievement Test. The Wide Range Achievement Test (WRAT) is a frequently used brief measure of academic functioning.[63] Currently in its third edition (WRAT3), the test consists of three subtests: reading, spelling, and arithmetic, and it is available in two forms. Norms are provided in the manual for the ages 5–74. Because the reading subtest measures word recognition rather than reading comprehension, neuropsychologists sometimes supplement this test with other measures, such as the reading comprehension subtest from the Peabody Individual Achievement Test[38] (PIAT) or the Kauffman Test of Academic Achievement[32] (KTEA).

VISUAL PERCEPTION

Rey-Osterrieth Complex Figure Test. The Rey-Osterrieth Complex Figure Test (ROCFT) is a measure of perceptual-organizational and constructional abilities.[42] It involves presenting the patient with a drawing of an abstract figure consisting of vertical, horizontal, diagonal, and curved lines. The patient is asked to copy the design freehand with paper and pencil. The initial copy is usually followed by a delayed recall(s), with different authors providing norms for different recall intervals.[37]

The ROCFT or a similar constructional task is appropriate in all evaluations with patients who have adequate sensorimotor abilities. These types of tasks have the advantages of being sensitive to the presence of brain injury and cognitive dysfunction in general, being generally brief to administer, and not requiring any cumbersome or expensive equipment. The quality of the ROCFT copy and recall and the strategy the patient uses can indicate the location and nature of brain dysfunction.

Trail Making Test. The Trail Making Test is usually incorporated into the HRNB, but it is frequently used on its own.[20] It was originally part of the Army Individual Test Battery. The Trail Making Test consists of two sections. In Part A, the patient is instructed to draw lines to connect 24 numbered circles in numerical order as quickly as possible. Part B has the same general format, except that the circles contain a number from 1 to 13 or a letter from A to L. The patient is again instructed to draw lines connecting the circles but also is told to alternate between numeric and alphabetical order (1 to A, A to 2, 2 to B). Errors are corrected by the examiner as they occur, and the score is based on time to completion. Successful performance of this test requires letter and number recognition, mental flexibility, visual scanning, and motor function.[7]

Like the ROCFT, the Trail Making Test has the advantages of being sensitive to the effects of brain impairment in general, being brief, and not requiring any equipment. Therefore, it is appropriate for use in the evaluation of patients with adequate sensorimotor abilities. This commonly used test is described as "highly vulnerable to the effects of head injury"[37] and has been demonstrated to be sensitive to a host of neurologic conditions, including dementia, mild traumatic brain injury, psychiatric disturbance, Huntington's disease, drug abuse, multiple sclerosis, and toxic exposure.[22,37] The Trail Making Test also may be useful in screening patients for visual perceptual difficulties that may interfere with driving.

Symbol Digit Modalities Test. The Symbol Digit Modalities Test (SDMT) is a coding task in which the patient is required to follow a key to write the appropriate numbers beneath a series of symbols presented on a piece of paper.[52] Following the written administration, the patient is given an identical form and asked to say the appropriate numbers aloud. The score for each modality is the correct number of substitutions made in 90 seconds.

The SDMT was originally designed to be a quick method for screening for cerebral pathology. Similar to the Trail Making Test, this task taps visual scanning and visual attention functions. The comparison of the scores on the two response modalities can be useful in isolating dysfunction.

The SDMT is sensitive to brain impairment in general. As with the Trail Making Test, it is brief and highly portable, making it appropriate for inclusion in a screening battery.

Hooper Visual Organization Test. The Hooper Visual Organization Test (HVOT) is a motor-free measure of visual synthetic and analytic skills.[28] It consists of 30 fragmented pictures of simple objects. The patient is requested to name each object. The score is the total number of correct identifications, with partial credit given for specific near misses.

The HVOT is a motor-free test of visual perception, and, as such, is appropriate for use with patients with motor impairments. It is quite easy for most patients, and its game-like quality is engaging. Many neurologically involved patients do well on the HVOT, but poor performance is almost always indicative of pathology.

REASONING AND PROBLEM SOLVING

Category Test. The Category Test[21] is an integral component of the HRNB: however, like the Trail Making Test, it is frequently administered separately. It consists of 208 figures grouped into seven subtests and presented to the patient one at a time. Each figure can be assigned a number from 1 to 4 based on a principle. The patient is asked to determine which number corresponds with each figure. The principle is not announced to the patient, although he or she is given immediate feedback as to the correctness of his or her answer. The task of the patient is to figure out the correct principle essentially by trial and error. The first six subtests contain one principle each, while the seventh contains items from the previous subtests. Successful performance requires abstract thinking, cognitive flexibility, and memory.

The Category Test itself is a cumbersome apparatus that includes a carousel slide projector and a frosted glass screen onto which the designs are projected. It is therefore difficult to transport and is prone to malfunctions. The Booklet Category Test is a more portable version that consists of two loose-leaf binders.[8] Normative data for the Category Test adjusted for age, gender, and education are available.[26]

The Category Test is reported to be the most sensitive test in the HRNB to the presence of brain impairment[45] and is therefore appropriate for use as a screening test. When the test is used in a battery, it is useful to compare performance on this less-structured, novel task with scores on measures of more automatic and overlearned abilities. This comparison may reveal the presence of deficits in adaptive functioning that are not obvious. For example, in a relatively structured hospital setting, many brain-injured patients may appear cognitively intact to staff. However, some of these patients lose this characteristic when they are discharged and return to a more demanding work setting. These types of patients tend to do poorly on the Category Test. However, the repeated negative feedback for patients who are having difficulty on this task can be extremely frustrating and disheartening, and its length is onerous for elderly and severely impaired patients.

The Wisconsin Card Sorting Test. The Wisconsin Card Sorting Test (WCST) is similar to the Category Test in that it is a measure of abstract thinking, including the ability to generate and test hypotheses and profit from feedback.[25] Four stimulus cards are laid out in front of the patient, each with a different design: one red triangle, two green stars, three yellow crosses, and four blue circles. The patient is given 128 response cards. On each of these cards are printed figures of varying numbers (one to four), colors (red, green, yellow and blue), and shapes (triangles, stars, crosses, and circles). The patient is instructed to match each response card with one of the stimulus cards (the actual manipulation of the cards can be done by the examiner if the patient is unable to do so). Initially, color is the correct principle; after ten correct consecutive responses, the sorting principle is unannouncedly changed to shape; and, after ten more consecutive responses, to number. The cycle is repeated. Verbal feedback of "right" or "wrong" is provided by the examiner; however, the patient is not informed of the correct sorting principle. The test continues until all the cards have been used or the patient has completed the six categories.

The manual provides norms for ages 6–89. The adult norms are corrected for education from 8 or fewer years to 18 or more years.

Although they seem to tap similar functions, patients tend to find the WCST easier than the Category Test, and thus it can be used for patients who cannot tolerate the latter measure; however, there is a danger of false negatives. The WCST is extremely portable and is sensitive to brain impairment in general.

LANGUAGE

Boston Naming Test. This test of word-finding ability consists of a series of 60 line drawings of common objects.[30] The patient is asked to name each object. If the patient has difficulty, a stimulus cue is provided (for example, the stimulus cue of "It's an animal" for a picture of a beaver). If the patient is still unable to name the object, a phonemic cue is provided, consisting of the first sound of the word (for example, "bea"). The score is the total number of spontaneous identifications and identifications following a stimulus cue.

This test is sensitive to word-finding problems in aphasia, mild traumatic brain injury, dementia, and multiple sclerosis.[37] It can also detect perceptual difficulties in patients with right hemisphere damage.

Verbal Fluency for F-A-S. Verbal Fluency for F-A-S, also called the Controlled Oral Word Association Test (COWAT), is a test of expressive language function. It is part of the Neurosensory Center Comprehensive Examination for Aphasia.[53] The patient is instructed to say as many words as he or she can that begin with the letter "F," after being cautioned against using proper nouns, numerals, and the same word with different suffixes. One minute is allowed. The same procedure is then used with the letters "A" and "S." Variations of this task are available using different letters and categories.[37]

This test has much to recommend it. It is brief, simple, requires no special equipment or forms, and is sensitive to a variety of brain dysfunctions. It is frequently used as part of an evaluation of dementia. Normative data are available adjusted for age, gender, and education.[37] For the results to be meaningful, the patient must be fluent in the language in which the test is administered.

Revised Token Test. The Revised Token Test[40] is a measure of auditory deficits arising from brain dysfunction and is one of several versions of the Token Test available. It is primarily a test of receptive language functions, as opposed to the Boston Naming Test and Verbal Fluency, which are primarily tests of expressive language functions.

The patient is presented with 20 plastic tokens, which come in four colors, two shapes, and two sizes. The test consists of 100 commands that direct the patient to do something with the tokens. The commands are initially simple ("Touch the black circle") but become increasingly more complex ("Unless you have touched the little white square, touch the big green circle"). The scoring system of the RTT incorporates five dimensions: correctness or accuracy, responsiveness, completeness, promptness, and efficiency.

Lezak describes the Token Test as being "remarkably sensitive to the disrupted linguistic processes that are central to the aphasic disability."[37] Therefore, a version of this test can be used when language deficits are suspected.

SENSORY AND MOTOR TESTS

Sensory and motor tests are frequently used to provide some indication of a lesion's laterality. In general, impaired performance may indicate dysfunction in the contralateral cerebral hemisphere. However, these types of findings should be viewed with caution because other factors, such as spinal or peripheral injuries, also can interfere with the performance of these tasks.

The Finger Tapping Test and Sensory-Perceptual Examination are representative sensory and motor tests. Both are part of the HRNB,[45] but they are sometimes used outside of this battery.

Finger Tapping Test. Also referred to as the Finger Oscillation Test, this test requires the patient to rapidly tap a counter with his or her index finger for 10 seconds. This is usually done for five trials first using the preferred and then the non-preferred hand. The score is the mean number of taps using each hand.

This test is primarily used for lateralizing dysfunction, but it may have some utility in vocational testing for jobs that require rapid motor movements.

Sensory-Perceptual Examination. This group of tasks assesses sensation and perception in tactile, auditory, and visual modalities. It includes double simultaneous stimulation in all modalities to detect extinctions. It is essentially a standardization of a neurologic exam.

ATTENTION AND CONCENTRATION

Adequate attentional abilities are a prerequisite for successful performance of any task, with the demands for attention and concentration generally increasing as the complexity of the task increases. Many test batteries incorporate measures that are particularly sensitive to deficits in attention and concentration. These include the arithmetic and digit span subtests from the Wechsler Intelligence Scales; the digit span, visual memory span, and mental control subtests from the Wechsler Memory Scale–Revised; and the seashore rhythm test from the Halstead-Reitan Neuropsychological Battery. Tests such as Part B of the Trail Making Test require *divided* attention: the ability to rapidly shift from one idea to another and back again. In addition, there are specific individual tests of attention and concentration.

Paced Auditory Serial Addition Test. The Paced Auditory Serial Addition Test (PASAT) is a commonly used test of concentration.[19] It consists of a taped voice reciting 60 randomized one-digit numbers. The patient is requested to add the number just heard to the one heard before and say the sum out loud. The series of numbers is repeated at four increasingly fast speeds.

This test is sensitive to subtle difficulties in concentration, such as may be manifested in mild traumatic brain injury[54] and solvent exposure.[1] However, this test is stressful, even for cognitively intact subjects, and the neuropsychologist should be aware of the possible emotional consequences.

TESTS OF EMOTIONAL FUNCTIONING

Minnesota Multiphasic Personality Inventory. The Minnesota Multiphasic Personality Inventory-2 (MMPI-2) is a restandardization of the original MMPI.[23] The MMPI-2 is the most widely used instrument for the measure of personality. It consists of 567 items but is often given in an abbreviated form using the first 370 items, which include all of the component items in the basic scales. The patient is asked to respond either "true" or "false" to each item as it applies to him or her.

The basic scoring of the MMPI provides 14 indices: the "Cannot Say" score, three validity scales, and ten clinical scales. The Cannot Say (denoted as "?") score is the total number of items that were omitted or double-marked. A high score on this index may reflect defensiveness or a "none of your business" attitude, or the patient may have been unable to comprehend the item. The validity scales address whether the clinical scales accurately reflect the personality of the patient. The L scale is designed to identify gross efforts to avoid answering the items honestly to give an inordinately good impression. The F scale is the opposite, measuring infrequently endorsed items, which may indicate a patient's attempt to appear more pathologic than he or she actually is. The K scale measures more subtle forms of defensiveness and is used to adjust some of the clinical scales.

The 10 clinical scales were developed empirically for their power to distinguish between various patient groups and normals. Patients who score high on scale 1 (hypochondriasis or Hs) typically present with numerous vague physical complaints and are overconcerned about their health. High responders to scale 2 (depression or D) manifest a depressed mood. Scale 3 (conversion hysteria or Hy) is sensitive to patients who may develop sensory or motor symptoms in response to stress. Scale 4 (psychopathic deviate or Pd) measures antisocial behavior. Scale 5 (masculinity-femininity or Mf) reflects traditional male-female interests. High responders to scale 6 (paranoia or Pa) are overly suspicious. Scale 7 (psychasthenia or Pt) is a measure of anxiety. Elevations on scale 8 (schizophrenia or Sc) indicate poor reality contact and idiosyncratic thought patterns. Scale 9 (mania or Ma) is a measure of impulsivity and psychic energy. Scale 0 (social introversion-extraversion or Si) is a measure of social interaction.

The MMPI-2 is interpreted by converting the raw scores for each scale into T scores, with a mean of 50 and a standard deviation of 10. A T score of 65 or above is judged to be clinically elevated. The scores from the validity and clinical scales are typically plotted and presented as a graph. The individual scales are not interpreted; rather, the psychologist examines the complete profile. In addition to the basic scales, a number of supplementary scales can be calculated that may augment the clinical profile. Various software packages are available to facilitate this process.

The MMPI-2 is appropriate in neuropsychological evaluations in which the patient is capable of the task demands and time permits. The MMPI-2 is especially helpful in detecting deviant response sets, such as would be seen in malingering. It is also helpful in investigating the possibility of conversion disorder. However, because some of the items refer to possible symptoms of neurologic conditions, the MMPI-2 should be interpreted with caution in patients seen in the course of a neuropsychological evaluation. "Canned" computerized narratives should not be used; they may incorrectly attribute the presence of sensory, motor, or cognitive symptoms to psychiatric illness.

Other Personality Tests. Even in its 370-item version, the MMPI-2 is sometimes too demanding for many impaired patients, particularly the elderly. Briefer measures of emotional function are available. The Symptom Checklist-90–R[11] (SCL-90–R) is a 90-item checklist that contains common symptoms of psychiatric and medical illness. This measure has been used with patients with a number of different neuropsychological disorders.[37]

The Beck Depression Inventory (BDI)[6] is another frequently used instrument that documents the presence and intensity of depressive symptomatology.

Like the MMPI-2, these measures contain items concerning sensory, motor, and cognitive changes that may be associated with neurologic conditions. An item-by-item analysis is necessary to ensure that these symptoms are not mistakenly attributed to emotional or psychiatric conditions. Likewise, "canned" computerized narratives should not be used.

Projective Tests. Projective tests are a group of techniques for eliciting a patient's response to ambiguous stimuli. The rationale is that the patient will "project" some salient aspect of his or her emotional functioning into the response. Commonly used projective tests include the Rorschach, Thematic Apperception Test (TAT), and human figure drawings.[4] Most of these tests are not empirically based and lack demonstrated validity and reliability.[67] Exner has attempted to standardize the Rorschach.[15] However, psychometric criticisms have been raised about his system.[14,65,66] In addition, projective techniques may not be admissible in court in the United States based upon a new standard of expert testimony.[39] Most clinical neuropsychologists do not routinely use projective tests in their evaluations.[55]

TOPICS OF SPECIAL INTEREST TO OCCUPATIONAL MEDICINE PHYSICIANS

Relatively minor blows to the head can result in neuropsychological deficits. Confusion exists as to the correct terminology for these events. The terms mild head injury (MHI) or postconcussion syndrome (PCS) are often used. However, **mild traumatic brain injury** (MTBI) is the most precise term.[33]

MTBI is usually defined as an external trauma to the head that results in a loss of consciousness of 20 minutes or less, Glasgow Coma Scale scores of 13–15, no mass lesions, and hospitalization of 48 hours or fewer.[46] The neurologic and physical deficits associated with MTBI typically include difficulties with attention and concentration, impaired verbal retrieval, and emotional distress.[37] Most patients with MTBI become symptom-free within months of the injury, a few report difficulties 1 year after the trauma,[33] and for some patients the deficits may be permanent.[47]

The mechanism and course of these deficits is a matter of controversy in the neuropsychology literature. Some researchers attribute longstanding deficits associated with MTBI to patient expectation rather than any physiologic process.[41] However, other researchers have documented the presence of PET scan abnormalities in patients with persisting deficits.[47]

Levin, Eisenberg and Benton discuss MTBI in detail.[36]

Exposure to a number of **industrial and environmental toxins**, including metals, solvents, and insecticides, can cause brain impairment.[62] The neuropsychological consequences of such an exposure are variable and affected by such factors as the substance, length and intensity of exposure, and patient characteristics. Hartman provides a comprehensive treatment of this subject.[22]

Electrical injuries can result in neuropsychological deficits and emotional disturbance.[34,43] However, no consistent pattern of psychological sequelae has been detected in patients with electrical injury. This may be due to the heterogeneous nature of these injuries, with a failure to control for the nature of the injury and characteristics of the patient.[43]

In referring a patient for a neuropsychological evaluation, the occupational medicine physician can take several steps to help ensure quality care for the patient:

1. Refer to a qualified neuropsychologist. When in doubt, ask to examine a copy of the neuropsychologist's curriculum vitae. Be suspicious of anyone who refuses to provide this document.
2. Provide a specific, concise reason for referral. You probably won't get the information that you need if you don't ask for it. In addition, if the neuropsychological evaluation would not provide the information you need, the neuropsychologist can let you know that prior to this costly and time-consuming procedure.
3. Make records available. As a general rule, the more records, the better.

ACKNOWLEDGMENT

The author would like to thank Julie Karcis, Christopher J. King, PsyD, and Ann Genetta, PsyD, for their helpful comments on this manuscript.

REFERENCES

1. Allison WM, Jerrom DWA: Glue sniffing: A pilot study of the cognitive effects of long-term use. Int J Addict 19:453–458, 1984.
2. American Psychiatric Association: Diagnostic and Statistical Manual of Mental Disorders. 4th ed. Washington, DC, APA, 1994.
3. American Psychological Association: Guidelines for providers of psychological services to ethnic, linguistic, and culturally diverse populations. Am Psychol 48:45–48, 1993.
4. Anastasi A: Psychological Testing. 6th ed. New York, Macmillan, 1988.
5. Barona A, Reynolds CR, Chastain R: A demographically based index of premorbid intelligence for the WAIS–R. J Consult Clin Psychol 52:885–887, 1984.
6. Beck AT: Beck Depression Inventory. San Antonio, Harcourt Brace Jovanovich, 1987.
7. Corrigan JD, Hinkeldey NS: Relationships between Parts A and B of the Trail Making Test. J Clin Psychol 43:402–409, 1987.
8. DeFilippis NA, McCampbell EA: The Booklet Category Test Manual. Odessa, FL, Psychological Assessment Resources, 1991.
9. Delis DC, Kramer JH, Kaplan E, Ober BA: California Verbal Learning Test Manual—Research Edition. San Antonio, Harcourt Brace Jovanovich, 1987.
10. DeLuca JW, Putman SH: The professional/technician model in clinical neuropsychology: Deployment characteristics and practice issues. Prof Psychol 24:100–106, 1993.
11. Derogatis LR: SCL-90–R: Administration, Scoring and Procedures Manual. 3rd ed. Minneapolis, National Computer Systems, 1994.
12. Division 40, American Psychological Association: Definition of a clinical neuropsychologist. Clin Neuropsychol 3:22, 1989.
13. Division 40, American Psychological Association: Guidelines regarding the use of nondoctoral personnel in clinical neuropsychology assessment. Clin Neuropsychol 3:23–24, 1989.
14. Exner JE: A comment on "The comprehensive system for the Rorschach: A critical examination." Psychol Sci 7:11–13, 1996.
15. Exner JE: The Rorschach: A Comprehensive System: Vol 1. Basic Foundations. 3rd ed. New York, Wiley, 1993.

16. Folstein MF, Folstein SE, McHugh PR: Mini-mental state. J Psychiatr Res 12:189–198, 1975.
17. Fridlund AJ, Delis DC: California Verbal Learning Test IBM User's Guide. Version 1. San Antonio, Harcourt Brace Jovanovich, 1987.
18. Golden CJ, Purisch AD, Hammeke TA: Luria-Nebraska Neuropsychological Battery: Forms I and II. Los Angeles, Western Psychological Services, 1985.
19. Gronwall DMA: Paced Auditory Serial-Addition Task: A measure of recovery from concussion. Percept Mot Skills 44:367–376, 1977.
20. Guilmette TJ, Faust D, Hart K, Arkes HR: A national survey of psychologists who offer neuropsychological services. Arch Clin Neuropsychol 5:373–392, 1990.
21. Halstead WC: Brain and Intelligence. Chicago, University of Chicago Press, 1947.
22. Hartman DE: Neuropsychological Toxicology: Identification and Assessment of Human Neurotoxic Syndromes. 2nd ed. New York, Plenum Press, 1995.
23. Hathaway SR, McKinley JC: Minnesota Multiphasic Personality Inventory-2 Manual. Minneapolis, University of Minnesota Press, 1989.
24. Heaton RK: Comprehensive Norms for an Expanded Halstead-Reitan Battery: A Supplement for the Wechsler Adult Intelligence Scale–Revised. Odessa, FL, Psychological Assessment Resources, 1992.
25. Heaton RK, Chelune GJ, Talley JL, et al: Wisconsin Card Sorting Test Manual. Revised and Expanded. Odessa, FL, Psychological Assessment Resources, 1993.
26. Heaton RK, Grant I, Matthews CG: Comprehensive Norms for an Expanded Halstead-Reitan Battery: Demographic Corrections, Research Findings, and Clinical Applications. Odessa, FL, Psychological Assessment Resources, 1991.
27. Heaton RK, Grant I, Matthews CG, PAR Staff: HRB Norms Program. Vol 2. Odessa, FL, Psychological Assessment Resources, undated.
28. Hooper HE: Hooper Visual Organization Test Manual. Los Angeles, Western Psychological Services, 1958.
29. Kane RL, Parsons OA, Goldstein G: Statistical relationships and discriminative accuracy of the Halstead-Reitan, Luria-Nebraska, and Wechsler IQ scores in the identification of brain damage. J Clin Exp Neuropsychol 7:211–223, 1985.
30. Kaplan E, Goodglass H, Weintraub S: Boston Naming Test. Revised Edition. Philadelphia, Lea & Febiger, 1983.
31. Katz MM, Lyerly SB: Methods for measuring adjustment and social behavior in the community: I. Rationale, description, discriminative ability and scale development. Psychol Rep 13:503–535, 1963.
32. Kaufman AS, Kaufman NL: Kaufman Test of Educational Achievement Comprehensive Form Manual. Circle Pines, MN, American Guidance Service, 1985.
33. Kay T, Newman B, Cavallo M, et al: Toward a neuropsychological model of functional disability after mild traumatic brain injury. Neuropsychology 6:371–384, 1992.
34. Kelley KM, Pliskin N, Meyer G, Lee RC: Neuropsychiatric aspects of electrical injury: The nature of psychiatric disturbance. Ann N Y Acad Sci 720:213–218, 1994.
35. Lees-Haley PR, Dunn JT: The ability of naive subjects to report symptoms of mild brain injury, post-traumatic stress disorder, major depression, and generalized anxiety disorder. J Clin Psychol 50:252–256, 1994.
36. Levin HS, Eisenberg HM, Benton AL (eds): Mild Head Injury. New York, Oxford University Press, 1989.
37. Lezak MD: Neuropsychological Assessment. 3rd ed. New York, Oxford University Press, 1995.
38. Markwardt FC Jr: The Peabody Individual Achievement Test–Revised. Circle Pines, MN, American Guidance Service, 1989.
39. McDonald JJ, Lees-Haley PR: Avoiding "junk science" in sexual harassment litigation. Employee Relat Law J 21:51–71, 1995.
40. McNeil TR, Prescott TE: Revised Token Test Manual. Austin, Pro-Ed, 1978.
41. Mittenberg W, DiGuilio DV, Perrin S, Bass AE: Symptoms following mild head injury: Expectation as aetiology. J Neurol Neurosurg Psychiatry 55:200–204, 1992.
42. Osterrieth RA: Le test de copie d'une figure complex [The complex figure drawing test]. Arch Psychol 30:206–356, 1944.
43. Pliskin NH, Meyer GJ, Dolske MC, et al: Neuropscyhiatric aspects of electrical injury: A review of neuropsychological research. Ann N Y Acad Sci 720:219–223, 1994.
44. Purisch AD, Sbordone RJ: Forensic Neuropsychology: Going Beyond the Test Data. Irvine, CA, Neuropsychological Associates of California, undated.
45. Reitan RM, Wolfson D: The Halstead-Reitan Neuropsychological Test Battery: Theory and Clinical Interpretation. 2nd ed. S. Tucson, Arizona, Neuropsychology Press, 1993.

46. Rimel RW, Giordani B, Barth JT, et al: Disability caused by minor head injury. Neurosurgery 9:221–228, 1981.
47. Ruff RM, Crouch JA, Tröster AI, et al: Selected cases of poor outcome following a minor brain trauma: Comparing neuropsychological and positron emission tomography assessment. Brain Inj 8:297–308, 1994.
48. Sattler JM: Assessment of Children. 3rd ed. San Diego, JM Sattler, 1988.
49. Sbordone RJ: Neuropsychology for the Attorney. Orlando, FL, Paul M. Deutsch Press, 1991.
50. Schinka JA: Neuropsychological Status Examination (NSE). Odessa, FL, Psychological Assessment Resources, 1983.
51. Shelly C, Goldstein G: Psychometric relations between the Luria-Nebraska and the Halstead-Reitan Test Batteries in a neuropsychiatric setting. Clin Neuropsychol 4:128–133, 1982.
52. Smith A: The Symbol Digit Modalities Test: A neuropsychological test for economic screening of learning and other cerebral disorders. Learn Disord 3:83–91, 1968.
53. Spreen O, Benton AL: Neurosensory Center Comprehensive Examination for Aphasia Manual. Victoria, BC, University of Victoria Neuropsychology Laboratory, 1977.
54. Stuss DT, Stethem LL, Hugenholtz H, Richard MT: Traumatic brain injury. Clin Neuropsychol 3:145–156, 1989.
55. Sweet JJ, Moberg PJ, Westergaard CK: Five-year follow-up of practices and beliefs of clinical neuropsychologists. Clin Neuropsychol 10:202–221, 1996.
56. Taylor EM: Psychological Appraisal of Children with Cerebral Deficits. Cambridge, MA, Oxford University Press, 1959.
57. Terrell F, Terrell SL, Taylor J: Effects of race of examiner and cultural mistrust on the WAIS performance of black students. J Consult Clin Psychol 49:750–751, 1981.
58. Wechsler D: A standardized memory scale for clinical use. J Psychol 19:87–95, 1945.
59. Wechsler D: Manual for the Wechsler Adult Intelligence Scale. New York, The Psychological Corporation, 1955.
60. Wechsler D: Manual for the Wechsler Adult Intelligence Scale–Revised. New York, The Psychological Corporation, 1981.
61. Wechsler D: Manual for the Wechsler Memory Scale–Revised. New York, The Psychological Corporation, 1987.
62. White RF, Feldman RG, Travers PH: Neurobehavioral effects of toxicity due to metals, solvents, and insecticides. Clin Neuropharmacol 13:392–412, 1990.
63. Wilkinson GS: Wide Range Achievement Test 1993 Edition Administration Manual. Wilmington, DE, Wide Range, Inc., 1993.
64. Williams JM: The Cognitive Behavior Rating Scales Manual. Odessa, FL, Psychological Assessment Resources, 1991.
65. Wood JM, Nezworski MT, Stejskal WJ: The comprehensive system for the Rorschach: A critical examination. Psychol Sci 7:3–10, 1996.
66. Wood JM, Nezworski MT, Stejskal WJ: Thinking critically about the comprehensive system for the Rorschach: A reply to Exner. Psychol Sci 7:14–17, 1996.
67. Ziskin J, Faust D: Coping with Psychiatric and Psychological Testimony. 5th ed. Vol II: Special Topics. Los Angeles, Law and Psychology Press, 1995.

ROBERT T. SATALOFF, MD, DMA
JOSEPH SATALOFF, MD, DSc

AUDIOLOGIC TESTING: AN OVERVIEW FOR OCCUPATIONAL PHYSICIANS

From Thomas Jefferson University
Philadelphia, Pennsylvania

Reprint requests to:
Robert T. Sataloff, MD, DMA
1721 Pine Street
Philadelphia, PA 19103

This chapter has been adapted from Sataloff RT, Sataloff J: Occupational Hearing Loss, 2nd ed. New York, Marcel Dekker, 1993.

Occupational hearing loss has been recognized since the industrial revolution and is currently our most prevalent occupational malady. The federal government showed its concern for this problem by including noise and hearing regulation in the Occupational Safety and Health Act and a subsequent hearing conservation amendment. The law mandates hearing conservation measures in every work environment in the United States that produces more than 85 dBA of noise for 8 hours daily. Hearing conservation programs and otologic diagnosis depend, in part, upon accurate audiologic testing. A comprehensive review of hearing tests is beyond the scope of this chapter. Reliable, valid testing requires considerable skill and training, and accurate interpretation of audiograms requires even more.[6] No diagnosis (including occupational hearing loss) can be made on the basis of an audiogram alone. This chapter provides an overview of the more common and important tests that may be encountered by occupational physicians caring for workers with hearing loss complaints.

AUDIOMETRIC TESTING

Definitions

An audiogram is a written record of a person's hearing level measured with certain pure tones. The pure tones generally used clinically are the frequencies 250, 500, 1000, 2000, 3000, 4000, 6000, and 8000 Hz; these tones are generated electronically by the audiometer. This frequency range includes the speech spectrum. Although testing at 250 Hz is performed routinely in otologists' offices, it is often omitted in occupational settings since it is not required by OSHA or included in most formulas used to calculate hearing impairment disability. Testing at 8000 Hz is not mandated by OSHA but should always be performed because the response at this frequency is often helpful in differentiating occupational hearing loss from presbycusis. If 0 dB represents ideal normal hearing, a 60 dB hearing threshold level also can be called a 60 dB "hearing loss." Though both terms describe the same condition, the term "hearing level" is currently more popular in otology because it emphasizes the hearing that the patient has remaining rather than the hearing lost. Furthermore, it recognizes that normal hearing is not simply 0 dB, but rather is represented by a range of hearing levels from 0–25 dB. Also, because a -5 dB level is a gain rather than a loss among persons with normal hearing, the "level" avoids the confusion of "negative losses" and contributes to a more positive approach in helping patients with deficient hearing. However, the terms "hearing loss" and "hearing level" are used interchangeably in common practice.

The reader should be aware that the term decibel (dB) implies the use of a logarithmic ratio scale. Decibels are used to measure many phenomena in nature including not only sound, but also heat, light, and others.[6] In otology, a few different decibel scales are used. The dB referred to in the previous paragraph are dBHL referring to hearing level. They are different from dBSPL (sound pressure level) used in physics to measure the sound pressure level of a given noise relative to 0.0002 microbar. Rather, dBHL on the audiometer are normalized at each frequency so that the hearing threshold of a population of young, healthy individuals with no otologic pathology is 0 dB at each frequency. Hence, 0 dBHL on the audiometer at 500 Hz and 4000 Hz represents different sound pressure levels and dB as measured by a sound level meter. Another term used commonly is dBA, which refers to dBSPL measured through the A-filtering network on a sound level meter. For a more complete explanation of this complex subject, the reader is referred to other literature.[6]

Reference Hearing Level

The original American Standards Association (ASA 1951) 0 dB reference level was established from data obtained in 1935 and 1936. Older audiograms performed using the ASA standard frequently produced normal hearing levels of -10 dB and -5 dB. Newer data obtained some 30 years later indicated that the human ear was approximately 10 dB more sensitive. This information led to the International Standards Organization (ISO 1964) reference level, which was later adopted by the American National Standards Institute (formerly ASA) and is now known as ANSI 1989. Tables showing the differences are available in many standard references.[6] The change in standard resulted in audiograms of 0 dB for most people with normal hearing, with much fewer people achieving levels of -5 dB or -10 dB.

Horizontal and Vertical Variables in a Graphic Audiogram

Ideally, one should measure a patient's ability to hear speech, but because of several difficulties, pure tones are still used. For simplicity, only specific frequencies were selected for routine use. They are called *octave frequencies* because each successive tone is an octave above the one immediately below it, and the number of cycles per second from one tone to the next is doubled. Octave frequencies constitute the horizontal variable in an audiogram: how well the patient hears at each frequency. Does the patient hear the tone as well as a person with normal hearing, or does it have to be made louder; if so, how much louder? To make this comparison, one must have a normal baseline for each frequency. There are certain shortcomings inherent in any system that relies on sampling of this sort. To improve the tests, frequencies between the usual octaves are also often tested, particularly 3000 Hz and 6000 Hz because hearing changes due to noise are most likely to occur in the 3000 Hz to 6000 Hz range. Frequencies above the usual test range may also be useful, including 10,000 Hz, 12,000 Hz, and sometimes higher frequencies.

What Is Normal Hearing?

The threshold at the various frequencies of a person with normal hearing ability originally was obtained by testing a large number of young people between the ages of 20 and 29 and determining the intensities of the thresholds at the various frequencies. It was found that the thresholds fluctuated over approximately a 25-dB range even in subjects with normal hearing. An average was reached at 0 dB of hearing. Some subjects heard better than 0; many of them heard tones as weak as -10; others did not hear a sound until it was amplified to a level between 0 and 15 dB. This variation indicated that the range between -10 and +15 dB could be considered normal for the average young person (ASA). The range for the ANSI scale is 0–25 dB, and this is the current standard level.

The reference level on the audiometer is 0 dB. A hearing loss at some specific frequency is expressed and recorded as the number of decibels required for the individual to hear it.

What the Audiometer Measures

Commercial audiometers are calibrated and recording methods are standardized in such a way that what is recorded is not a patient's ability to hear, but rather the hearing *level* in the frequencies tested. If one can hear 0 dB, there is no hearing loss; but if one cannot hear until the tone is 30 dB louder than 0 dB, there is a hearing loss. The pure-tone audiometer offers the most valid, reliable means yet devised for routine hearing measurement. That is why pure-tone threshold testing has been accepted as the preferred method for hearing screening and for medicolegal purposes.

Forms of the Audiogram

The audiogram, which shows a patient's hearing threshold for the standard range of frequencies, can be recorded in several ways. The most common is a graph on which the frequencies are marked off from left to right, and the tone intensities range up and down. A statement that O represents the right ear and X the left should appear at the bottom of each graph for standardization. One of the chief disadvantages of using this type of graph in industry and otology is that if eight or ten audiograms are done in a year on a certain subject, the record becomes bulky, and it becomes difficult to compare one curve with another performed on a different date.

Serial audiogram recording is recommended for industry, schools, and otologic practice. Instead of using a symbol for the right and left ears, the number of decibels designating the threshold is recorded at each frequency. Serial audiograms make it easier to record all thresholds obtained independently and to compare the results of tests performed at different times.

Audiograms are remarkably consistent in cooperative subjects from test to test. Although variations of up to ± 5 dB are considered acceptable, even this slight variation is not usually seen provided that audiograms are performed by a trained, expert tester using calibrated equipment in a sound-controlled environment. The standard of medical care mandates the use of sound-treated test environments and frequent equipment calibration, and OSHA specifies requirements for both audiometer calibration and test room ambient noise levels. There are many pitfalls in testing technique that can produce misleading audiogram results. The complexities of testing technique are covered in greater detail elsewhere.[4,5] The audiogram is a medical and legal record, and the importance of accuracy cannot be overemphasized. In occupational settings, the first audiogram will serve as the baseline against which future tests are compared. Since hearing changes (and OSHA reporting requirements) depend on deviations from the baseline in many cases, the practical importance of accuracy in acquisition of every test is obvious. OSHA provides guidelines for changing the baseline audiogram used as a reference over time to account for expected aging changes and other factors that may result in stable hearing change requiring an adjustment of the "baseline" used for future test comparisons.

COMPONENTS OF THE TYPICAL AUDIOGRAM

Air Conduction

Air conduction denotes the ability of the ear to receive and conduct sound waves entering the external ear canal. Normally, these waves cause the eardrum to vibrate, and the vibrations are transmitted through the chain of ossicles to the oval window. When air conduction is impaired as a result of damage to the outer or the middle ear and the sensorineural mechanism of the inner ear is intact, the maximum difference between air and bone conduction thresholds is about 60 dB. This is so because when the sound is louder than 60 dB, it will be conducted by the bones of the skull directly to the cochlea.

Bone Conduction

To some extent bone conduction is a measure of the patient's ability to hear sound vibrations that are transmitted directly to the cochlea through the bones of the skull, bypassing the outer and the middle ear. Bone conduction is unimpaired in simple conductive hearing loss. Thus, conductive hearing loss (mechanical loss in the outer or middle ear) can be distinguished from sensorineural hearing loss by tuning forks or bone conduction audiometry. Before audiometry was available, hearing testing used to be done with a set of tuning forks that vibrated at different frequencies. They were placed next to the ear or against the skull (mastoid, nasal bridge, or teeth), and subjective judgments were made by the physician. The audiometer provided a way to quantify this kind of hearing assessment.

Tuning fork tests[6] always should be done to confirm the audiometric findings. When inconsistencies occur, the tuning fork test often turns out to be correct. The physician should be familiar with basic testing techniques. In general, a 512-Hz tuning fork should be used. It is struck firmly against a solid object (such as an elbow) but not hard enough to create audible overtones. For the Weber test, the tuning fork is placed on the forehead, nasal bridge or teeth, and the patient is asked whether the sound is louder in the right ear, left ear, or whether it seems to be in the center of the head. In a symmetric conductive hearing loss, the tuning fork lateralizes to the worse ear. In sensorineural hearing loss, it is louder in the better ear. The Rinne test compares bone conduction with air conduction by placing the tuning fork on the mastoid, nasal bridge or teeth (bone conduction), and next to the ear. In conductive hearing loss, bone conduction will be louder than air conduction. In normal hearing or sensorineural hearing loss, air conduction will be better.

Although sounds up to about 50 dB directed to one ear by air conduction through an earphone usually are heard by that ear alone, this is not the case with bone conduction. Bone-conducted sounds are heard almost equally well by both ears regardless of where the vibrations are impressed upon the skull. This holds true of both the tuning fork and the audiometer vibrator because they vibrate the whole skull. The proper way to minimize confusion is to mask the opposite ear by introducing enough neutral sound into it to occupy its auditory pathway and prevent the test from reaching it. Such masking must be used for all bone conduction testing and for specific circumstances in air conduction testing.

Speech Reception Threshold

Speech reception threshold is a measure of a person's ability to hear speech—not pure tones—using a speech audiometer that controls the intensity of the speech output. This test uses human speech rather than frequency-specific tones. One can test the speech reception threshold (SRT) by means of simple two-syllable words or sentences to determine the weakest intensity at which the subject can hear well enough to repeat half the spoken words or the sentences. A person who hears normally can hear and repeat these words at a level of about 15 dB. For hard-of-hearing individuals, the SRT is higher (i.e., the speech has to be louder to enable them to repeat it). The higher the number of decibels required, the greater the hearing loss. The SRT should be approximately equal to the pure-tone average in the speech frequencies. That is, if the hearing level in decibels at 500, 1000, 2000, and 3000 Hz are added and the result is divided by 4, the value should be approximately the same as the SRT.

Discrimination Score

The discrimination score does not measure the weakest intensity at which the patient hears speech sounds, but rather how well one can repeat correctly certain representative words delivered to the ear at about 40 dB above the SRT. A person with normal hearing discriminates 90–100% of the words. Patients with sensorineural losses may have anywhere from normal to severely decreased discrimination scores. Patients with acoustic neuromas, for example, may have discrimination scores as low as 0%.

Recruitment

To a patient with recruitment, compared to someone without it, a tone that sounds soft becomes louder much more suddenly and rapidly when its intensity is increased. This abnormally great and abrupt increase in the sensation of loudness, especially marked in patients with sensory hearing loss, generally is absent in patients with conductive and neural hearing loss. Recruitment testing can be done with a tuning fork or audiometrically using the alternate binaural loudness balance test, short-increment sensitivity test, and other methods. The tuning fork is crude but may be helpful especially in patients with asymmetric sensorineural hearing loss. For example, in a patient with sensorineural hearing loss on the right and little or no hearing loss on the left, the tuning fork can be struck very softly and placed next to each ear. The person is asked in which ear the sound is louder and confirms that the tuning fork is louder on the left. The tuning fork can then be struck forcefully and the test repeated. If the tuning fork now sounds louder on the right, this suggests recruitment in the right ear, a sign of cochlear (sensory) pathology.

Abnormal Tone Decay or Pathologic Adaptation

Abnormal tone decay occurs predominantly in neural hearing loss. It helps distinguish neural hearing (caused by lesions such as acoustic neuroma) from sensory (cochlear) hearing loss (caused by conditions such as occupational noise exposure). A patient who exhibits abnormal tone decay is unable to continue hearing a tone at threshold when it is prolonged at a uniform level of intensity; hearing fatigues rapidly. The phenomenon is called pathologic fatigue or abnormal tone decay.

Someone who has normal hearing continues to hear a very weak threshold tone for several minutes, but an individual with abnormal tone decay may hear the sound only for several seconds. The person then will ask that the sound be made louder. When this is done, the patient will hear the sound again for a few seconds, only to lose it again quickly and request that the volume be increased, and this pattern will be repeated.

Quantifying Hearing Levels for Medicolegal Purposes

For otologic purposes, audiograms are reviewed, and hearing levels at various frequencies are evaluated individually. Hearing is ordinarily not converted to "percentages" of hearing level or loss. However, percentages of loss are commonly calculated to quantify impairment for compensation purposes. For medicolegal matters involving occupational hearing loss, all calculations are based on pure-tone air conduction thresholds. The methods for determining hearing impairment and disability vary from jurisdiction to jurisdiction.[5] However, the most widely accepted formula has been promulgated by the American Academy of Otolaryngology (AAO), and it forms the basis of the majority of laws in the United States.

The ultimate test in any formula for determining hearing disability is the ability to understand speech, but because speech audiometry has certain limitations for practical use, pure-tone audiometry is used. Formerly, the most commonly used frequencies for calculating hearing impairment were 500, 1000, and 2000 Hz. Recently the AAO has recommended that 3000 Hz also be included. A so-called "low fence" has been determined, below which a hearing loss is considered insufficient to warrant compensation. There is a difference of opinion as to precisely where this low fence should be. The committee on hearing and bio-acoustics (CHABA), a subcommittee of the National Academy of Sciences National Research Council, had recommended that the low fence be placed at 35 dB. The AAO recommends that the low fence be maintained at 25 dB. Each state has its own method of paying disability and uses its own formula and provides a method for measuring and calculating binaural hearing impairment. The hearing level for each frequency is the number of decibels at which the listener's threshold of hearing lies above the standard audiometric 0 for that frequency. The hearing level for speech is a simple average of the hearing levels at the frequencies 500, 1000, 2000 and now 3000 Hz. The following is an example of how to calculate hearing impairment for compensation purposes[2] (AAO guidelines, 1979):

1. The average of the hearing threshold levels at 500, 1000, 2000, and 3000 Hz should be calculated for each ear.
2. The percent impairment for each ear should be calculated by multiplying by 1.5% the amount by which the above average hearing threshold level exceeds 25 dB (low fence) up to a maximum of 100%, which is reached at 92 dB (high fence).
3. The hearing handicap, a binaural assessment, should then be calculated by multiplying the smaller percentage (better ear) by 5, adding this figure to the larger percentage (poorer ear), and dividing the total by 6.

Example 1.
Mild Hearing Loss

	500 Hz	1000 Hz	2000 Hz	3000 Hz
Right Ear	15	25	45	55
Left Ear	20	30	50	60

AAO Method: 25 dB Fence

1. Right ear $\dfrac{15 + 25 + 45 + 55}{4} = \dfrac{140}{4} = 35$ dB average
2. Left ear $\dfrac{20 + 30 + 50 + 60}{4} = \dfrac{160}{4} = 40$ dB average

Monaural Impairment
1. Right ear   35 - 25 = 10 dB × 1.5% = 15%
2. Left ear   40 - 25 = 15 dB × 1.5% = 22.5%
3. Better ear 15 × 5 = 75
4. Poorer ear 22.5% × 1 = 22.5
5. Total   97.5 ÷ 6 = 16.25%

Model Legislation Method used to calculate the above loss:

1. Right ear $\dfrac{15 + 25 + 45 + 55}{4} = \dfrac{140}{4} = 35$ dB average
2. Left ear $\dfrac{20 + 30 + 50 + 60}{4} = \dfrac{160}{4} = 40$ dB average
3. Better ear threshold = 35 db = 5%

Example 2.
Severe Hearing Loss

	500 Hz	1000 Hz	2000 Hz	3000 Hz
Right Ear	80	90	100	110
Left Ear	75	80	90	95

AAO Method: Average Hearing Test Level

1. Right ear $\dfrac{80 + 90 + 100 + 110}{4} = \dfrac{380}{4} = 95$ dB (use 92 maximum)
2. Left ear $\dfrac{75 + 80 + 90 + 95}{4} = \dfrac{340}{4} = 85$ dB

Monaural Impairment
1. Right ear   92 - 25 = 67 dB × 1.5% = 100.5% (use 100%)
2. Left ear   85 - 25 = 60 dB × 1.5% = 90%
3. Better ear 90 × 5 = 450
4. Poorer ear 100 × 1 = 100
5. Total   550 ÷ 6 = 91.7%

New Jersey Method used to calculate the above loss:

1. Right ear $\dfrac{80 + 90 + 100 + 110}{4} = \dfrac{380}{4} = 95$ dB (use 92 maximum)
2. Left ear $\dfrac{75 + 80 + 90 + 95}{4} = \dfrac{340}{4} = 85$ dB
3. Better ear > 81 dB = 100%

SPECIAL TESTING

Using Speech to Detect Central Hearing Loss

Special tests using modified speech are becoming useful in the determination of whether a hearing loss is caused by damage in the central nervous system. Lesions in the cortex do not result in any reduction in pure-tone thresholds, but brainstem lesions may cause some high-frequency hearing loss. Routine speech audiometry is almost always normal in cortical lesions. Sometimes it is impaired in brainstem lesions, but without a characteristic pattern. Since neither pure-tone nor routine speech tests help to localize damage in the central nervous system, more complex tests have been developed to help provide this information.

A chief function of the cortex is to convert neural impulses into meaningful information. Words and sentences acquire their significance at the cortical level. Because quality, space, and time are factors governing the cortical identification of a verbal pattern, the tests are designed so that they explore the synthesizing ability of the cortex when one or more of these factors is purposely changed.

Binaural Test of Auditory Fusion

One such test of central auditory dysfunction is the binaural test of auditory fusion. Speech signals are transmitted through two different narrow-band filters. Each band by itself is too narrow to allow recognition of test words. Subjects who have normal hearing show excellent integration of test words when they receive the signals from one filter in one ear and the other filter in the other ear. Poorer scores are made by patients with brain lesions and are indications of a functional failure within the cortex.

Sound Localization Tests

Sound localization tests are also being used in the diagnosis of central lesions. Deviation of the localization band to one side points to a cerebral lesion on the contralateral side or to a brainstem lesion on the ipsilateral side.

Other Tests

Distorted-voice, interrupted-voice, and accelerated-voice tests likewise are used in detecting central lesions. In the **distorted-voice test**, PB (phonetically balanced) words are administered about 50 dB above SRT through a low-pass filter that is able to reduce the discrimination to about 70–80% in normal subjects. Patients with temporal lobe tumors present an average discrimination score that is poorer in the ear contralateral to the tumor.

The **interrupted-voice test** presents PB words at about 50 dB above thresholds, interrupting them periodically 10 times per second. Subjects with normal hearing obtain about 80% discrimination; those with temporal lobe tumors have reduced discrimination in the ear contralateral to the tumor.

In the **accelerated-voice test**, when the number of words per minute is increased from about 150 words to about 350 words, the discrimination approaches 100% in subjects who have normal hearing, but threshold is raised by 10–15 dB. In patients with tumors of the temporal lobe, there is a normal threshold shift, but the discrimination never attains 100% in the contralateral ear. In cortical lesions, the impairment always seems to be in the ear contralateral to the neoplasm and moderate (roughly 50–75%) in extent. Brainstem lesions exhibit ipsilateral or bilateral impairments.

Ipsilateral and contralateral stapedius reflex tests also provide useful information.[5]

TESTING FOR FUNCTIONAL HEARING LOSS

Whenever a patient claims to have a hearing loss that does not seem to be based on organic damage to the auditory pathway, or whenever test responses and the general behavior of the patient appear to be questionable, a variety of tests can be performed to help determine whether the loss is functional rather than organic.

The most suggestive findings are inconsistencies in the hearing tests. For example:

1. A patient has a hearing threshold level of 70 dB in one test and a 40 dB threshold when the test is repeated several minutes later.

2. The audiogram of a patient shows a 60-dB average hearing loss bilaterally, but the patient inadvertently replies to soft speech behind his back.

3. The patient has an SRT of 20 dB in contrast to a 60-dB pure-tone average.

4. The patient gives poor or no responses in bone conduction tests, indicating severe sensorineural involvement, but has suspiciously good discrimination ability for the alleged degree and type of loss.

However, care must be exercised. Certain organic conditions, such as Meniere's disease, multiple sclerosis, and severe tinnitus also may cause inconsistent responses.

Lombard or Voice-Reflex Test

When a patient claims deafness in one ear but it is suspected of being functional, several simple tests are available to determine the validity of the loss. The patient is given a newspaper or a magazine article to read aloud without stopping. While he is reading, the tester presents noise to the good ear. This may be done by rubbing a piece of typing paper such as onionskin paper over the patient's good ear. If the patient's voice does not get significantly louder, it is highly suggestive that he can hear in his supposedly "bad" ear. Because hearing involves a feedback mechanism that informs the speaker how loud he or she is speaking, a person with normal hearing will speak more loudly in a noisy area to hear himself or herself and be heard above the noise. If the patient does not raise his voice when noise is applied to one ear, it means that the patient is hearing himself speak in the other ear, and consequently that ear does not have the marked hearing loss indicated on the pure-tone or speech audiogram. Instead of rubbing paper against the patient's ears as the source of noise, a Bárány noise apparatus or the noise from an audiometer noise generator is extremely effective in this test, because the level of the noise can be controlled. It can be started at about 60 dB above threshold and then adjusted. This type of test is called the Lombard or voice-reflex test, and although it does not help to establish thresholds, it does give the examiner some idea of whether the loss is exaggerated.

Stenger Test

The Stenger test is also used for detecting unilateral functional hearing loss and evaluating the approximate amount of residual hearing. This test can be done with tuning forks or with an audiometer, the latter being the more reliable.

The Stenger test depends on a given pure tone presented to both ears simultaneously. The tone will be perceived only in the ear where it is louder. If the sound in one ear is made louder, the listener will hear it in that ear and will not realize that a weaker sound exists in the other ear.

A tone is presented to the good ear about 10 dB above threshold and, at the same time, 10 dB below the admitted threshold in the bad ear. If the patient responds, the test is a negative Stenger because he heard the tone in the good ear without realizing there was a weaker tone in his bad ear. If the patient does not respond, it is a positive Stenger because he heard the sound in his assumed bad ear without realizing a tone of weaker intensity was presented to his good ear.

This test can be done with speech as well as pure tones. There must be a difference of at least 30 dB between thresholds of the good and bad ear for the test to be effective. Also, a two-channel audiometer is needed to administer the test.

The Stenger test also enables the examiner to obtain an approximation of the patient's true thresholds in the bad ear.[5] This is done by presenting the pure tone 10 dB above threshold in the good ear and presenting a pure tone at 0 Hz in the bad ear. The tone in the bad ear is increased in 5-dB steps until the patient stops responding. (Remember, he is hearing the tone in his good ear at first.) The Stenger pure-tone threshold of the bad ear is approximately 15 dB above his true threshold.

Repetition of Audiogram without Masking

Still another test to indicate whether a patient really has a total unilateral hearing loss or may be malingering is to repeat the audiogram, but this time without masking the good ear. Since a pure tone presented to the test ear can be heard also in the non-test ear, when the loudness of the tone is 50–55 dB above the threshold of the non-test ear, at least some shadow curve should be present in the absence of masking. If the patient does not respond when the intensity levels reach this point, the chances are that he has a functional deafness in the test ear. If the patient does not report hearing the tone, he should be questioned carefully about its location. Again, total lack of response is an indication of the dilemma that the functional patient faces when he feels that his claim is threatened with exposure.

Delayed Auditory Feedback Test

The monitoring of an ear also can be disrupted if a person listens to himself speak through earphones while the return voice is delayed in time. A delay of 0.1–0.2 seconds causes symptoms similar to stuttering. If this occurs when the feedback level is lower than the admitted threshold, functional loss is present. In the delayed auditory feedback test (also called the delayed talk-back test), which is done through a modified tape recorder, it is possible to detect hearing losses of sizable degree, but not the minor exaggerations that occur occasionally in medicolegal situations. This is because delayed feedback affects the rhythm and the rate of the patient's speech at levels averaging 20–40 dB above threshold.

BERA in Malingering

Brainstem evoked-response audiometry (BERA) is discussed later in this chapter. However, because BERA testing is objective, the technique may provide valuable information in malingerers and patients with functional hearing loss.[1] Although in its present state of development BERA threshold testing has shortcomings, it is often helpful in assessing auditory function in patients who are unable or unwilling to cooperate. The shortcomings include an extremely long test time, relatively limited availability of appropriate test equipment, high test equipment cost, and numerous technical difficulties and controversies regarding the optimal nature of the stimulus and test technique. Nevertheless, in the hands of professionals with appropriate expertise and experience, BERA testing (also called ABR testing for auditory brainstem response) can provide valid, reliable threshold information.

IMPEDANCE AUDIOMETRY

Impedance audiometry is an objective method for evaluating the integrity and function of the auditory mechanism. It includes four separate types of measurements and has the potential for a much wider role as research in its use continues. The procedures most often used are (1) tympanometry, (2) static compliance, (3) acoustic reflex thresholds, and (4) acoustic reflex decay test.

Tympanometry

The eardrum and connecting ossicles constitute a mechanism that should transfer vibrating energy efficiently. Tympanometry measures the mobility of this system. It is analogous to pneumatic otoscopy. If the system becomes stiffer and more resistant because some condition impedes its free movement, we are able to measure the abnormal impedance (or its reciprocal "compliance"). The compliance or impedance of the middle ear system is measured by its response to variations in air pressure on the eardrum. The entrance of the ear canal is sealed with a probe tip containing three holes: one for supply of air pressure, one for a low-frequency probe tone (usually of 220 Hz), and the third opening connected to a pick-up microphone. As controlled degrees of positive and negative air pressure are introduced into the sealed ear canal, the resulting movement (or reduced movement) of the mechanism is plotted or automatically graphed on a chart called a tympanogram.

Static Compliance

Static compliance is a measure of middle ear mobility. It is measured in terms of equivalent volume in cubic centimeters, based on two volume measurements: (1) C1 is made with the tympanic membrane in a position of poor compliance with a pressure of +200 mm H_2O in the external canal, (2) C2 is made with TM at maximal compliance. C1 - C2 = static compliance, which cancels out the compliance due to the column of air in the external canal. The remainder is the compliance due to the middle ear mechanisms.

Static compliance is low when the value is less than 0.28 cc and high when greater than 2.5 cc. Its major contribution is to differentiate between a fixed middle ear bone and an ossicular discontinuity.

Physical Volume

The physical volume (PV) test uses a signal of fixed intensity in the ear canal. With an intact tympanic membrane, the meter will balance at a cc value of 1.0–1.5 in an adult and 0.7–1.0 in a child. If the eardrum is not totally intact, the PV measures will be large, often exceeding 5.0 cc. It is helpful in ruling out a nonobservable perforation, or it also can help to identify obstruction of a ventilating tube.

Acoustic Reflex Thresholds

Acoustic reflex thresholds determine the level in dB at which the stapedius muscle contracts. Normally, the reflex for pure tones is elicited at about 90 dB above the hearing threshold. For broad band noise, it occurs at about 70 dB above threshold. The contraction occurs bilaterally, even when only one ear is stimulated. In patients with cochlear damage and associated recruitment, the reflex may occur at sensation levels less than 60 dB above the auditory pure-tone threshold (Metz recruitment). In bilateral conductive losses and in some unilateral losses, the acoustic reflex may be absent bilaterally. In a unilateral cochlear loss not exceeding 80 dB, acoustic reflexes may appear unilaterally when the stimulation earphone is on the "dead ear" side. These factors then can be diagnostically important, especially when masking is impractical.

Acoustic Reflex Decay Test

In the normal ear, contraction of the middle ear muscles to a sound 10 dB above the acoustic reflex threshold can be maintained for at least 45 seconds without detectable decay or adaptation. In the presence of an acoustic neuroma or other retrocochlear lesion, however, the middle ear muscle contraction may show fatigue or decay in less than 10 seconds. In some cases, it may be entirely absent.

Other impedance tests include the **ipsilateral reflex test** for the differential diagnosis of brainstem lesions; **facial nerve test** for localizing the site of a lesion in facial paralysis; **eustachian tube tests** for determining eustachian tube function; **fistula test** in which positive air pressure will cause dizziness and deviation of the eyes if a fistula into the inner ear exists; and a test for presence of a **glomus tumor** in which meter variations in synchrony with the pulse beat can be observed.

Impedance audiometry is especially useful in difficult-to-test patients such as very young children, the mentally impaired, the physically impaired, and the malingerer. Like all other tests, it is not 100% accurate and must be interpreted with expertise.

Continuous Frequency Audiometry

Audiograms merely sample hearing at selected frequencies, leaving many frequencies between them untested. In some cases, it is helpful to test these frequencies. This can be done with a Békésy audiometer or with several commercially available audiometers that permit either continuous frequency testing or testing at approximately 60-Hz intervals. This kind of test may be useful, for example, in a person who complains of ringing tinnitus and fullness in one ear but whose routine audiogram is normal. Continuous frequency testing may reveal a dip at an in-between frequency, e.g., 6450 Hz, that helps establish the cause of the symptom.

Tinnitus Matching

Several devices are available to help quantify tinnitus, and some newer audiometers include tinnitus-matching capabilities. These tests allow reasonably good quantifications of tinnitus pitch and loudness. Interestingly, even very loud tinnitus is rarely more than 5–10 dB above threshold.

High-Frequency Audiometry

It is often useful to test frequencies above 8000 Hz. Testing to 12,000 or 14,000 Hz provides the desired information in most cases, and testing at frequencies above 14,000 Hz presents special difficulties. High-frequency testing is especially valuable for differentiating presbycusis from occupational hearing loss, detecting early effects of ototoxic drugs, and potentially in selected trauma cases, such as those with tinnitus and normal routine audiograms.

ELECTROCOCHLEOGRAPHY

Electrocochleography, a method of assessing difficult-to-test patients, involves placing an electrode in the ear and measuring directly the ear's electrical response to a sound stimulus. Most commonly, the electrode is placed through the eardrum into the promontory. In children, this may require a short general anesthetic. Newer electrodes permit high-quality testing with the electrodes placed in the ear canal rather than through the tympanic membrane. Electrocochleography has proven clinically valuable particularly for confirming wave I in the brainstem response if the BERA results are equivocal and, also, for confirming endolymphatic hydrops in patients with Meniere's disease.

Promontory Stimulation

The promontory stimulation test is suitable for patients with profound deafness and is rarely appropriate in patients with occupational hearing loss. The test involves placement of an electrode through the tympanic membrane. The electrode is placed against the promontory, and the cochlea is stimulated electrically. The test is used most commonly when assessing patients for possible cochlear implant candidacy.

EVOKED-RESPONSE AUDIOMETRY

Accurate hearing testing in infants, persons with limited mental capacity, neurologically disabled patients, and others who cannot or will not volunteer accurate responses is a special problem. A few objective tests (those requiring no patient cooperation) are now available. Impedance audiometry is objective, but it is difficult to determine hearing thresholds from it in some cases.

Evoked-response audiometry is similar to electroencephalography or brainwave testing. Painless electrodes are attached to the patient. A darkened, "soundproof" room is used. A computer is required to isolate the auditory responses from the rest of the electrical activity from the brain. Pure-tone or broad-band stimuli can be used. There are two types of evoked-response audiometry, cortical evoked-response audiometry and brain-stem evoked-response audiometry.

Cortical Evoked-Response Audiometry

Cortical evoked-response audiometry focuses on electrical activity at the cerebral cortex level. It allows measurement not only of auditory signals, but also of other brain-wave variations that are associated with the perception of sound. Therefore, it may prove a valuable tool in evaluating not only thresholds, but also whether a sound actually reaches a level of perception in the brain. Cortical evoked responses occur at approximately 200 ms after the stimulus. Unfortunately, they are of limited value for threshold testing because they can be affected volitionally. For example, responses are better if a patient concentrates on an auditory signal than if he attempts to ignore it. Cortical evoked responses may also be altered substantially by drugs and state of consciousness.

Middle Latency Responses

Middle latency responses are electrical potentials whose origins are still uncertain. They are thought to be generated by sites central to the brainstem generators, such as the primary auditory cortex, association cortex, and thalamus. Although responses around 40 ms are considered most common, middle latency responses may be observed between 8 and 50 ms following stimulus onset. Middle latency responses appear to be somewhat more amenable to use for special testing than brainstem responses, but they are also more subject to extraneous influence. Although middle latency response testing still appears to hold promise for special populations who are difficult to test by traditional means, shortcomings of this procedure have limited its routine clinical application.

Brainstem Evoked-Response Audiometry

Brainstem evoked responses occur within the first 10 ms, and they are unaffected by behavior, attention, drugs, or level of consciousness. In fact, they can be measured under general anesthesia or during deep coma. They give information about the ear and central auditory pathways at the brainstem level, although not about cortical perception of hearing. BERA has become popular because it is objective, consistent, and provides a great deal of valuable information. The test measures electrical peaks generated in the brainstem along the auditory pathways. The sites or origin of the waves are still controversial. Traditionally, the following scheme has been believed: wave I is actually generated at the junction of the hair cells and VIII nerve, but the measured peak occurs in the distal auditory nerve where it leaves the bone and enters the CSF and the internal auditory canal; wave II comes from the proximal portion of the auditory nerve, although previously it was believed to originate at the cochlear nucleus; wave III, at the superior olive; wave IV, probably at the level of the lateral lemniscus in the pons; wave V, at the inferior colliculus; wave VI, probably at the thalamus; and wave VII, possibly at the cortical level. Although good research supports these beliefs, other opinions have been offered. The most common alternate schema is as follows: wave I, as above; wave II, proximal portion of the auditory nerve; wave III, cochlear nucleus; wave IV, contralateral superior olivary complex; wave V, lateral lemniscus. At present, only waves I–V are used clinically for audiologic purposes, and waves I, III and IV are most easily defined. Absence or distortion of peaks, or delay between peaks, can help localize lesions in the auditory pathway. For example, difference in latency between a patient's two ears of greater than 0.2 ms currently appears to be the most sensitive audiologic test for detecting acoustic neuromas. However, BERA can have other localizing value. The presence of wave I with absence of later waves may occur following a brainstem vascular accident with normal peripheral hearing and damaged central pathways. Increasing interwave latencies with clear separation of waves IV and V (which usually overlap) occurs in conditions that cause conduction delay, classically multiple sclerosis. In demyelinating disease, one also sees degradation of later waves aggravated by higher rates of stimulation. Testing can be done with pure tones, broadband noise, logons, or clicks. Approximate threshold levels can be determined.[1] The tests can be used on infants and children and have even been advocated for routine screening in nurseries for newborns.

Otoacoustic Emissions

The study of otoacoustic emission (OAE) is a growing area of interest in the scientific community. In 1977, Kemp discovered that the cochlea was capable of producing sound emissions.[3] Specifically, Kemp proposed that a biomechanical amplifier within the organ of Corti underlies these properties. This amplifier is the origin of otoacoustic emissions that are apparently generated as a byproduct of the traveling wave initiated amplitude enhancement of basilar membrane vibration. There are four categories of otoacoustic emissions: spontaneous, evoked, stimulus frequency, and distortion product of otoacoustic emissions, which may be conceptualized as an echo in response to a sound stimulus. They may produce consistent patterns in cochlear pathology with involvement of the outer hair cells such as noise-induced hearing loss, ototoxicity, and hereditary hearing loss. These emissions are also generally absent in hearing loss greater than 30 dB and thus may be a good hearing screening tool for infants.

Distortion product otoacoustic emissions (DPOAE) are generated in response to paired pure tones and are felt to be more frequency specific. Some researchers feel that DPOAEs can accurately assess boundaries between normal and abnormal hearing with losses up to 50 dB. This category of OAEs may be useful clinically in monitoring changes in the cochlea due to hereditary hearing loss, progressive disease, and ototoxic agents. Research in the area of OAEs is still young, and many proposed theories have yet to be widely accepted and used in a clinical setting.[4]

CONCLUSION

This chapter reviews only a small number of the many hearing tests available to patients with real or alleged hearing impairments. Occupational physicians should be familiar with the principles of audiologic testing and the complexities involved in obtaining valid, reliable hearing tests. Interpretation requires information from a history, physical examination, noise exposure history (vocational and nonvocational), and many other factors. In many cases, the needs of the worker, company, and occupational physician are best served by close collaboration with an otologist who has practical expertise in occupational hearing loss.

REFERENCES

1. Frattali MA, Sataloff RT, Hirshout D, et al: Audiogram construction using frequency-specific auditory brainstem response thresholds. Ear Nose Throat J 74:691–700, 1995.
2. American Academy of Otolaryngology: The Guide for Conservation of Hearing in Noise, revised ed. Rochester, MN, AAO—Head and Neck Surgery Foundation, Inc., 1982.
3. Kemp OT: Stimulated acoustic emissions from within the human auditory system. J Acoust Soc Am 64:1386–1391, 1978.
4. Lonsbury-Martin BL, Harris FP, Stanger BB, et al: Distortion product emissions in humans. I: Basic problems in normally hearing subjects. Ann Otol Rhinol Laryngol 99:3–14, 1990.
5. Rintelmann W (ed): Hearing Assessment. Baltimore, University Park Press, 1979.
6. Sataloff RT, Sataloff J: Occupational Hearing Loss. 2nd ed. New York, Marcel Dekker, 1993.

LAWRENCE G. GRAY, OD

TESTING THE AFFERENT VISUAL SYSTEM

From the Departments of
  Neurology and Ophthalmology
Allegheny University of the Health
  Sciences
Philadelphia, Pennsylvania

Reprint requests to:
Lawrence G. Gray, OD
Departments of Neurology and
  Ophthalmology
Allegheny University of the Health
  Sciences
1427 Vine Street
Philadelphia, PA 19102

When a patient presents with reduced acuity, the clinician should determine if the reduced acuity is due to refractive error, functional amblyopia, ocular media opacity, retinal disease, or disease of the optic nerve or chiasm. Monocularly reduced acuity means that the cause must be in front of the optic chiasm. This chapter describes tests that help to determine the source of reduced acuity.

"QUALITATIVE" SNELLEN ACUITY

Snellen acuity is a powerful diagnostic tool. How the patient reads the Snellen acuity chart is often an untapped resource of diagnostic information. If the 20/40 acuity line "FZBDE," is read as "FZB--" with the right eye and "--BDE" with the left eye, this is characteristic of bitemporal hemianopia or bilateral caecocentral scotomas. If the line is read backwards, or the patient has difficulty finding the beginning of the next line, or reads the letters "--BDE" with each eye, a left homonymous hemianopia should be suspected. If there is difficulty in completing the line or the patient reads "FZB--" with each eye, a right homonymous hemianopia should be suspected as the probable diagnosis.

Remember that a reduced visual acuity represents a "blunting" of the peak of the hill of vision. The eye's greatest resolution is at the foveola and decreases with retinal eccentricity. When a patient's visual acuity is reduced, the clinician should suspect a central scotoma and may be able to determine its size. Based upon the range of eccentric retinal locations at which a given acuity is expected, a reading of 20/50 suggests an absolute central scotoma of 1.5–4.5°, a 20/100 reading represents a scotoma of 4–11°, and 20/200 correlates with a scotoma of 9–18°.[22] An easy way to remember this is to divide the denominator of the Snellen fraction by a factor of 10 to get a rough estimate of the size of the absolute scotoma; thus 20/50 ≈ 5° central scotoma, 20/100 ≈ 10° central scotoma, and 20/200 ≈ 20° central scotoma.

One can take advantage of three Snellen optotypes as high-contrast targets to probe for visual field loss on each side of the vertical hemianopic line. Isolating on the acuity projector three different letters on the 20/100 line tests the visual field at about 1–1.5° on each side of fixation. As the patient occludes one eye, he fixates on the middle letter and then judges whether the nasal or temporal letter appears more clear. The Troxler effect may cause the surrounding letters to fade away, but a small refixation movement, or blink, allows the patient to recover the optotype clarity.

Most clinicians test Snellen visual acuity using a projector in a darkened room. This may not be practical if the testing is done as part of a screening examination by non-eyecare professionals. The Snellen acuity chart measures high spatial frequency and high contrast. One can challenge the visual system by increasing the ambient room illumination. This converts the Snellen optotypes into high spatial frequency, low-contrast targets. An eye that sees 20/20 with the lights off but drops to 20/40 with the lights on may have an afferent system defect.

A dull or faded temporal letter implies a temporal visual field defect or caecocentral scotoma. If the patient has difficulty viewing the middle letter, there may be a central scotoma. Functional amblyopes may see the optotypes at the ends of the line more clearly than those in the center. If the optotypes are seen above or below fixation, an altitudinal hemianopia or paracentral scotoma may be present. Distorted letters mean a metamorphopsia is present, which indicates retinal disease.

A chronicle of reduction in visual acuity may be important in establishing the tempo of the visual loss and the behavior of the disease process.

Unilateral or bilateral reduced visual acuity accompanies some diseases and excludes others. For example, toxic nutritional diseases and cone dystrophies can cause symmetric, bilateral reduced visual acuity.[4] Compressive lesions of the anterior visual system cause asymmetric visual loss.

The acuity in an amblyopic eye is generally poorer during binocular than monocular viewing conditions, better when one optotype is presented at a time, and improves under dim illumination.

Diseases such as glaucoma, retinitis pigmentosa, and retrochiasmal visual pathway disorders spare the central acuity, while others such as optic neuritis and ischemic optic neuropathy often affect central acuity.

Matching the distant and near acuity may be revealing. The causes of a disparity between distance and near acuity include functional vision loss, visual field deficits, downbeat nystagmus, and vertical gaze palsies.

PINHOLE ACUITIES

The pinhole occluder has endured into the era of "high-tech" ocular instrumentation and continues to serve as an instrument that can quickly determine the patient's best refractable acuity (Fig. 1).

A multiple pinhole occluder improves reduced acuity that is otherwise blurred by refractive error. By reducing the blur circles on the retina, the occluder sharpens the retinal image. One can actually determine if the patient is myopic, hyperopic, or emmetropic by moving the occluder back and forth from left to right. If objects move with the occluder, the patient is myopic. If the objects move against the movement of the occluder, the patient is hyperopic. No movement suggests emmetropia.

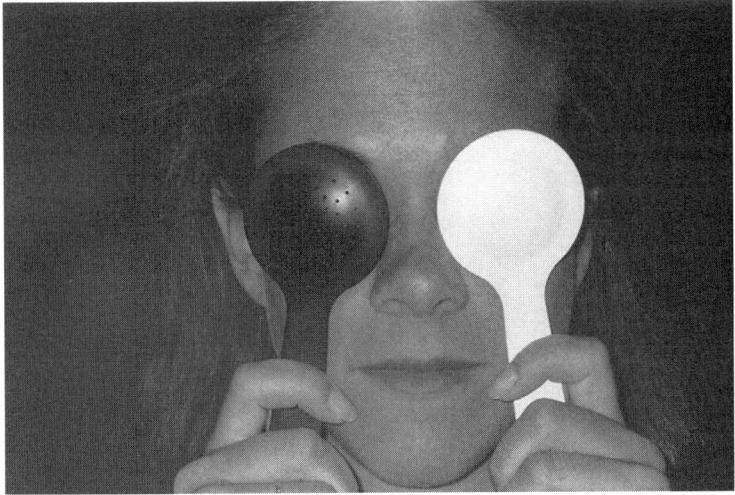

FIGURE 1. Patient covers her right eye with a multiple pinhole occluder to determine the best correctable Snellen acuity.

Corrective lenses almost always create a clearer retinal image than does the pinhole occluder. Exceptions include keratoconus, corneal or lens opacities, and irregular astigmatism, in which pinhole acuity is better than spectacle lens acuity.

Pinholes reduce the amount of light entering the eye. Decreasing illumination in impaired eyes from whatever cause reduces visual acuity. It worsens the acuity in patients with diffuse opacification of the ocular media, with central scotomas from retinal or optic nerve disease, and with amblyopia. In aphakic or highly myopic eyes, one must use a +10 D or –10 D lens, respectively, in combination with the pinhole to obtain optimal visual acuity.

NEUTRAL LENS DENSITY FILTER

The 2.0 logarithmic, neutral lens density filter (Kodak #96) is another means of investigating reduced visual acuity (Fig. 2). It is a less precise means of determining whether reduced vision is caused by amblyopia or by organic disease.

This commercially available filter reduces all visible wavelengths of light equally. Placing the filter before a normal eye may cause minimal reduction in visual acuity, by about one or two lines on the Snellen chart. However, in an eye with retinal or optic nerve disease, the filter "washes out" the acuity chart, causing a reduction in visual acuity. The diagnostic "surprise" occurs in an amblyopic eye, when visual acuity remains unchanged (if the amblyopia is profound, then the results are unreliable). This happens because diseased eyes have better resolution under higher illumination and amblyopic eyes have better resolution under lower illumination. Degrading acuity with a neutral lens density filter is a "soft" diagnostic test since certain optic neuropathies such as toxic nutritional amblyopia perform similarly.

PUPIL TESTING

With rare exceptions, the presence of a direct pupillary response is objective proof that an eye has some vision. In a monocularly blind patient, the pupil will not respond to light in the blind eye or respond consensually in the other eye. However,

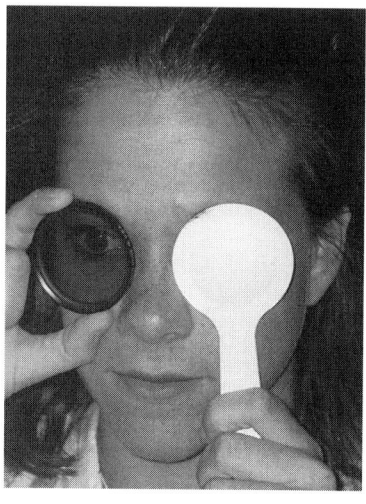

FIGURE 2. A 2.0 logarithmic, neutral density filter is placed before the right eye to distinguish between amblyopia and organic disease.

direct illumination of the good eye will create a pupillary response and a consensual response in the blind eye. Both pupils will react to near fixation.

If the pupil of a seeing eye does not react to light, but the consensual response of the opposite eye is intact, one should consider the differential of a pharmacologically dilated pupil, a posterior synechia, a tonic pupil, a fixed pupil (associated with a palsy of cranial nerve III), and a pupil in aberrant regeneration of the third cranial nerve. Both a tonic pupil and a pupil in aberrant regeneration of the third cranial nerve would react at near.

A patient who claims to have a completely blind eye, with a preserved direct pupillary response, should be viewed with suspicion because the afferent pupillomotor fibers and the visual fibers are routed together. The pupillomotor fibers are routed through the brachium of the superior colliculus to the pretectal nuclei. These nuclei innervate the Edinger-Westphal nuclei, which drive the pupillary response. The visual fibers are channeled via the optic tract to the lateral geniculate body. Therefore, the presence of a direct pupillary response to light means that an action potential generated from the optic nerve has reached the lateral geniculate body. There are creative ways to challenge functional patients, which are discussed later.

Relative afferent pupillary defect (RAPD) testing is one of the most important tests of visual function and a means to distinguish optic nerve disease from retinal disease. There are a number of tests that distinguish macular from optic nerve dysfunction (Table 1).

TABLE 1. Characteristics of Retinal and Optic Nerve Dysfunction

	Macula	Optic Nerve
Color vision	Normal	Abnormal
Sense of brightness	Minimally impaired	Impaired
Field defect	Central scotoma	Central scotoma plus enlarged blindspot
Amsler grid	Metamorphopsia	Negative scotoma
Photostress	Abnormal	Normal
Relative afferent pupillary defect	Normal	Abnormal

However, an RAPD is an "objective probe" of the anterior afferent visual system. Because the eyes are paired, one pupil's response to light can be matched against the other's, and the examiner can objectively discover defects in the anterior visual system. Evaluating the pupil in an eye with impaired vision requires that the clinician determine the pupil's response to direct light and whether an RAPD is present. To evaluate a direct response to light, the patient must fixate on a target across a dark room. A bright light source can be applied three or four times to assess the briskness of the response. In normal eyes, both pupils will briskly constrict. In an afferent pupillary defect, the direct response of the pupil to light is less than its consensual response. For example, if the left eye is affected, light presented rhythmically to the left eye will lead to dilation of both pupils (Fig. 3).

Afferent visual system defects can cause a diminished pupillary response to direct light. However, these abnormal pupillary responses may be subtle. The search for an afferent pupillary defect is performed by matching the direct and consensual responses in the same eye. In the affected eye, miosis created by the direct response is compared to the miosis caused by the consensual response from the opposite eye.

Testing conditions must be correct to ensure the accuracy of the test. A dark room is preferable because a brightly illuminated room reduces the amount of pupillary movement, leading to difficulty in determining subtle defects. To prevent false positives and to determine all defects, the examiner should use a bright, cool, hand-held light and conduct the test in a dark room.

Next, anisocoria should be identified. RAPDs do not cause anisocoria. When one pupil is larger than the other, the larger pupil might be mistakenly identified as abnormally dilating. Furthermore, an anisocoria greater than 1 mm may be associated with a false positive finding. A smaller pupil shades the retina, and a larger one exposes the retina to proportionately more light. Retinal exposure decreases light sensitivity and promotes a physiologically-induced RAPD in the eye with the larger pupil. Neutral lens density filters can be used to compensate for the unequal retinal illumination using 0.1 log units for every millimeter of anisocoria.[27] This means that 1 mm of anisocoria requires placement of a 1.0 neutral lens density filter before the eye with the larger pupil before proceeding with the test.

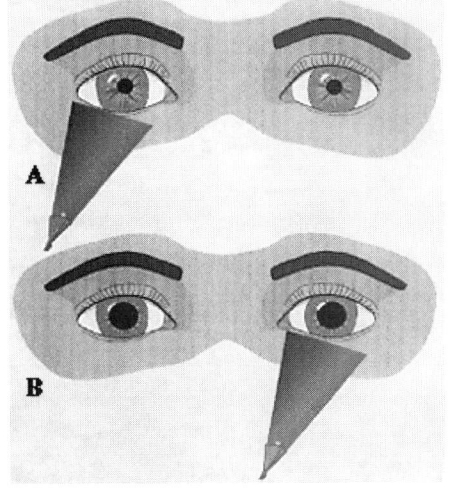

FIGURE 3. *A*, A patient with left optic nerve disease. A bright light illuminates the normal right eye. The right, direct pupillary response and the left, consensual pupillary response generate miosis. *B*, The light is aimed at the left pupil. When the left eye is illuminated, the pupils fail to "hold" the miosis and both pupils dilate. Thus the left direct pupillary response is less than its consensual response, induced by the right eye. The clinician who watches only the illuminated pupil, as he rhythmically swings the light source between the two eyes, sees the pupil of the abnormal left eye dilate.

Third, the patient should not be exposed to bright lights before testing because bleaching of the photoreceptors can occur, creating a false positive. One can induce a physiologic afferent pupillary defect by shining a bright light in one eye for a few minutes. Eyedrops might interfere with the pupil's reactions and should not be used prior to the testing procedure.

A patient who is ready for testing should maintain distance fixation to prevent miosis of the near response. The light source is directed at either pupil, and the eye is observed for miosis. After 2 seconds, the light source is shifted to the other pupil for another 2 seconds, and that pupil is observed for miosis. The clinician then rhythmically shifts the light back and forth three or four times to compare how each pupil holds the miosis or which pupil dilates. The test is then stopped to ensure against photoreceptor bleaching. There is a great temptation for the clinician searching for an abnormal pupillary dilation to linger on a suspect eye and thus overexpose that eye, inducing a pseudo-afferent pupillary defect. Testing may resume after 30 seconds without extraneous light exposure.

When a normal eye is exposed to bright light for more than a few seconds, the pupil constricts, redilates, and begins to oscillate. As the light source is swung back and forth between the eyes, the constriction and redilation should appear symmetric. Normal dilation should not be interpreted as an afferent pupillary defect. If the "swing" of the light is "out of rhythm," a "normal constriction" of one eye might be matched with a "normal dilation" of the other and subsequently misinterpreted.

If the conduction defect is marked, the pupils of both eyes dilate as the light source is directed at the affected eye. In an eye with a subtle conduction defect, the pupil may initially constrict but redilate more quickly than when light is directed into the opposite eye. It appears as if the pupil of the affected eye fails to "hold the miosis." These responses are rated on an arbitrary scale of 1+ to 4+ based on the direction of pupil movement. A rating of 1+ is early release of the pupil; 2+ shows no initial movement, followed by early release; 3+ is associated with immediate release of the pupil; and 4+ is an amaurotic response associated with no light perception vision.

However, the amount of pupil reactivity is not proportional to the degree of axonal damage. Elderly patients have less pupillary mobility than younger patients. If the starting size of the pupil is small, there is less pupillary excursion to evaluate. The same degree of axonal damage in a younger patient may reflect a more obvious pupillary defect because of greater pupillary movement. For this reason, it is more accurate to use a logarithmic neutral density filter to "balance out" an afferent pupillary defect.[6,26,28] Neutral density filters calibrated in log units are used during the swinging flashlight exercise placed before the good eye. Filters are added at 0.3 logarithmic steps, with 5- to 10-second breaks while the pupils are "washed" with equal exposures to light. This is performed until no afferent pupillary defect can be seen. One should next try to exceed the endpoint and create an RAPD in the filtered eye. Six filters that are clinically useful are 0.3, 0.6, 1.0, 1.5, 2.0, and 3.0 log units. Beyond a 1.2 log unit neutral density filter, it may become more difficult to observe the pupillary response, and one may have to glance behind the filter. A 0.3 log unit neutral density filter is particularly helpful in flushing out a subtle RAPD. If the physician is unsure whether an early pupillary release has occurred, a 0.3 log unit filter can be placed in front of the suspected abnormal eye. If a small or sluggish pupil creates an equivocal response, a 0.6 unit filter can be used. A 0.3 log unit neutral density filter should not produce an RAPD in a normal eye; however, if there is a preexisting conduction defect, the early release of the pupil will be enhanced.

When one pupil is immobile due to a synechia, anterior segment inflammation, mydriatic drops, or paresis, conduction defects can be assessed by observing the normal pupil of the opposite eye.[24] Under these conditions, the consensual response of the eye with the fixed pupil can be compared with the direct response of the non-affected eye. For example, a patient with a complete third cranial nerve palsy has a fixed, dilated pupil. When light is directed at the fixed pupil, the consensual response causes a constriction in the opposite eye.

If optic nerve function is normal in the eye with the fixed pupil, then light directed into the other eye should not cause an increase in miosis. However, if the normal pupil seems to constrict to a more miotic position, a conduction defect in the ophthalmoparetic eye is probable. Thus, the consensual response of the paretic is poorer than the direct response of the normal eye. Involvement of the optic nerve (cranial nerve II) and cranial nerve III anatomically localizes a lesion to the superior orbital tissue.

An afferent pupillary defect can be elicited when there is a reduction in nerve impulse or action current in the axonal pathway. For example, axons are "insulated" with myelin sheaths. When there is loss of myelin, such as in demyelinating optic neuritis, action current "leaks out" or dissipates at the denuded area. When light is directed into the uninvolved eye, both the affected and uninvolved eye appear to dilate.

An afferent pupillary defect is not a diagnosis but rather signals a need for thorough investigation of optic nerve function. The RAPD is directly proportional to the amount of visual field loss.[29] One can quantitatively match the central standard mean deviation of a central threshold visual field with the neutral lens density log value used to tilt an RAPD.[13]

Afferent pupillary defects do not occur bilaterally. If there is bilateral optic neuropathy, there may be bilaterally deafferented pupils. There has to be a relatively greater amount of axonal death in one eye to create a (relative) afferent pupillary defect. A marked afferent pupillary defect is most likely caused by optic nerve dysfunction and usually signals a lesion anterior to the chiasm.

Before one can label a pale disc "atrophic," optic nerve dysfunction must be substantiated with poor visual acuity, a visual field defect, associated nerve fiber layer dropout, and an afferent pupillary defect. Similarly, the RAPD is the hallmark of traumatic optic neuropathy and accompanies idiopathic optic neuritis and ischemic optic neuropathy.

Certain retinal diseases can create subtle conduction pupil defects, including extensive retinal detachments and advanced, or age-related, macular degeneration. However, there is more RAPD per line of visual acuity reduction in optic nerve disease than with macular disease.[33] Anterior chiasmal lesions may cause afferent pupillary defects. Optic tract lesions with asymmetric visual field defects may cause an RAPD between 0.3 and 0.6 log units.[3] If there is poor visual acuity, without an afferent pupillary defect, one should suspect some cause other than optic nerve disease.

The near response does not need to be routinely tested. However, the time to test the near response is when the direct response is poor or absent. The near response is not really a reflex but an inseparable triad of miosis, accommodation, and convergence. The neuroanatomic pathway remains incompletely delineated.

One way to test the near response is to ask the patient to fixate on one number on a wristwatch. Because it may be easier to observe dilation than constriction, the pupil's redilation can be observed as the patient refixates on a distant target. Often, when locating the near-point of convergence, observing pupillary dilation will reveal the "break" finding.

The near response may be quite variable, depending on the patient's cooperation and effort. It is probably for this reason that the direct response appears to be more brisk than to near. It is also for this reason that the patient needs encouragement for the maximal response.

A pupillary near reaction greater than the direct light reflex is called a "light-near response disassociation pupil." There are five causes of a light-near disassociation response. They include: (1) amaurotic pupil, (2) tonic pupil, (3) Argyll-Robertson pupil, (4) tectal pupils, (5) aberrant regeneration of the third cranial nerve.

COLOR VISION

Color vision is one of the first optic nerve functions to deteriorate and the last to recover in optic nerve disease.[5,11] The presence of a dyschromatopsia is essential in the diagnosis of optic atrophy. Most commercial color vision plate tests were designed to investigate congenital red/green confusion. Nevertheless, used monocularly, these tests identify and quantitate a dyschromatopsia. The American Optical Hardy-Rand-Rittler pseudoisochromatic plates seem to be more sensitive in identifying optic nerve disease.[15] A routine search for a dyschromatopsia should be performed by alternatively occluding each eye as the patient views a confusion color plate. The sorting or arrangement color vision tests (Farnsworth Munsell 100 hue test, Farnsworth Dichotomous Test for Color Blindness [D-15]) offer finer resolution of a patient's color discrimination and facilitate classifying a congenital color vision defect.

Can color vision testing help sort disease of the retina from optic nerve disease? The controversial Koellner's rule equates blue/yellow defects with macular disease and red/green defects with optic nerve disease.[7] Macular disease creates a marked peak in the color circle in the blue-purple area, with a smaller peak in the yellowish area. In optic nerve disease, there is a broader peak centered in the blue-purple area combined with a green peak.[20] But, in fact, optic nerve disease desaturates colors more than retinal disease. Poor acuity with good color vision implies retinal disease, while poor acuity with poor color vision suggests optic nerve disease. The progressive cone degenerations are the exception.[16] Good acuity and poor color vision occur with congenital color vision deficiencies–so-called colorblindness, which is often sex-linked.

Acquired color vision defects are associated with an apparent change of hue. Cross comparison of a red object with each eye screens for a dyschromatopsia. A pure red target will appear more yellowish to an eye with an optic neuropathy. As the optic neuropathy progresses, the redness will fade to orange, yellow, and then be perceived as colorless.[8]

The design of color confusion plates offers an unadvertised testing advantage. Rarely, if a patient is unable to detect a number or figure in a color confusion plate, this may suggest simultanagnosia, a disorder of higher cortical function. Cerebral achromatopsia, the inability to name colors while color acuity is normal, also implies a disorder of higher cortical function. This rare disorder is seen with bilateral superior quadrantic defects, and occasionally prosopagnosia, a form of visual agnosia in which face recognition, including the recognition of one's own face in a mirror, is abnormal or absent.[12,19] This is probably due to damage to the anteromedial aspect of the occipital lobe at the occipito-temporal junction.[33]

BRIGHTNESS SENSE

A subjective way to detect or confirm a conduction optic nerve defect is to ask the patient to compare "brightness" perceived with each eye. Patients with optic nerve disease have a significantly reduced brightness sense that is disproportionate to the severity of their visual acuity loss.[23] The eye with the suspected optic nerve defect is occluded, and a numerical value is assigned to the brightness of the light seen by the unaffected eye. The patient is told that the light to the normal eye is worth 100 points in brightness. The normal eye is then occluded, and the patient is asked to assign a numerical rating to the light perceived by the affected eye. A red target may be used in the same way, substituting redness for brightness. Small differences in brightness perceived by normal eyes may be due to dominant-eye luminance and should not be mistaken as a conduction defect. Polaroid lenses may be used to quantitate the difference between the two eyes.

PHOTOSTRESS RECOVERY TEST

The phenomenon of being momentarily "blinded" by a flashbulb afterimage has been harnessed for clinical use to differentiate between macular disease and optic nerve conduction defects.[10] Cone opsin is bleached from the cone when intense light is concentrated on the foveola. This creates a "flashbulb-like" afterimage, i.e., a positive scotoma with a reduction in visual acuity. How quickly vision returns depends on the remanufacturing of cone photosensitive pigment, cone opsin. This process depends on the integrity of the photoreceptors and the retinal pigment epithelium, the source of nourishment and maintenance.

When the photosensitive pigment is depleted with a bright light, damaged photoreceptors or retinal pigment epithelium delay resynthesis of photosensitive pigment and a return to normal acuity. This photochemical process operates independently of any neural mechanism, which makes it ideal to separate optic nerve disease from retinal disease.

The photostress recovery test begins by obtaining the best corrected acuities in each eye. The test is invalid for patients with less than 20/80 visual acuity. The eye with impaired vision is occluded, and the patient is asked to stare directly into a bright penlight for 10 seconds. The light is removed, and the patient is asked to read the next larger line of optotypes while the recovery is timed. Recovery time is recorded when the patient can read any three optotypes larger than the best corrected acuity. The same procedure is repeated on the opposite eye, and the recovery times are compared. A normal eye or an eye with optic nerve disease will recover vision in less than 50 seconds, but an eye with a retinopathy has a recovery time of 120–480 seconds.

CONFRONTATION VISUAL FIELD TESTING

Confrontation visual field testing is used to determine if the reduced visual function is due to chiasmal or retrochiasmal disease.

Lesions located behind the optic chiasm rarely cause reduced acuity. Chiasmal disease asymmetrically decreases acuities. Performing confrontation fields routinely offers a quick screening of every patient for insidious field loss. It also directs the quantitative or computerized perimeter to the important portion of the visual field. Performing confrontation fields also allows the questioning or confirming of the plotted findings of more sophisticated quantitative testing.

Performing a reliable confrontation field is an artful technique.[32] The clinician's face should be positioned about 25 inches from and level with the patient's face (Fig. 4). Unless the patient is wearing an aphakic lens or has high minus correction, the patient's eyeglasses should be removed. At this distance, the circumference of the clinician's face outlines a 20° visual field. The distance from the nose to chin or ear is about half this, or 10°. The patient is asked to cover the left eye with the

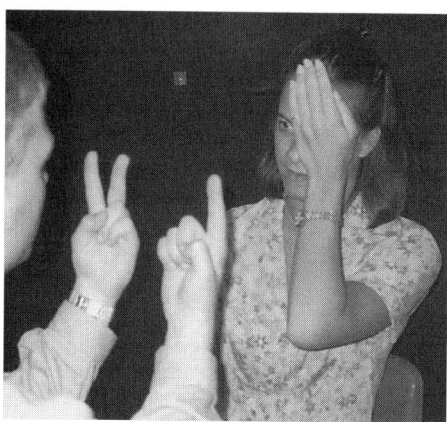

FIGURE 4. Confrontation fields are performed by presenting finger targets in the four quadrants of the visual field as the patient fixates on the clinician's nose. Finger counting, simultaneous finger counting, and simultaneous hand comparison are routine visual field investigation techniques.

palm and to look at the clinician's nose. Questions to the patient should be phrased in a forced choice format, with "yes" or "no" suffix at the end of the question. If the patient is allowed to point, the clinician might get poked in the face. The clinician should ask, "Can you see my nose, yes or no?" If the patient cannot see the nose, there is a dense central scotoma. The patient is next asked if something is missing or blurry on the clinician's face. If the patient cannot see an eye, eyebrow, or mouth, the patient may have a paracentral scotoma. You may even challenge patients by closing an eye and asking if both of your eyes are open or if your mouth is open or closed. You can literally check the vertical hemianopic line in a "wink of an eye" by alternatively closing each eye and asking if both eyes are open.

Next, the clinician's face is described as divided into four quadrants, with the nose continuing to function as the fixation point. The targets are one, two, three, and five fingers presented to each of the four quadrants. Bringing the fingers closer to your face decreases the isopter size, increases the sensitivity of the test, and enlarges the visual field defect. Placing fingers closer to the patient's face increases the isopter size, decreases the sensitivity of the test, and reduces the size of the visual field defect.

Once finger-counting has been performed in all four quadrants, simultaneous finger-counting is performed. Two targets are presented in two quadrants and the patient is asked for the total number of fingers. This tests the "extinction phenomenon," in which the patient may count fingers correctly in each quadrant but will miss them when simultaneously presented in both visual fields. It also tests the patient's ability to perform simple calculations, which assesses parietal lobe function.

The third step is for the clinician to present both hands simultaneously in each hemifield to check for bitemporal field loss. The clinician asks, "As you look at my nose, and allow for the room lighting, is one hand more clear than the other, yes or no?" Orienting the clinician's hands above and below the nasal horizontal raphé checks the nasal step. One must be careful that the room illumination does not make one hand brighter than the other.

Targets should be kept in the central 20–30° visual field, which approximately matches the circumference of the face. Almost all neurologic visual field defects affect the central 30° of the visual field. A common mistake is to present targets too far into the periphery. You can be assured of presenting the targets correctly in the central field by keeping your elbows snugly against your sides and placing your fingers in front of your face.

Advanced confrontation techniques include mapping out the blind spot in the air. Reduced Snellen acuity with a normal blindspot suggests retinal disease while an enlarged blindspot implies optic nerve disease. The patient is asked to look at the clinician's eye (right eye to left eye, and left eye to right eye), and the clinician uses his fingertip to plot his blind spot against the patient's. Once the common blind spot is found, a "missing" fingertip ensures that the patient is fixing properly. Fingertips or nails can be used as targets to check the arcuate zones by asking, "Is my fingernail as clear above (superior arcuate), as it is below (inferior arcuate), yes or no?"

Relative central scotomas can be detected by using the "pinkness" of fingernails. One fingernail is placed in front of the clinician's nose and the other to the side, and the patient is asked which nail appears "more pink."

Finally, red targets (such as caps to mydriatic medications, red swizzle sticks, or pens) can be used as lower threshold stimuli in any of these confrontation techniques.

Probing for visual field defects in children and aphasic patients is difficult. However, a gross assessment of their field can be obtained with visually elicited eye movements. Keep their attention directed at your face and noiselessly introduce an interesting object in the peripheral field to be tested. If the field is intact, the eyes will first saccade and the head will turn toward the object.

Another technique is to approach the patient from behind and place your face in the field in question. Response to threat can also elicit eye movement into an intact visual field. Children from ages 3–5 years, who cannot count, will enjoy making a game of finger mimicking in all four quadrants. Ask the child, "Can you make me one of these?" and quickly present your finger targets before the child can fixate them. A child who fails to cooperate and continues to look toward the finger target can be turned so that his eye is in an abducting position and he cannot turn his head any further. Then his hemifield can be easily checked.

When evaluating a binasal or bitemporal visual field loss, one should not forget that when a patient converges to fixation point, overlapping nasal fields fall in front of fixation and temporal fields superimpose behind fixation. This explains postfixational blindness in a complete bitemporal hemianopia. One can check binasal or bitemporal visual field loss by asking the patient to fixate on your finger, introducing another finger from below, and encouraging fixation until the patient sees two fingers. This assures that there is not an absolute scotoma in the nasal or temporal field. A neat trick is to place a red target first in front, and then behind, the finger on which the patient is fixating. Assuming that the illumination is controlled, the patient is asked to compare color saturation in front of and behind the clinician's finger. A red target that seems to be desaturated in front of the finger would support a relative scotoma in the nasal fields and vice versa for temporal fields.

AMSLER GRID

An inexpensive and efficient screening device for the central 20° of visual field is the Amsler grid, a chart composed of grids with a fixation dot at its center.[1] The sides of the squares on the grid are approximately 5 mm and subtend a visual angle of 1° at 13 inches. Once one eye is occluded and the proper corrective lens is in place, the patient is asked a series of questions. While the test looks easy to perform, don't be fooled. The way the grid is presented and the questions that are asked are critical to gaining the maximum amount of information.

For subtle defects, a red grid on a black background (a low-contrast testing pattern) offers a suprathreshold test. However, if the patient has difficulty seeing this, one can switch to white on a black grid. Beginning with the abnormal eye prevents the patient from being intimidated into saying he sees something that he really does not see.

The patient is first asked the color of the grid. If the patient answers "gray" for the white grid or "washed-out orange" for the red grid, this is the first clue for optic nerve disease. The patient is then asked if he sees anything besides squares and, if so, what. The answer should be "a red dot." If not, there may be a central or paracentral scotoma. The patient is next asked to stare at the fixation dot and asked whether any squares are missing or distorted. This test checks for central or paracentral scotoma and for metamorphopsia of retinal disease. If the patient has difficulty describing what is seen, the patient should be asked to "snap a mental photograph" and draw it. Finally, the patient is asked whether he can see all four corners of the large square while simultaneously staring at the dot. This test checks for arcuate bundle defects.

If everything appears normal, the patient can be challenged with a cross-comparison between eyes. One should ask whether both eyes can see the color, the dot, and the grid in the same way. Barring refractive error or media problems, there should be little difference.

The "big pumpkin test" is another variation on this theme used to test the papillomacular bundle.[31] The patient stares at a 2-foot square piece of elliptical, orange poster board with an eccentrically placed fixation dot. The fixation point is designed so that the test covers at least 7° of nasal visual field and 20° of temporal visual field, encompassing the physiologic blindspot. The question is simply whether any part of the orange color is washed out as if there is a "watermark" on the page. This finding directs the clinician to the location of a scotoma, if present.

CONTRAST SENSITIVITY

A patient's contrast sensitivity is delineated by how little contrast is required to see. For example, decreasing the contrast on a television set so that the picture is barely visible yields a low-contrast image. A person who is still able to discern the picture has good or high-contrast sensitivity. However, a person who needs to maximize the television set's picture contrast control to see the image—so that there is the greatest possible difference between the brightest and darkest regions, creating a high-contrast image—has low or poor contrast sensitivity. Snellen acuity charts measure vision with high-contrast targets.

Commercial tests that measure a patient's contrast sensitivity function include Vector Vision's CSV-1000, Vistech System, Vision Contrast Test System, and Arden Gradings. Contrast sensitivity function (CSF) is usually plotted out in a CSF graph with the sensitivity plotted along the vertical axis and the spatial frequency (size of the bars in the testing grading) assigned to the horizontal axis. CSF is measured in "cycles/degree" or the number of bar pairs (one bright bar and one dark bar) that fill in 1° of visual angle. Both the CSV-1000 and Vistech System use a forced-choice chart using spatial frequencies of 3, 6, 12, and 18 cycles/degree. To help appreciate the spatial equivalent of this measurement, the above frequencies are equivalent to 20/200, 20/100, 20/50, and 20/30, respectively, on a Snellen chart.[21]

Performing this test monocularly allows comparison between eyes and to the normal population. A drop in the contrast sensitivity curve occurs with amblyopia, cataracts, macular disease, glaucoma, and optic neuropathies.[2] While contrast sensitivity does not sort out the causes of reduced visual function, it does identify more subtle visual loss than traditional Snellen optotypes, which test only one point on the contrast sensitivity curve. This is particularly helpful in a patient with optic neuritis who has recovered 20/20 Snellen acuity but continues to complain about "washout" of vision. Contrast sensitivity is valuable in monitoring the progression of diseases that damage nerve fiber bundles, such as the chronic papilledema of pseudotumor cerebri, the optic nerve compression of dysthyroid optic neuropathy, optic neuritis, ischemic optic neuropathy, and glaucoma. It should be included as an essential part of the optic nerve function work-out routine.

TESTS OF FUNCTIONAL (NONORGANIC) VISUAL LOSS

Tests of functional visual loss identify decreased vision in one eye and functional blindness in one or two eyes.

Different strategies to detect functionally **decreased vision in one eye** can be used. The manner of presentation of optotypes to the patient can be revealing. For example, instead of beginning with the largest optotypes and asking the patient to read down the chart, one can start by isolating a 20/10 line of optotypes. Then present enlarging lines of optotypes to 20/15 and, later, 20/20. Some projector charts have a few 20/20 lines that allow the clinician to tell the patient that the optotype is being enlarged when a 20/20 optotype line is actually being maintained.

In a patient with true visual loss, halving the testing distance improves the Snellen acuity fraction twofold because the Snellen optotypes are designed with an overall 5° angle and 1° angle of detail at a 20-foot testing distance. Each letter's size is calculated using the tangent of the 5° angle at a given distance. The 5° angle remains the same so that halving the testing distance doubles the visual angle or doubles the denominator of the Snellen fraction. A 20/20 Snellen optotype at 20 feet converts to double the denominator at 10 feet.

A patient who is able to see 20/100 at 20 feet should be able to see 20/50 at 10 feet. An acuity that fails to improve violates laws of physiologic optics, confirming functional visual loss.

The patient suspected of having decreased vision is placed behind the phoropter. Tell the patient that you are going to "improve the vision" in the good eye by using corrective lenses. Both of the patient's eyes must be looking through the phoropter. As the patient reads the acuity chart, plus lenses are slowly introduced to "fog" the good eye. As the patient continues to read the 20/20 acuity, the plus lenses are continually increased. Finally, acuity is tested in the unaffected eye that was fogged. If the vision in the fogged eye is, for example, 20/200, one can assume that the vision in the affected eye is as good as what the patient had read with the fogging lens in place. This proves that the patient was seeing clearly out of the "defective" eye.

Another technique uses combinations of neutralizing plus and minus trial lenses, such as +6.0 D and –6.0 D. One should occlude the good eye, tell the patient that these lenses offer a "powerful magnification" that will clear the vision, and coax the patient into reading increasingly smaller optotypes.

A 6-8 prism diopter lens is then placed base-down before the affected eye. The prism causes a vertical diplopia, and the image is displaced upward in the eye with the prism before it. The patient is asked if he can see both lines of print and if he can read the higher line of print. Not understanding the principle behind prisms may beguile the patient into reading the line of print in the eye with functional visual loss. Use of a vectographic projection slide with polarized glasses in binocular refraction techniques allows each eye to be tested individually while both eyes remain open. The Titmus stereoacuity test also is helpful in measuring functional visual loss. In fact, the Polaroid vectographic test of stereopsis has a linear relationship with Snellen acuity.

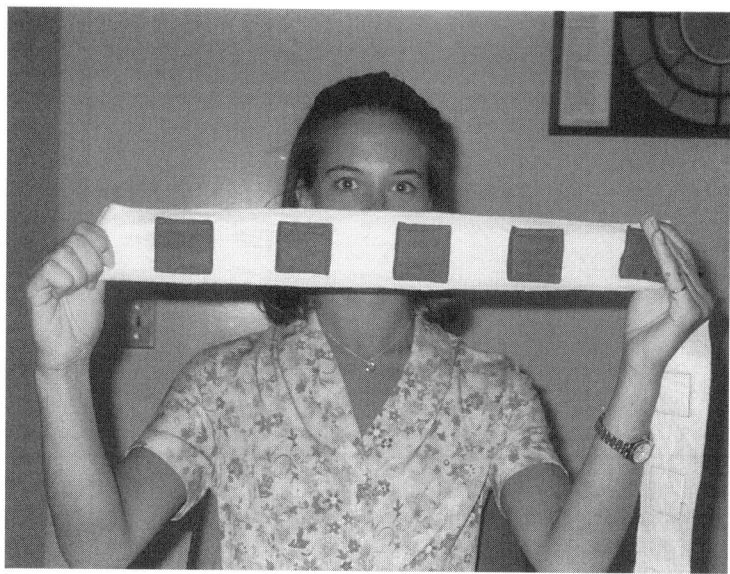

FIGURE 5. Patient's view of a clinician's pulling of optokinetic tape from the patient's right to left. A patient with functional blindness would find it difficult to suppress the induced optokinetic nystagmus.

An amaurotic pupil is the hallmark of a blind eye. If the pupil works to light, one should be suspicious of functional visual loss. When evaluating **functional blindness in one eye**, some use threat, shocking images, and optokinetic nystagmus. If optokinetic nystagmus is present, some vision is present. One can estimate the minimal visual acuity by rotating a striped drum (or pulling a cloth tape with 2-inch squares, each separated by 2 inches) at 2–4 feet (Fig. 5). If nystagmus is present, the acuity is at least finger-counting at 3–5 feet. If nystagmus can be induced with a tailor's tape, acuity is at least 3/200 to 20/400.[9]

Use of red-green glasses with the duochrome filter on the acuity projector allows testing of each eye with both eyes open. The eye with the red lens sees the red portion of the acuity line, and the eye with the green lens sees the green portion of the chart. It is probably prudent to place the red lens over the "blind eye" in question.

Occluding the good eye, the clinician pulls an optokinetic tape or moves a large mirror horizontally and vertically before the "blind" eye. Any eye movement suggests some level of vision. One then introduces a 6-8 prism diopter lens base-out in front of the patient's "blind" eye as the patient binocularly stares at an optotype across the room. While removing the prism, the clinician should look for refixational movement, which supports vision in the "blind" eye.

There is another role for prisms in the testing of a "blind" eye. Placing a rimless 8 diopter prism lens base-down before the good eye—bisecting the pupil—should cause a monocular diplopia. The clinician carefully watches the patient's "blind" eye to see if it squints shut. A malingerer may do this to discover whether the diplopia is monocular. Once monocular diplopia is created, the prism is moved upward to create binocular diplopia. The patient is asked if he still sees double. This confirms that the "blind" eye sees. Having the patient read the upper diplopic line gives the level of acuity in the "blind" eye.[14]

If one eye is completely blind, the clinician should be able to plot the blindspot in the good eye without occlusion. Inability to find the blindspot is indirect evidence that the patient is using the "blind" eye.[25]

It pays to perform binocular confrontation fields in a patient who feigns a blind eye. The peripheral 30° of each eye is monocularly represented at the contralateral, anterior portion of the calcarine cortex. If a patient really has a blind eye, the 30° of temporal visual field of the blind eye should be depressed under binocular viewing conditions as well.

Optokinetic nystagmus, mirrors, and prisms work equally well in **bilateral blindness**. In addition, the patient can be asked to sign his name. Blind patients have no difficulty performing this task with their eyes closed. The patient can be asked to touch his nose or right thumb with left index finger. These tasks are performed on the basis of proprioception and do not require sight.

REFERENCES

1. Amsler M: Earliest symptoms of disease of the macula. Br J Ophthalmol 37:521, 1953.
2. Arden GB: The importance of measuring contrast sensitivity in cases of visual disturbance. Br J Ophthalmol 62:198, 1978.
3. Bell RA, Thompson HS: Relative afferent pupillary defect in optic tract hemianopias. Am J Ophthalmol 85:538, 1978.
4. Clark FJJ: A study of Troxler's effects. Optica Acta 7:219, 1960.
5. Cruysberg JRM, Pinkers A: Acquired color vision defect in compressive optic neuropathy. Neuro-ophthalmology 2:169, 1982.
6. Fineberg E, Thompson HS: Quantitation of the afferent pupillary defect. In Smith JL (ed): Neuro-ophthalmology Focus 1980. New York, Masson Publishing, 1980.
7. Francois J, Verriest G: On acquired deficiency of color vision. Vision Res 1:201, 1961.
8. Frisen L: Clinical Tests of Vision. New York, Raven Press, 1990.
9. Glaser JS: Neuro-ophthalmology. New York, Harper & Row, 1978.
10. Glaser JS, Savino PJ, Sumers KD, et al: The photostress recovery test in the clinical assessment of visual function. Am J Ophthalmol 83:255, 1977.
11. Griffen JF, Wray SH: Acquired color vision defects in retrobulbar neuritis. Am J Ophthalmol 86:193, 1978.
12. Green GL, Lessell S: Acquired cerebral dyschromatopsia. Arch Ophthalmol 95:121, 1977.
13. Kardon RH, Hauper CL, Thompson HS: The relationship between static perimetry and the relative afferent pupillary defect. Am J Ophthalmol 104:351, 1993.
14. Kestenbaum A: Clinical Methods of Neuro-ophthalmologic Examination. New York, Grune & Stratton, 1946.
15. Kirkham TH, Coupland SG: Multiple regression analysis of diagnostic predictors in optic nerve disease. J Can Sci Neurol 8:67, 1981.
16. Krill AE, Deutman AF, Fishman M: The cone degenerations. Doc Ophthalmol 35:1, 1973.
17. Levitan P: Pupillary escape in disease of the retina or optic nerve. Arch Ophthalmol 62:768, 1959.
18. Levy NS, Glick EB: Stereoscopic perception and Snellen acuity. Am J Ophthalmol 78:722, 1974.
19. Meadows JC: Disturbed perception of colours associated with localized cerebral lesions. Brain 97:615, 1974.
20. Plant GT, Mullen KT: Anomalies in the appearance of colours and of hue discrimination in optic neuritis. Clin Vision Sci 1:303, 1987.
21. Rabin J: Spatial frequency and letter size. Optom Monthly July:386–387, 1982.
22. Randall HG, Brown DJ, Sloan LL: Peripheral visual acuity. Arch Ophthalmol 75:4, 1966.
23. Sadun AA, Lessell S: Brightness-sense and optic nerve disease. Arch Ophthalmol 103:39, 1985.
24. Smith JL: The Pupil. Miami, 1974.
25. Szily AV: D blinde flect in dienste d. entarvung simulation einseitiger blindheit. Klin Monatabl Augenheilkd 65:1, 1920.
26. Thompson HS: Putting a number on the relative afferent pupillary defect. In Thompson HS (ed): Topics in Neuro-ophthalmology. Baltimore, Williams & Wilkins, 1979.
27. Thompson HS: Pupillary signs in the diagnosis of optic nerve disease. Trans Ophthalmol Soc U K 96:279, 1976.
28. Thompson HS, Corbett JJ, Cox TA: How to measure the relative afferent pupillary defect. Surv Ophthalmol 26:39, 1981.

29. Thompson HS, Montague P, Cox TA, Corbett JJ: The relationship between visual acuity, pupillary defect and visual loss. Am J Ophthalmol 93:681, 1982.
30. Thompson HS, Watzke RC, Weinstein JM: Pupillary dysfunction in macular disease. Trans Am Ophthalmol Soc 78:311, 1980.
31. Walsh T: Paracentral scotoma testing. Ophthalmic Surg 4:72–79, 1973.
32. Welsh RC: Finger counting in the four quadrants as a method of visual field gross screening. Arch Ophthalmol 66:678, 1961.
33. Zeki SM: Colour coding in rhesus monkey prestriate cortex. Brain Res 53:422, 1973.

BEVERLY J. COWART, PhD
I. M. YOUNG, MD
ROY S. FELDMAN, DDS, DMSc
LOUIS D. LOWRY, MD

CLINICAL DISORDERS OF SMELL AND TASTE

From Monell Chemical Senses
  Center (BJC)
Thomas Jefferson University (BJC, IMY, LDL)
  and
Veterans Affairs Medical Center (RSF)
Philadelphia, Pennsylvania

Reprint requests to:
Beverly J. Cowart, PhD
Monell Chemical Senses Center
3500 Market Street
Philadelphia, PA 19104-3308

This chapter is from Beauchamp GK, Bartoshuk LM (eds): Tasting and Smelling. San Diego, Academic Press, Inc., 1997. It is reproduced here with the permission of Academic Press, Inc.

Throughout most of this century, disorders of smell and taste have received relatively little attention from the medical community. This was not always the case, however. For example, in an 1884 medical test on diseases of the nose and throat,[61] Mackenzie devoted as much space to a consideration of chemosensory (primarily smell) dysfunction as to allergic rhinitis, citing medical references going back to 1700, and well over a dozen case reports and general articles on this topic that had appeared in the 19th century medical literature to that point.

The past decade has seen a renewed medical interest in disorders of these so-called minor senses. Although chemosensory dysfunction is not as obvious to the observer as is dysfunction in vision or audition, nor does it have the broad lifestyle implications, it can impact substantially on quality of life, impede performance in some occupations (e.g., food preparation, perfumery), lead to nutritional difficulties,[63,64,65] and render individuals more vulnerable to the hazards of fire, chemical toxins in the environment, and spoiled food. Moreover, it is becoming increasingly clear that these types of dysfunction are not rare, but affect a substantial portion of the population at some point in their lives. At the very least, many if not most individuals experience measurable loss in olfactory sensitivity with aging.[13,20,27,41,92,102] In addition, a number of common medical conditions are associated with long-term, permanent, or recurrent chemosensory dysfunction.

For example, it has been shown that clinically significant diminutions in olfactory sensitivity are present in over 23% of patients suffering from allergic rhinitis.[21] Because nasal allergies are estimated to afflict 10–15% of the general population,[33,90] 2.5–3.5% of the population could be expected to suffer from smell loss as a result of this etiologic factor alone.

One manifestation of the renewed clinical interest in the chemical senses has been the appearance of numerous reviews of chemosensory disorders in medical journals and texts in the past 15 years.[32,40,69,83,84,89,95,96] It would be impossible not to replicate those efforts to some extent in a chapter on this topic. In an attempt to present the subject in a somewhat different perspective, however, the present review will focus more on unanswered questions, and tentative but intriguing observations made in clinical settings, than on providing a comprehensive overview of the conditions and medications that have been associated with chemosensory dysfunction. In most cases, the observations will be drawn from the authors' own experiences in the Monell-Jefferson Chemosensory Clinical Research Center (MJC) and those of researchers affiliated with the University of Pennsylvania Smell and Taste Center (UPenn), and the Connecticut Chemosensory Clinical Research Center (CCCRC). In addition, repeated reference will be made to the Mackenzie 1884 text in order to compare and contrast our current understanding of chemosensory dysfunction with that of a century ago.

SMELL VERSUS TASTE: CONFUSION AND RELATIVE VULNERABILITIES

"The recognition of the bitter, sweet, salt, and acid characters of food by the tongue and fauces constitutes taste. The appreciation of the *savor* of meat, the *flavor* of fruit, and the *bouquet* of wine, depends entirely on smell. It is necessary to call attention to these facts, because the mistake is not unfrequently [*sic*] made by medical writers, of describing cases as loss of taste, when it is clear from the context that they mean loss of smell."[61] Although medical writers of today are probably somewhat more sensitive to this distinction, the confusion Mackenzie describes is still commonly observed among patients presenting with chemosensory complaints, underscoring the need for careful sensory evaluation of these complaints.[24,39,42,69] Mackenzie goes on to remark that "while taste is rarely impaired, smell is often altogether lost," a point that has been largely confirmed in the major chemosensory clinical centers.

For example, figures from UPenn[24] indicate that although approximately 66% of their patients present with a complaint of taste loss ($N = 750$), fewer than 4% are found to have a measurable gustatory deficit; in contrast, 71% are found to have absent or diminished smell function. Similarly, at MJC 65.7% of 833 patients have presented with a taste loss complaint, but we have found only 8.8% to suffer from a clinically significant taste deficit, and only 2 to have a complete loss, compared with almost 67% found to have measurable smell dysfunction (31.8% are considered to suffer from a complete loss). The frequency with which taste loss is diagnosed at the CCCRC (~30% of 441 cases, with 2 cases of ageusia) is substantially higher than at either UPenn or MJC, but still much lower than the frequency of either complaint of taste loss (~60%) or diagnosed smell deficits (which is also somewhat higher than at the other two centers: 86%, with 51% considered to suffer from anosmia).[42]

A cursory consideration of the anatomies of these two sensory systems provides one obvious explanation for the apparent difference in their relative vulnerabilities. Whereas olfaction is subserved by a single cranial nerve (I), branches of three cranial nerves (VII, IX, and X) carry gustatory information. Moreover, the olfactory nerve is located in a somewhat vulnerable position in that the axons must pass through the cribriform plate of the ethmoid bone prior to dissemination on the surface of the olfactory bulb. They are therefore potentially subject to tearing or severing as a result of coup contra coup forces that may be associated with head injury.[18]

In addition, olfactory receptors are localized in a relatively small patch of tissue high in the nasal cavity, and any number of factors producing changes in nasal patency or air flow patterns could potentially limit the access of stimulus molecules to those receptors. In contrast, gustatory receptors are found on a large portion of the tongue dorsum, and a significant number may also be found on the soft palate, larynx, pharynx, and epiglottis.

Finally, the olfactory neurons *are* the receptor cells and are uniquely exposed to the external environment, extending cilia along the epithelial surface, rather than being protected by epithelial and receptor cells as are gustatory neurons. Of course, receptor elements in both of these systems are subject to a constant barrage of chemical stimuli, some of which are potentially toxic, as well as being susceptible to direct injury from microbes. Although in both systems there is ongoing regeneration of these elements, in olfaction this process requires reinnervation of the olfactory bulb.

In short, it is not really surprising that smell dysfunction would be more common than taste dysfunction or that, in the words of Mackenzie, smell might often be "altogether lost."[61]

SMELL DISORDERS

Terminology

There are inconsistencies in the literature in the use of terms describing olfactory dysfunction. In general, *anosmia* is used to refer to an absence of smell function, and *hyposmia* to diminished smell sensitivity. Occasionally, however, the term *anosmia* seems to be used more broadly to encompass both of these conditions, and the term *specific anosmia* (deficit in olfactory sensitivity to a specific odorous compound or limited class of compounds, with intact general olfactory abilities) is often used to refer to relative as opposed to absolute insensitivity. A large number of specific anosmias have been described, and these hold considerable interest in terms of their implications for both the genetic involvement in olfaction and olfactory receptor mechanisms;[1] they do not, however, typically present as clinical problems and will not be considered further here. A final point that should be made in this context is that, even when used in its more restricted sense, anosmia does not necessarily imply a complete inability to detect the presence of a volatile odorous compound at any concentration, because most odorous compounds, at least at high concentrations, also stimulate nasal fibers of the trigeminal (V) nerve.[26]

The terms *dysosmia* and *parosmia* are widely used to refer both to cases in which the patient experiences an odor sensation in the absence of an odorous stimulus and to those in which there are distortions in the perceived qualities of odorous stimuli. The former condition is often referred to more specifically as *phantosmia*. Although Henkin[45] proposed an elaborate classification system that included three terms (cacosmia, heterosmia, and parosmia) to describe different forms of odor distortions, there is no generally agreed upon term to refer specifically to distortions. In the present review, therefore, use of the term dysosmia will be restricted to odor quality distortions, and phantosmia will be used to refer to spontaneous (unstimulated) odor sensations. [It should perhaps be noted that at least one modern author has used dysosmia to refer generally to any disruption in olfactory function that manifests in reduced ability to identify common odorants.[111]]

Assessment of Smell Disorders

Both implicitly in his comment on the frequent confusion of taste with smell by medical writers and more explicitly in his criticism of a case report because the patient's *"sense of smell was never actually tested,"* Mackenzie seemed to recognize that one of the weaknesses of the 19th century medical literature on chemosensory disorders was the lack of standardized assessment procedures to document both the nature and the degree of dysfunction.[61] To a large extent, this problem has been remedied in recent years, at least in the case of olfactory assessment.

Researchers at MJC, UPenn, and the CCCRC have each developed measures of olfactory function that have been administered to large samples of healthy volunteers to establish normative values.[11,20,28] In each case the test battery includes a measure of threshold sensitivity and a multiple-choice odor identification test. Both MJC and UPenn assess threshold sensitivity using phenyl ethyl alcohol (PEA), an odor compound that elicits little or no nasal trigeminal response at any concentration,[26,57] and administer 40-item, four-alternative, forced-choice identification tests [the test used at UPenn, the University of Pennsylvania Smell Identification Test (UPSIT), employs microencapsulated odors and is commercially available]. MJC also obtains a measure of threshold sensitivity to pyridine.[91] The battery employed by the CCCRC differs in that threshold for butanol is assessed, and the identification measure is not forced-choice and is based on responses to only 7 items.

The similar rates of diagnosis of olfactory dysfunction in the three centers (see page 466) suggest that variations in the stimuli presented and procedural details may have little impact on the results of olfactory testing in a clinical setting, although the lack of a forced-choice format in their identification test may contribute to the somewhat higher rate of olfactory diagnosis reported by the CCCRC than by MJC and UPenn. Nonetheless, the composite score obtained from the CCCRC tests has been shown to correlate well with UPSIT scores alone.[94] Moreover, all three centers have reported high correlations between their measures of threshold sensitivity and odor identification ability,[11,20,28] and it has been suggested that both types of test measure essentially the same property (sensitivity) and are redundant.[11]

At MJC, however, we have observed that this correlation breaks down in individuals complaining of dysosmia.[22] For example, in our current sample of 797 patients who have completed both the PEA threshold and odor identification tests, the correlation between these two measures is 0.75 among patients with no complaint of odor quality distortions ($n = 621$), indicating that in this group the score on one test accounts for 56% of the variance on the other. Among patients who report distortions ($n = 176$), however, the correlation falls to 0.45, accounting for only 20% of the variance. The difference between these two correlations is statistically reliable ($z = 5.67, p < .0001$). The relatively poor correlation between threshold and identification measures in patients reporting dysosmia reflects the fact that most of these patients evidence reasonably good absolute sensitivity to the presence of odorous stimuli but have substantial difficulty identifying those stimuli, presumably due to the quality distortions they experience.[116] At MJC, we now use a discrepancy in performance on threshold and identification measures, in conjunction with patient report of distortions, to assign a primary olfactory diagnosis of dysosmia (as opposed to hyposmia or anosmia), and of those patients with measurable smell dysfunction, 14.1% (78/554; 9.4% of the total sample) meet these criteria for dysosmia. As described on pages 472–473, there is preliminary evidence that this diagnostic distinction may have prognostic significance, at least in terms of patients' subjective reports.

No performance measure has been found to distinguish phantosmia, and all of the clinical centers continue to rely exclusively on patient report of this form of dysfunction. Most patients who complain of odor phantoms do, however, evidence measurable olfactory dysfunction; for example, of 128 such patients seen at MJC, 73.4% produced aberrant scores on olfactory testing, with 41 being diagnosed as hyposmic, 33 as anosmic, and 20 as primarily dysosmic.

Finally, Mackenzie suggested that when patients present with a complaint of smell impairment, function should be tested separately in each nostril to determine "whether the sense is destroyed on one side, or blunted on both," although his rationale for this is questionable ["in loss of smell dependent on injury to the seventh or fifth nerves the affection is almost always unilateral"].[61] Both UPenn and the CCCRC routinely administer either a threshold test or both threshold and identification tests unilaterally, but neither has reported the frequency with which unilateral olfactory dysfunction is observed, or its etiologic/prognostic significance. Thus, the utility of routine unilateral clinical assessment of olfaction has yet to be established. On the other hand, Leopold has proposed, based on clinical experience, that phantosmias and, perhaps, dysosmias that arise from peripheral damage to the olfactory epithelium may almost always be unilateral (D. A. Leopold, personal communication, May, 1993). Because this could have implications for treatment, or at least for recommendations to aid patients in coping with their dysfunction, it deserves further study and documentation.

Etiologies of Smell Disorders

Mackenzie suggested that the "most common cause of anosmia is prolonged catarrh," with the term *catarrh* being used to refer to inflammation of the nasal membrane with associated changes in mucous discharge and, thus, to any form of rhinitis.[61] Consistent with this observation, modern chemosensory clinical centers[23a,69] have found diseases of the nose and/or paranasal sinuses to contribute to the plurality of cases of documented smell dysfunction (~30%; 15–29% of all presenting cases in the same centers). (It is, however, noteworthy that Mackenzie does not mention the paranasal sinuses, much less sinus disease, anywhere in his text.) Smell losses associated with nasal/sinus disease (NSD) can be profound; indeed, the majority of NSD patients who present to chemosensory clinical centers are found to be anosmic.[11,23a] Reports of phantom odors, sometimes in association with odor quality distortions, are not uncommon in this patient group;[69] at MJC 15.2% of patients with NSD-related dysfunction ($n = 151$) present with such complaints (11.3% with phantoms alone)—but quality distortions by themselves are relatively rare (reported by fewer than 6% of these patients at MJC).

Mechanical obstruction of the access of molecules to the olfactory receptors in rhinitis (and/or nasal polyposis) would seem to provide an easy explanation for this form of loss, and although he mentions that as a potential contributing factor, Mackenzie seemed to favor, with no specific evidence, an explanation based on changes in the normal moisture of the olfactory neuroepithelium, and possible destruction of the receptor cell processes by the "inflammatory exudation."[61] It now seems clear that pathologic mechanisms other than mechanical obstruction are involved in NSD-related smell loss. For example, obstruction of the nasal airway in patients with allergic rhinitis has not been found to be associated significantly with olfactory sensitivity.[21] Moreover, at least some patients with NSD and diminished olfactory function can be shown through modern endoscopic and computerized tomography (CT) scanning techniques to be free of significant obstruction, but they nonetheless recover olfaction with treatment of their NSD.[69] Although damage to the olfactory receptors by products of inflammation is theoretically possible, the fact that this form of loss often responds rapidly to the anti-inflammatory effects of systemic corticosteroid therapy[11,51,69] suggests that is not the major underlying mechanism; in addition, the few available histologic studies of the olfactory mucosa in patients with NSD-related anosmia have found it to be essentially normal.[29,113] Alternatively, edema of the neuroepithelium could stretch the olfactory neurons and impede synaptic transmission.[69]

Finally, Mackenzie placed early, insightful emphasis on the critical importance to olfaction of the "normal moisture of the [neuroepithelial] surface."[61] Changes in the composition of the mucous overlaying the olfactory receptor cilia could interfere with transport of odorant molecules to the receptors and/or with receptor binding. The possible role of such changes in NSD-related olfactory loss deserves further study.

Mackenzie seemed unaware of what now appears to be the second most common etiologic basis for smell dysfunction, prior upper respiratory infection (URI)—or at least he did not distinguish these dysfunctions from those secondary to ongoing inflammatory diseases of the nose and/or sinuses. The chemosensory clinical centers report that prior URI is implicated in 14–26% of all presenting cases.[23a,69] Because viral URI can precede and incite secondary bacterial sinusitis,[68] patients with these two forms of smell dysfunction may, in fact, present with similar histories. A number of characteristics of URI-related smell dysfunction do, however, clearly differentiate it from NSD-related loss.

First, URI-related dysfunctions tend to occur less frequently in young individuals than do NSD-related losses.[60,69] At MJC, for example, 12.3% of our patients with apparent URI-related dysfunction have been under 40 years of age (18 of 146 patients), whereas over 18% of those whose smell dysfunction appeared to be related to ongoing NSD have been that young (28 of 151 patients); this difference is not statistically significant, however. The post-URI patient group also includes proportionately more women than does the NSD group (MJC data: 68.5% vs. 51%, respectively; Fisher's Exact Test, $p = .003$).[60,69] In addition, URI-related dysfunctions are significantly less likely to manifest as anosmia than are NSD-related dysfunctions (MJC data: 20.5% vs. 58.9%, respectively; Fisher's Exact Test, $p < .0001$). Other authors address these points, as well.[11,60,69]

On the other hand, several authors have reported that dysosmia and phantosmia are frequent components of URI-related olfactory dysfunction,[89,116] with approximately half of the patients reporting one or both of those symptoms.[46] (See ref. #60 for a contradictory report.) At MJC, we have found dysosmia in particular to distinguish URI and NSD patients. Odor quality distortions with no phantom experience are reported by 32.2% of our URI patients (8.9% report phantoms alone and 15.8% report both), and significantly more URI than NSD patients receive a primary olfactory diagnosis of dysosmia (27.4% vs. 3.3%, respectively; Fisher's Exact Test, $p < .0001$).

Finally, and most basically, in URI-related dysfunction there appears to be damage to peripheral olfactory receptors.[29,50,113] In the largest histopathological study of postviral olfactory dysfunction to date, Jafek, Hartman, et al.[50] observed varying degrees of olfactory epithelial destruction in these patients, ranging from virtually total destruction of olfactory receptor neurons to reductions in the number of receptors with patches of epithelium having a relatively normal appearance. Furthermore, the severity of histopathologic change was found to be correlated with the observed olfactory deficit. The authors speculate that either abnormal axonal reconnection of regenerating neurons or the patchy degeneration (and/or incomplete regeneration) they observed, which could alter the sorptive characteristics of the receptor sheet, might underlie the odor quality distortions often reported by URI patients.

The third major etiologic basis for smell dysfunction at chemosensory clinical centers is head trauma, accounting for 10–19% of all presenting cases.[23a,69] The first reports of posttraumatic anosmia appeared in the medical literature in the latter half of the 19th century,[103] and Mackenzie noted that these types of cases "are by no means rare."[61] Current estimates suggest that 20–30% of head trauma patients sustain some degree of olfactory impairment (anosmia, hyposmia, or dysosmia).[18] The likelihood of posttraumatic olfactory loss appears to increase with the severity of the injury,[18] although it can occur after trivial injuries with no associated posttraumatic amnesia, and blows to the occipital region may be most likely to produce smell dysfunction.[103] As is the case in NSD-related loss, the majority of trauma patients who present to chemosensory clinical centers are found to be anosmic.[11,23a] Phantosmia and dysosmia are more common in trauma-related than in NSD-related dysfunctions, however; at MJC, 23.3% of trauma patients with smell dysfunction ($n = 86$) report distortions, 18.6% report a phantom smell, and 5.8% report both, with 16.3% meeting our diagnostic criteria for dysosmia.

Mackenzie postulated that the basis for olfactory loss in trauma cases was a separation of the olfactory bulbs from the brain. Although damage to higher neural pathways is possible, it is now believed that the most common mechanism is tearing or severing of the olfactory neuron axons at the point at which they pass through the small openings in the cribriform plate, as a result of the coup contra coup forces associated with head injury.[18] Jafek, Eller, Esses, & Moran have reported that observations from the ultrastructural examination of olfactory epithelium biopsies from five patients with posttraumatic anosmia seem to be consistent with traumatic severing of the olfactory filaments at the cribriform plate, followed by regeneration of the neuropeithelium and a failure of regenerating axons to reach the olfactory bulb (possibly as a result of fibrotic healing of the lamina cribrosa of the cribriform plate and closure with scar tissue).[48] Specifically, they consistently observed disruption in the epithelial organization consonant with a regenerating epithelium, large numbers of axon tangles throughout the epithelium, and few, if any, olfactory cilia projecting from the receptor cells, a condition that they postulated reflects the dependency of olfactory dendrite ciliogenesis on axonal contact with central nervous system tissue (but see the following discussion of Kallmann syndrome).

Mackenzie also specifically mentioned aging, exposure to "irritant vapors," and heredity or "congenital deficiency of the olfactory nerves" as etiologic factors in smell dysfunction.[61] Together with the three major factors discussed previously, these probably encompass most instances of olfactory dysfunction in which a causal condition can be identified, although a number of medical conditions (perhaps most notably Alzheimer disease) and some medications have also been associated with smell disorders. There are overviews of this literature.[69,83,85]

As noted on page 465, there is now extensive documentation of age-related decline in olfactory sensitivity, even in the healthy elderly. This form of loss apparently occurs gradually, is not typically complete, and often seems to go unnoticed by individuals experiencing it.[20,73,99] Nonetheless, it may be of magnitude sufficient to render them vulnerable to chemical hazards such as gas leaks[15,101,112] and to impact on food flavor perception.[12,70,81,82,100]

Given the relatively unprotected position of olfactory receptor neurons, it is not surprising they are susceptible to damage from pollutants in the ambient air. There are substantial animal toxicological data demonstrating damage to the olfactory neuroepithelium and bulb by airborne chemicals,[54,66,72,87] as well as a large but scattered literature on the adverse effects on the sense of smell of occupational exposures to industrial chemicals.[2] In humans, both acute and chronic exposures to a variety of chemical agents have been associated with olfactory dysfunction, which may be either temporary or permanent.[2] This factor may, in fact, play an important role in age-related smell loss.

There is still relatively little known about genetic/congenital olfactory dysfunction. The principal genetic syndrome associated with anosmia is **Kallmann syndrome**, which is also characterized by hypogonadotropic hypogonadism. These symptoms appear to be secondary to a failure during embryonic development of gonadotropin-releasing hormone-producing neurons to migrate to the brain from the olfactory placode,[79] and to insufficient or absent synaptic connections between olfactory neurons and cells in the olfactory bulb,[106] which is either aplastic or hypoplastic.[4,55,56,115] On the basis of histopathological studies of biopsy specimens from the olfactory region, Jafek, Gordon, Moran, and Eller reported an apparently complete absence of olfactory epithelium in one patient with Kallmann syndrome, as well as in six other cases of congenital anosmia with varying medical and family histories.[49] In a similar study of one anosmic Kallmann's patient, however, Schwob, Leopold, Szumowski, and Emko found olfactory epithelium similar to that observed in bulbectomized animals, with olfactory neurons that appeared to be structurally immature.[88] More recently, Rawson et al. demonstrated functional maturity (odorant-specific responsiveness) in isolated olfactory neurons from each of two anosmic patients with Kallmann syndrome.[75] Thus, anosmia in these patients was not due to a lack of functioning olfactory neurons, and differentiation of these neurons may not require contact with the olfactory bulb.

There are scattered reports of other forms of familial anosmia;[93] at MJC, however, fewer than 40% of the patients we have seen who did not recall ever being able to smell (11 of 29 patients) were aware of any family history of a similar problem. It is impossible to rule out early childhood loss secondary to a head injury or upper respiratory infection in these cases. Nonetheless, it is somewhat surprising that 3–4% of the patients presenting to chemosensory clinical centers report lifelong anosmia,[23a,24] suggesting that, although not common, this condition may not be extremely rare.

Finally, Mackenzie admitted "there are some cases of anosmia in which it is impossible to discover any cause for the loss."[61] This is unfortunately still true. Various centers for chemosensory evaluation have reported that no causative condition for chemosensory dysfunction can be identified in 10–24% of their patients,[69] although the higher estimates include at least a small proportion of individuals whose dysfunction is limited to taste, for which our understanding of causal factors is even poorer than is the case with smell.

Prognosis for Smell Disorders

The potent antibiotic and anti-inflammatory agents now commonly used in the medical treatment of NSD were not available in the 19th century, and as a result, Mackenzie was not altogether optimistic about the prognosis of NSD-related smell loss, although he did recognize it to be more favorable than in cases of traumatic lesion. In fact, this form of loss is now, to a large extent, defined by the fact that it reverses on treatment.[69] Long-term management is, however, complicated by the chronicity of the underlying disorders, and even patients who obtain effective treatment may be subject to recurring episodes of loss.

In cases of smell dysfunction secondary to peripheral nerve damage, such as is presumably the case in most instances of disorders that follow URI or toxin exposure, and in at least some cases of trauma-related disorder, gradual spontaneous recovery is theoretically possible due to the regenerative capacity of the olfactory neural receptors. Neither the time course of recovery nor factors affecting the likelihood of recovery have, however, been fully elucidated.

The most extensive prognostic studies have been conducted in patients suffering from posttraumatic smell dysfunction. Estimates of the incidence of full or partial recovery vary widely. In the two largest of these studies, however, Costanzo and Becker[17] and Sumner[103] both reported improvement in 30–40% of the patients examined. Data from both studies also suggest there is a decrease in the rate of recovery after 3–6 months, and thus, possibly more than one mechanism underlying the recovery process. Sumner speculated that rapid early recovery of olfaction may reflect the resolution of edema or blood clots, whereas the slower recovery rates observed at longer durations may reflect the regeneration and replacement of damaged olfactory neurons.

Data on spontaneous recovery in URI-related olfactory disorders are limited and conflicting. Mott and Leopold reported a longitudinal study of 40 post-URI patients at the CCCRC, in which 15% showed improvement in olfactory test scores of 40% or more after an average of 26 months, even though initial testing was performed, on average, 2 years after the onset of the problem.[69] In a similar study of 35 patients at the Olfactory Referral Center of the State University of New York (SUNY) Health Science Center, however, only 1 patient showed improvement of more than 15% on an odor identification test.[69] Similarly, Deems et al. reported no change in the mean odor identification scores (on the UPSIT) of an unspecified number of URI patients retested after an interval of 5 months to 6.4 years.[24] On the other hand, in a recent study of 21 URI patients, Duncan and Seiden reported that 67% (14) improved their UPSIT score by 4 points or more after an average of 3 years, with 13 of these patients also reporting subjective improvement.[30]

There is also some debate with regard to the prognostic significance of the development of dysosmic symptoms in head trauma and URI patients. It has been speculated that odor quality distortions could reflect either degenerative or regenerative changes in the olfactory epithelium. Leigh reported that in 72 cases of olfactory impairment following head injury, 3 of the 12 patients complaining of parosmia (25%) noted eventual recovery, whereas only 3 of 60 with complaints of simple loss (5%) reported recovery.[59] Retest data obtained by Deems et al.[24] and Duncan and Seiden[30] do not, however, support the hypothesis that recovery is more likely in patients with dysosmia, although the data also do not suggest these patients are more likely to evidence a decline in function.

In both of the latter studies, patients reporting phantom smells, as well as those whose test scores indicated they had no residual olfactory function even though they reported phantoms and/or distortions, were included in the "dysosmic" category. As described on page 468, at MJC patients are considered primarily dysosmic only if they evidence odor quality distortions in the absence of substantial loss in absolute olfactory sensitivity. On average, the odor identification performance of these patients is no better than that of patients diagnosed as hyposmic, although (by definition) their threshold sensitivity is greater. In follow-up interviews conducted with 268 patients (109 hyposmics, 115 anosmics, and 44 dysosmics), significantly more dysosmics (61.3%) than either anosmics (19.1%) or hyposmics (36.7%) reported having experienced improvement in smell function since their evaluation ($X^2 = 26.6; p < .0001$). Of course, subjective reports of improvement could reflect either a real change in olfactory function or the patient's having adapted to the problem, and firm conclusions must await objective testing in these patient groups.

No effective treatment for smell disorders other than those associated with nasal/sinus disease has been identified. Zinc is often prescribed, but has been shown to be no more effective than placebo in a double-blind study.[47] A number of other treatments have been suggested, especially for problems secondary to URI, but controlled clinical trials have not been conducted. Perhaps the most intriguing of these is vitamin A therapy. In a reasonably large study, although not one that was blinded or included an untreated control group, Duncan and Briggs reported that 50 of 56 anosmic patients treated with intramuscular injections of vitamin A alcohol in oil regained full or partial olfactory function.[31] The plurality of these patients had suffered a URI-related loss; neither the one patient with a congenital loss nor the three with losses secondary to head trauma responded to this treatment. More recently, Roydhouse also reported responsiveness to oral retinoid therapy in two patients, one whose dysfunction was secondary to URI, the other whose etiology was unknown.[78] Because vitamin A is present in the olfactory epithelium[31] and may play a role in neural regeneration, there is some rationale for this therapy and further research into its efficacy would seem to be warranted.

TASTE DISORDERS

Terminology

The terms commonly applied to taste dysfunction parallel those for smell disorders, and there is somewhat greater consistency in their usage; however, they fail to make some distinctions that probably should be made. As might be expected, *ageusia* refers to a complete absence of gustatory function and *hypogeusia* to diminished taste sensitivity. The difficulty here is that in the gustatory system fundamentally different transduction sequences underlie the perception of different taste qualities, and probably, at least in the case of bitter, that of different compounds with the same quality. Thus, an individual could potentially experience either a total but isolated loss in sensitivity to compounds eliciting a specific quality, or a more generalized diminution in sensitivity to compounds eliciting a variety of taste qualities, and in both cases be classified simply as hypogeusic. Some instances of specific gustatory insensitivity, such as genetic insensitivity to the bitter taste of phenylthiocarbamide (PTC) and its structural analogs,[53] are (like specific anosmias) unlikely to present as clinical problems; a specific loss in sensitivity to sweets might well, however.

As is also the case in smell loss, it should be noted that even a completely ageusic patient will be able to detect high concentrations of some gustatory stimuli through stimulation of fibers of the trigeminal (V) nerve. For example, both sodium chloride (salt) and sour acids can elicit oral irritation/trigeminal responses.[9,44] Whether sweet and bitter compounds do as well is unclear, although neither of the two ageusic patients who have been evaluated at MJC consistently reponded to high concentrations of either sucrose or quinine sulfate (markedly elevated, but stable, thresholds for salt and citric acid were obtained in both cases).

For the most part, the term *dysgeusia* is used in the clinical taste literature essentially as a synonym for *phantogeusia*, to refer to the experience of a taste sensation in the apparent absence of a gustatory stimulus. Primary distortions in the perceived qualities of gustatory stimuli are, unlike olfactory distortions, not well documented in clinical settings, although they may occur. Phantom tastes are sometimes accompanied by oral burning sensations, or such symptoms may appear alone in what is often referred to as *burning mouth syndrome*. This symptom complex will not be considered here, but a concise and balanced review of the relevant clinical literature may be found in Forman and Settle.[34,35]

Assessment of Taste Disorders

Clinical assessment of taste is not as well developed or standardized as that of olfaction. Because of the possibility of clinically significant, quality-specific loss, it is probably important to obtain some measure of responsivity to representatives of the four generally agreed-upon taste qualities (sweet, salty, sour, bitter). The most common choices are sucrose, sodium chloride, citric or hydrochloric acid, and quinine (sulfate or hydrochloride) or caffeine. This, obviously, creates logistical difficulties, especially given the necessity of preparing fresh taste stimuli frequently. An alternative to the use of chemical stimuli is measurement of electric taste via electrogustometry.[37] Although not sensitive to quality-specific loss, this form of assessment offers advantages not only in terms of simplicity and portability, but also in the degree of precision with which the stimulus may be applied. It has not, however, been widely used in the United States, and none of the chemosensory clinical research centers here relies exclusively, or even primarily, on electrogustometric assessment in taste evaluations.

Gent, Frank, and Mott reviewed and provided detailed descriptions of many of the taste assessment procedures used in clinical practice.[38] Of the three centers on which this review has focused, MJC and UPenn both rely primarily on measures of whole-mouth threshold sensitivity to the basic tastes in the diagnosis of taste loss (although UPenn does not include a bitter stimulus in this assessment). In addition, both utilize suprathreshold quality identification and category scaling of taste intensity as screening measures and to supplement the interpretation of threshold results. [Although quality identification has proved to be a very useful clinical tool in olfaction, its utility in gustatory assessment is limited by the fact that taste quality confusions (particularly sour–bitter, but also sour–salty and salty–bitter) are not uncommon in the general population.] As indicated, both MJC and UPenn also report very low rates of diagnosis of taste loss. The CCCRC, on the other hand, does not assess threshold sensitivity, but relies on a suprathreshold intensity scaling task that employs the psychophysical technique of magnitude matching to allow for the direct comparison of intensity ratings across subjects.[5] Presumably, this marked difference in assessment procedures accounts for the substantially higher rate of taste diagnosis that has been reported at the CCCRC.

In the context of the potential for quality-specific loss in taste, it is interesting to note that, in olfaction, not only are threshold measures highly correlated with identification measures (see pages 468–469), but at MJC we have found that the two olfactory thresholds we obtain (for odors that are qualitatively very different) are also highly correlated. In a sample of 740 patients who completed both odor threshold tests as well as all four measures of taste threshold, the correlation between the odor thresholds is .67; in contrast, correlations among taste thresholds are significantly lower, ranging from .25 (for sucrose and quinine) to .46 (for salt and citric acid) ($p < .0001$ in all comparisons with the odor threshold correlation). Indeed, among those patients considered to evidence taste loss on the basis of their threshold test results, almost half (36 of 73) showed clinically significant elevation in only a single taste threshold (in 19 of these cases, salt sensitivity was affected), and in only 6 cases (8.2% of those with any loss) were thresholds for all four tastes elevated.

As is the case with phantosmia, no performance measure clearly distinguishes phantogeusia. At MJC, we have found that only about 18% of the patients complaining of taste phantoms evidence measurable, whole-mouth taste loss, which is substantially lower than the frequency with which measurable smell dysfunction is observed in patients with phantom smell complaints (~73%). Nonetheless, diminished taste sensitivity is significantly more common among patients reporting taste phantoms than among those who do not (only 7% of whom evidence taste loss; Fisher's Exact Test, $p = .0015$).

Finally, because the gustatory system is bilaterally innervated by three cranial nerves, there is the possibility of loss localized to one or more receptor fields as a result of peripheral or central lesions. MJC, UPenn, and the CCCRC all employ regional gustatory testing to supplement whole-mouth testing in some patients. In all clinics, suprathreshold concentrations of chemical stimuli are swabbed or pipetted onto discrete regions of the tongue (and, when swabs are used, the palate), and patients rate the intensity of the resulting taste and label its quality; left-right and anterior-posterior differences in responsiveness are then examined. UPenn also utilizes electrogustometry in regional testing, which makes assessment of left-right thresholds feasible. In fact, regional losses often are not associated with any subjective change in taste experience; they may, however, underlie some instances of taste phantoms (see below).

Etiologies of Taste Disorders

Detailed reports of etiologic factors contributing to taste dysfunction in patients presenting to chemosensory clinics are largely lacking. Thus, the most common causes of such dysfunctions cannot be identified with any confidence. Indeed, at MJC, no clear precipitating event or readily identifiable underlying pathology has been evident in over 60% of the cases of taste loss and/or phantoms we have evaluated.

Based on the sheer number of clinical reports in the literature,[69,77,83,85] one might argue that the single most common etiologic factor contributing to taste dysfunctions is probably medication usage. One summary report from a Japanese taste clinic is consistent with this.[105] In the United States, however, cases of drug-related taste disturbances seem to be underrepresented among clinical research center patients, possibly because of their widespread recognition by medical practitioners and patients' ability to tie changes in taste to the use of specific medications. Different mechanisms undoubtedly underlie the gustatory effects of different medications. For example, taste perception could be affected through the alteration of salivary constituents, through vascular tastes, through disruption of transduction/receptor mechanisms, and through alterations in the central processing of gustatory input. In very few cases, however, have the specific mechanisms underlying taste effects of a given medication been elucidated. A better understanding of these effects might shed light on both normal gustatory function and the vulnerabilities of this system.

Oral health problems in the form of poor oral hygiene or periodontal disease are obvious potential sources of phantogeusias. Xerostomia, whatever its etiology, might also be expected to be associated with phantogeusia and/or taste loss as a result of its adverse impact on oral clearance and on the integrity of the teeth and oral mucosa; however, even severe, chronic failure of all salivary glands does not necessarily lead to taste complaints or abnormalities in taste function, a finding that attests to the remarkable resilience of the taste receptors.[108,109]

Xerostomia is also one of several factors, including the use of dentures, antibiotics, or corticosteroids and immunological deficiencies, that can predispose to the overgrowth of oral *Candida*.[34] Brightman, Guggenheimer, and Ship found that subclinical elevations in oral *Candida* (i.e., without clinically evident thrush or angular cheilitis) produced bad tastes and burning sensations in a third of subjects in whom fungal overgrowth was induced by an oral tetracycline rinse.[8] At MJC, we now routinely perform oral yeast cultures in patients complaining of phantogeusia. To date, just under a third (14 of 44) have been positive, and of the 7 patients we know to have received antifungal therapy, 5 reported resolution of their phantom. Similarly, Osaki et al. reported oral candidiasis to underlie dysgeusia in 3 of 14 patients they evaluated.[74] Interestingly, these investigators also found candidiasis to contribute to simple taste loss in nearly a quarter of 25 hypogeusic patients.

Two of the most common causes of smell dysfunction, URI and head trauma, may also be associated with true taste problems, with both phantogeusias and losses having been reported.[17,18,46,60] In both cases, taste symptoms are much less common than smell symptoms, and the underlying pathophysiology is not well understood. At MJC, about a fifth of our patients with taste loss have linked that symptom to a prior URI or head injury; almost all of these individuals also evidenced olfactory dysfunction. A smaller proportion (5%) of our phantogeusic patients (with no measured taste loss) have indicated their symptom was precipitated by either of these factors.

Two common surgical procedures may result in damage to the chorda tympani, which mediates taste perception on the anterior tongue. This nerve is frequently severed, stretched, or crushed during middle ear surgery,[10,16,43] and chorda-lingual damage has been estimated to occur in as many as 11% of patients who undergo third-molar extractions.[7] In cases of bilateral chorda tympani section, patients are often aware of some diminution in taste function, but they only rarely report a loss following unilateral damage.[10,43] On the other hand, complaints of phantogeusia following surgical damage to the chorda appear to be common.[10,67] Taste phantoms may also be experimentally induced by anesthetization of the chorda tympani.[114] Disinhibition of responses from taste receptors innervated by the glossopharyngeal nerve has been proposed as a mechanism to explain both the limited impact of chorda damage on whole-mouth taste perception and the occurrence of phantoms.[14,58,114] A decrease in spontaneous activity at the level of the nucleus of the solitary tract has also been suggested as a mechanism for these phenomena.[25] Finally, abnormal functioning of the damaged nerve at the periphery may underlie phantoms in some cases.[6]

Since publication of an apparently successful, single-blind trial of the efficacy of zinc supplementation in reversing hypogeusia,[80] zinc deficiency has received considerable attention as a potential etiology for taste dysfunction, even though a subsequent double-blind trial failed to show any significant difference between the effects of zinc and placebo.[47] Some controlled studies of documented zinc deficiency in specific disease states do indicate it may be associated with taste loss that reverses on treatment with zinc,[3,62,110] although the mechanisms by which zinc affects gustatory function are not known. Nonetheless, it seems unlikely zinc deficiency underlies most, or even many, cases of hypogeusia. The results of the double-blind study by Henkin et al.[47] are consistent with this, as is the report by Deems et al.[24] of no difference between the taste scores of patients presenting to UPenn who were taking zinc and those who were not. It should perhaps be noted, however, that Tomita has reported that the majority of a large sample of patients presenting to a Japanese clinic with taste complaints evidenced zinc deficiency and/or responded to zinc therapy.[105] On the other hand, Osaki et al. found no evidence of zinc deficiency in their sample of Japanese patients with complaints of hypogeusia or dysgeusia (they did identify iron deficiency as a source of hypogeusia in 7 of 25 patients).[74]

Finally, aging itself may be associated with diminished taste sensitivity. In the healthy elderly, this loss is, on average, less pronounced than are declines in olfactory sensitivity[20,98] and may be quality or compound specific, at least in terms of the degree of change.[19,20,23,71,86,97,107] Thus, patients with simple age-related taste losses are probably even less likely than are those with age-related smell losses to present with a complaint in a clinical setting. Aging or factors associated with aging may, however, render individuals more vulnerable to taste dysfunctions that do lead them to seek medical assistance. For example, among patients presenting to MJC, the elderly ($\geq$ 65 years of age) are significantly more likely to complain of phantogeusia than are the middle aged (45–64 years) and young (< 45 years); the respective percentages of patients in each group with this complaint are 28.6, 14.9, and 12.6% ($X^2 = 24.7$; $p < .0001$). A similar relationship is not seen in complaints of phantosmia. Elderly patients are also more likely than middle-aged and young patients to evidence diminished taste sensitivity; taste loss is diagnosed in 13.2, 9.8, and 4.5% of each group, respectively ($X^2 = 11.5$; $p < .005$). Again, we do not see this relationship in the diagnosis of smell loss in clinic patients.

Prognosis for Taste Disorders

Of the identifiable etiologies associated with taste dysfunction, several are amenable to intervention. The type or dosage of medications a patient is receiving can often be altered, and in most cases, the prognosis for drug-related taste problems is excellent.[77] Both periodontal disease and oral candidiasis respond to therapy, although these problems may often recur in susceptible patients. Xerostomia is difficult to manage, but recent clinical studies have shown oral pilocarpine to be beneficial in a variety of forms of xerostomia,[36,52,76] and it has now been approved for this use.

As is the case with smell dysfunctions secondary to URI or head trauma, some proportion of taste dysfunctions with these etiologies evidence spontaneous recovery, although there are even fewer long-term, follow-up data available on taste than there are on smell. There are, however, indications that, at least in the case of trauma-related chemosensory dysfunction, taste is more likely than smell to recover.[104]

Spontaneous resolution of symptoms following damage to the chorda tympani nerve has also been reported. The Bull report suggests that taste phantoms typically last 3–4 months, although they may persist for more than a year in a minority of patients.[10] Both Bull and Chilla et al. indicate that taste loss in the affected taste field (of which, as noted, patients are rarely aware) never recovers following transection of the nerve during middle ear surgery, but almost always does when the nerve is only stretched.[16] More recently, Zuniga, Chen, and Miller, in a preliminary report, demonstrated recovery of taste sensitivity in one patient following surgical intervention and repair of chorda-lingual damage sustained during a third-molar extraction.[117]

Finally, as has been indicated, many if not most cases of taste dysfunction are idiopathic in origin. The prognosis for these does not appear to be good. Among such patients who have been followed at MJC over a period of at least 6 months, 39% of those complaining of a phantom taste ($n = 41$) did report full or partial resolution of this symptom; however, almost 15% reported worsening and the remainder indicated there had been no change. In 15 cases of simple taste loss, only one patient reported any improvement in taste sensitivity.

CONCLUSION

A surprising amount was known about olfactory dysfunctions over a century ago. Nonetheless, substantial progress has been made in the characterization of these disorders and in the treatment of those that are secondary to nasal/sinus pathology. A better understanding of the mechanisms underlying olfactory dysfunctions has also been gained, although there is still much to be learned in this area. Finally, we are still in the position of being unable to intervene in most cases of olfactory disruption. Increases in basic knowledge about the regenerative process in the olfactory epithelium may ultimately provide therapeutic direction.

Gustatory disorders remain relatively more obscure. Although they are also relatively less common, to the extent that their prevalence increases with age, we may expect a growing number of such cases. The development of standardized assessment techniques that can reasonably be applied in clinical settings is of critical importance in furthering the study of taste dysfunction.

Acknowledgments

This work was supported in part by NIH Grant P50 DC 00214. The authors thank Elizabeth Varga for her careful supervision of sensory testing and data management at the Monell-Jefferson Taste and Smell Clinic.

REFERENCES

1. Amoore JE: Specific anosmia and the concept of primary odors. Chem Senses Flavour 2:267–281, 1977.
2. Amoore JE: Effects of chemical exposure on olfaction in humans. In Barrow CS (ed): Toxicology of the Nasal Passages. Washington, DC, Hemisphere Publishing, 1986, pp 155–190.
3. Atkin-Thor E, Goddard BW, O'Nion J, et al: Hypogeusia and zinc depletion in chronic dialysis patients. Am J Clin Nutr 31:1948–1951, 1978.
4. Bajaj S, Ammini AC, Marwaha R, et al: Magnetic resonance imaging of the brain in idiopathic hypogonadotropic hypogonadism. Clin Radiol 48:122–124, 1993.
5. Bartoshuk LM, Gent JF, Catalanotto FA, Goodspeed RB: Clinical evaluation of taste. Am J Otolaryng 4:257–260, 1983.
6. Bartoshuk LM, Kveton J, Lehman C: Peripheral source of taste phantom (i.e., dysgeusia) demonstrated by topical anesthesia [abstract]. Chem Senses 16:499–500, 1992.
7. Blackburn CW, Bramley PA: Lingual nerve damage associated with the removal of lower third molars. Br Dent J 167:103–107, 1989.
8. Brightman VJ, Guggenheimer J, Ship I: Changes in the oral microbial flora during treatment of recurrent aphthous ulcers [abstract]. J Dent Res 47(suppl):126, 1968.
9. Bryant BP, Moore PA: Factors affecting the sensitivity of the lingual trigeminal nerve to acids. Am J Physiol 268:R58–R65, 1995.
10. Bull TR: Taste and the chorda tympani. J Laryngol Otol 79:479–493, 1965.
11. Cain WS, Gent JF, Goodspeed RB, Leonard G: Evaluation of olfactory dysfunction in the Connecticut Chemosensory Clinical Research Center. Laryngoscope 98:83–88, 1988.
12. Cain WS, Reid F, Stevens JC: Missing ingredients: Aging and the discrimination of flavor. J Nutr Elderly 9:3–15, 1990.
13. Cain WS, Stevens JC: Uniformity of olfactory loss in aging. Ann N Y Acad Sci 561:29–38, 1989.
14. Catalanotto FA, Bartoshuk LM, Östrom KM, et al: Effects of anesthesia of the facial nerve on taste. Chem Senses 18:461–470, 1993.
15. Chalke HD, Dewhurst JR: Accidental coal-gas poisoning: Loss of sense of smell as a possible contributory factor with old people. BMJ 2:915–917, 1957.

16. Chilla R, Nicklatsch J, Arglebe C: Late sequelae of iatrogenic damage to chorda tympani nerve. Acta Otolaryngol 94:461–465, 1982.
17. Costanzo RM, Becker DP: Smell and taste disorders in head injury and neurosurgery patients. In Meiselman HL, Rivlin RS (eds): Clinical Measurement of Taste and Smell. New York, Macmillan Publishing, 1986, pp 565–578.
18. Costanzo RM, Zasler ND: Head trauma. In Getchell TV, Doty RL, Bartoshuk LM, Snow JB Jr (eds): Smell and Taste in Health and Disease. New York, Raven Press, 1991, pp 711–730.
19. Cowart BJ: Development of taste perception in humans: Sensitivity and preference throughout the life span. Psychol Bull 90:43–73, 1981.
20. Cowart BJ: Relationships between taste and smell across the adult life span. Ann N Y Acad Sci 561:39–55, 1989.
21. Cowart BJ, Flynn-Rodden K, McGeady SJ, Lowry LD: Hyposmia in allergic rhinitis. J Allergy Clin Immunol 91:747–751, 1993.
22. Cowart BJ, Garrison B, Young IM, Lowry LD: A discrepancy between odor thresholds and identification in dysosmia [abstract]. Chem Senses 14:692, 1989.
23. Cowart BJ, Yokomukai Y, Beauchamp GK: Bitter taste in aging: Compound-specific decline in sensitivity. Physiol Behav 56:1237–1241, 1994.
23a. Cowart BJ, Young IM, Feldman RS, Lowry LD: Unpublished data, 1996.
24. Deems DA, Doty RL, Settle RG, et al: Smell and taste disorders, a study of 750 patients from the University of Pennsylvania Smell and Taste Center. Arch Otolaryngol Head Neck Surg 117:519–528, 1991.
25. Dinkins ME, Travers SP: Alternative mechanisms for taste compensation following chorda tympani anesthetization [abstract]. Chem Senses 21:595–596, 1996.
26. Doty RL, Brugger WE, Jurs PC, et al: Intranasal trigeminal stimulation from odorous volatiles: Psychometric responses from anosmic and normal humans. Physiol Behav 20:175–185, 1978.
27. Doty RL, Shaman P, Applebaum SL, et al: Smell identification ability: Changes with age. Science 22:1441–1443, 1984.
28. Doty RL, Shaman P, Dann M: Development of the University of Pennsylvania smell identification test: A standardized microencapsulated test of olfactory function. Physiol Behav 32:489–502, 1984.
29. Douek E, Bannister LH, Dodson HC: Recent advances in the pathology of olfaction. Proc R Soc Med 68:467–470, 1975.
30. Duncan HJ, Seiden AM: Long-term follow-up of olfactory loss secondary to head trauma and upper respiratory tract infection. Arch Otolaryngol Head Neck Surg 121:1183–1187, 1995.
31. Duncan RB, Briggs M: Treatment of uncomplicated anosmia by vitamin A. Arch Otolaryngol 75:116–124, 1962.
32. Estrem SA, Renner G: Disorders of smell and taste. Otolaryngol Clin North Am 20:133–147, 1987.
33. Fadal RG: The medical management of rhinitis. In English GM (ed): Otolaryngology. Vol 2. Philadelphia, JB Lippincott, 1987, pp 1–25.
34. Forman R, Settle RG: Burning mouth symptoms: A clinical review, part I. Compend Cont Ed Dent 11:74–82, 1990.
35. Forman R, Settle RG: Burning mouth symptoms, Part II: A clinical review. Compend Cont Ed Dent 11:140–146, 1990.
36. Fox PC, Atkinson JC, Macynski AA, et al: Pilocarpine treatment of salivary gland hypofunction and dry mouth (xerostomia). Arch Intern Med 151:1149–1152, 1991.
37. Frank ME, Smith DV: Electrogustometry: A simple way to test taste. In Getchell TV, Bartoshuk LM, Doty RL, Snow JB Jr (eds): Smell and Taste in Health and Disease. New York, Raven Press, 1991, pp 503–514.
38. Gent JF, Frank ME, Mott AE: Taste testing in clinical practice. In Seiden AM (ed): Taste and Smell Disorders. New York, Thieme Medical Publishers, 1997, pp 146–158.
39. Gent JF, Goodspeed RB, Zagraniski RT, Catalanotto FA: Taste and smell problems: Validation of questions for the clinical history. Yale J Biol Med 60:27–35, 1987.
40. Getchell TV, Doty RL, Bartoshuk LM, Snow JB Jr (eds): Smell and Taste in Health and Disease. New York, Raven Press, 1991.
41. Gilbert AN, Wysocki CJ: The smell survey results. National Geographic 172:514–525, 1987.
42. Goodspeed RB, Gent JF, Catalanotto FA: Chemosensory dysfunction: Clinical evaluation results from a taste and smell clinic. Postgrad Med 81:251–260, 1987.
43. Grant R, Miller S, Simpson D, et al: The effect of chorda tympani section on ipsilateral and contralateral salivary secretion and taste in man. J Neurol Neurosurg Psychiatry 52:1058–1062, 1989.
44. Green BG, Gelhard B: Salt as an oral irritant. Chem Senses 14:259–271, 1989.
45. Henkin RI: Taste and smell disorders. In Adelman G (ed): Encyclopedia of Neuroscience. Boston, Birkhauser, 1987, pp 1185–1187.

46. Henkin RI, Larson AL, Powell RD: Hypogeusia, dysgeusia, hyposmia, and dysosmia following influenza-like infection. Ann Otol Rhinol Laryngol 84:672–682, 1975.
47. Henkin RI, Schechter PJ, Friedewald WT, et al: A double blind study of the effects of zinc sulfate on taste and smell dysfunction. Am J Med Sci 272:285–299, 1976.
48. Jafek BW, Eller PM, Esses BA, Moran DT: Post-traumatic anosmia: Ultrastructural correlates. Arch Neurol 46:300–304, 1989.
49. Jafek BW, Gordon ASD, Moran DT, Eller PM: Congenital anosmia. Ear Nose Throat J 69:331–337, 1990.
50. Jafek BW, Hartman D, Eller PM, et al: Postviral olfactory dysfunction. Am J Rhinol 4:91–100, 1990.
51. Jafek BW, Moran DT, Eller PM, et al: Steroid-dependent anosmia. Arch Otolaryngol Head Neck Surg 113:547–549, 1987.
52. Johnson JT, Gerretti GA, Nethery WJ, et al: Oral pilocarpine for post-irradiation xerostomia in patients with head and neck cancer. N Engl J Med 329, 390–395, 1993.
53. Kalmus H: The genetics of taste. In Beidler LM (ed): Handbook of Sensory Physiology. Vol 4, Chemical Senses. Part 2, Taste. New York, Springer-Verlag, 1971, pp 165–179.
54. Keenan CM, Kelly DP, Bogdanffy MS: Degeneration and recovery of rat olfactory epithelium following inhalation of dibasic esters. Fundam Applied Toxicol 15:381–393, 1990.
55. Klingmüller D, Dewes W, Krahe T, et al: Magnetic resonance imaging of the brain in patients with anosmia and hypothalamic hypogonadism (Kallmann's syndrome). J Clin Endocrinol Metab 65:581–584, 1987.
56. Knorr JR, Ragland RL, Brown RS, Gelber N: Kallmann syndrome: MR findings. Am J Neurosci Res 14:845–851, 1993.
57. Kobal G: A new method for determination of the olfactory and the trigeminal nerve's dysfunction: Olfactory (OEP) and chemical somatosensory (CSEP) evoked potentials. In Rothenberger A (ed): Event-Related Potentials in Children. Amsterdam, Elsevier Biomedical Press, 1982, pp 455–461.
58. Kveton JF, Bartoshuk LM: The effect of unilateral chorda tympani damage on taste. Laryngoscope 104:25–29, 1994.
59. Leigh AD: Defects of smell after head injury. Lancet 244:38–40, 1943.
60. Leopold DA, Hornung DE, Youngentob SL: Olfactory loss after upper respiratory infection. In Getchell TV, Doty RL, Bartoshuk LM, Snow JB Jr (eds): Smell and Taste in Health and Disease. New York, Raven Press, 1991, pp 731–734.
61. Mackenzie M: A Manual of Diseases of the Throat and Nose. Vol II, Diseases of the Oesophagus, Nose, and Naso-pharynx. New York, Wood, 1884.
62. Mahajan SK, Prasad AS, Lambujon J, et al: Improvement of uremic hypogeusia by zinc: A double-blind study. Am J Clin Nutr 33:1517–1521, 1980.
63. Mattes RD, Cowart BJ: Dietary assessment of patients with chemosensory disorders. J Am Diet Assoc 94:50–56, 1994.
64. Mattes RD, Cowart BJ, Schiavo MA, et al: Dietary evaluation of patients with smell and/or taste disorders. Am J Clin Nutr 51:233–240, 1990.
65. Mattes-Kulig DA, Henkin RI: Energy and nutrient consumption of patients with dysgeusia. J Am Diet Assoc 85:822–826, 1985.
66. Min Y-G, Rhee C-S, Choo M-J, et al: Histopathologic changes in the olfactory epithelium in mice after exposure to sulfur dioxide. Acta Otolaryngol (Stockh) 114:447–452, 1994.
67. Moon CN, Pullen EW: Effects of chorda tympani section during middle ear surgery. Laryngoscope 73:392–405, 1963.
68. Mott AE: Topical corticosteroid therapy for nasal polyposis. In Getchell TV, Doty RL, Bartoshuk LM, Snow JB Jr (eds): Smell and Taste in Health and Disease. New York, Raven Press, 1991, pp 553–572.
69. Mott AE, Leopold DA: Disorders in taste and smell. Med Clin North Am 75:1321–1353, 1991.
70. Murphy C: Cognitive and chemosensory influences on age-related changes in the ability to identify blended foods. J Gerontol 40:47–52, 1985.
71. Murphy C, Gilmore MM: Quality-specific effects of aging on the human taste system. Percept Psychophys 45:121–128, 1989.
72. Nikula KJ, Lewis JL: Olfactory mucosal lesions in F344 rats following inhalation exposure to pyridine at threshold limit value concentrations. Fundam Appl Toxicol 23:510–517, 1994.
73. Nordin S, Monsch AU, Murphy C: Unawareness of smell loss in normal aging and Alzheimer's disease: Discrepancy between self-reported and diagnosed smell sensitivity. J Gerontol Psychol Sci 50B:P187–P192, 1995.
74. Osaki T, Ohshima M, Tomita Y, et al: Clinical and physiological investigations in patients with taste abnormality. J Oral Pathol Med 25:38–43, 1996.

75. Rawson NE, Brand JG, Cowart BJ, et al: Functionally mature olfactory neurons from two anosmic patients with Kallmann syndrome. Brain Res 681:58–64, 1995.
76. Rhodus NL, Schuh MJ: Effects of pilocarpine on salivary flow in patients with Sjögren's syndrome. Oral Surg Oral Med Oral Pathol 72:545–549, 1991.
77. Rollin H: Drug-related gustatory disorders. Ann Otol 87:37–42, 1978.
78. Roydhouse N: Retinoid therapy and anosmia. N Z Med J 101:465, 1988.
79. Rugarli EI, Ballabio A: Kallmann syndrome, from genetics to neurobiology. JAMA 270:2713–2716, 1993.
80. Schechter PJ, Friedewald WT, Bronzert DA, et al: Idiopathic hypogeusia: A description of the syndrome and a single-blind study with zinc sulfate. Int Rev Neurobiol Suppl 1:125–140, 1972.
81. Schiffman SS: Food recognition by the elderly. J Gerontol 32:586–592, 1977.
82. Schiffman SS: Changes in taste and smell with age: Psychophysical aspects. In Ordy JM, Brizzee K (eds): Sensory Systems and Communication in the Elderly. Vol 10, Aging. New York, Raven Press, 1979, pp 227–246.
83. Schiffman SS: Taste and smell in disease. Part I. N Engl J Med 308:1275–1279, 1983.
84. Schiffman SS: Taste and smell in disease. Part II. N Engl J Med 308:1337–1343, 1983.
85. Schiffman SS: Drugs influencing taste and smell perception. In Getchell TV, Doty RL, Bartoshuk LM, Snow JB Jr (eds): Smell and Taste in Health and Disease. New York, Raven Press, 1991, pp 845–850.
86. Schiffman SS, Gatlin LA, Frey AE, et al: Taste perception of bitter compounds in young and elderly persons: Relation to lipophilicity of bitter compounds. Neurobiol Aging 15:743–750, 1994.
87. Schwartz BS, Doty RL, Monroe C, et al: Olfactory function in chemical workers exposed to acrylate and methacrylate vapors. Am J Public Health 79:613–618, 1989.
88. Schwob JE, Leopold DA, Szumowski KEM, Emko P: Histopathology of olfactory mucosa in Kallmann's syndrome. Ann Otol Rhinol Laryngol 102:117–122, 1993.
89. Scott AE: Clinical characteristics of taste and smell disorders. Ear Nose Throat J 68:297–315, 1989.
90. Seebolm PM: Allergic and nonallergic rhinitis. In Middleton E, Reed C, Ellis E (eds): Allergy Principles and Practice. Vol 2. St. Louis, CV Mosby, 1978, pp 868–876.
91. Sherman AH, Amoore JE, Weigel V: The pyridine scale for clinical measurement of olfactory threshold: A quantitative reevaluation. Otolaryngol Head Neck Surg 87:717–733, 1979.
92. Ship JA, Weiffenbach JM: Age, gender, medical treatment, and medication effects on smell identification. J Gerontol Med Sci 48:M26–M32, 1993.
93. Singh N, Grewal MS, Austin JH: Familial anosmia. Arch Neurol 22:40–44, 1970.
94. Smith DV: Assessment of patients with taste and smell disorders. Acta Otolaryngol Suppl 458:129–133, 1988.
95. Smith DV: Taste and smell dysfunction. In Paparella MM, Shumrick DA, Gluckman JL, Meyerhoff WL (eds): Otolaryngology. Vol 3. 3rd ed. Philadelphia, WB Saunders, 1991, pp 1911–1934.
96. Snow JB Jr: Clinical problems in chemosensory disturbances. Am J Otolaryngol 4:224–227, 1983.
97. Stevens JC: Detection of tastes in mixture with other tastes: Issues of masking and aging. Chem Senses 21:211–221, 1996.
98. Stevens JC, Bartoshuk LM, Cain WS: Chemical senses and aging: Taste versus smell. Chem Senses 9:167–179, 1984.
99. Stevens JC, Cain WS: Age-related deficiency in the perceived strength of six odorants. Chem Senses 10:517–529, 1985.
100. Stevens JC, Cain WS: Smelling via the mouth: Effect of aging. Percept Psychophys 40:142–146, 1986.
101. Stevens JC, Cain WS, Weinstein DE: Aging impairs the ability to detect gas odor. Fire Technol 23:198–204, 1987.
102. Stevens JC, Dadarwala AD: Variability of olfactory threshold and its role in assessment of aging. Percept Psychophys 54:296–302, 1993.
103. Sumner D: Posttraumatic anosmia. Brain 87:107–120, 1964.
104. Sumner D: Post-traumatic ageusia. Brain 90:187–202, 1967.
105. Tomita H: Zinc in taste and smell disorders. In Tomita H (ed): Trace Elements in Clinical Medicine. Tokyo, Springer-Verlag, 1990, pp 15–37.
106. Truwit CL, Barkovich AJ, Grumbach MM, Martini JJ: MR imaging of Kallmann syndrome, a genetic disorder of neuronal migration affecting the olfactory and genital systems. Am J Neurosci Res 14:827–854, 1993.
107. Weiffenbach JM, Baum BJ, Burghauser R: Taste thresholds: Quality specific variation with human aging. J Gerontol 37:372–377, 1982.
108. Weiffenbach JM, Fox PC, Baum BJ: Taste and salivary function. Proc Natl Acad Sci U S A 83:6103–6106, 1986.

109. Weiffenbach JM, Schwartz LK, Atkinson JC, Fox PC: Taste performance in Sjögren's syndrome. Physiol Behav 57:89–96, 1995.
110. Weisman K, Christensen E, Dreyer V: Zinc supplementation in alcoholic cirrhosis: A double-blind clinical trial. Acta Med Scand 205:361–366, 1979.
111. Wright HN: Characterization of olfactory dysfunction. Arch Otolaryngol Head Neck Surg 113:163–168, 1987.
112. Wysocki CJ, Gilbert AN: National Geographic smell survey: Effects of age are heterogenous. Ann N Y Acad Sci 561:12–28, 1989.
113. Yamagishi M, Hasegawa S, Nakano Y: Examination and classification of human olfactory mucosa in patients with clinical olfactory disturbances. Arch Otorhinolaryngol 245:316–320, 1988.
114. Yanagisawa K, Bartoshuk LM, Karrer TA, et al: Anesthesia of the chorda tympani nerve: Insights into a source of dysgeusia [abstract]. Chem Senses 17:724, 1992.
115. Yousem DM, Turner WJD, Li C, et al: Kallmann syndrome: MR evaluation of the olfactory system. Am J Neurosci Res 14:839–843, 1993.
116. Zilstorff K, Herbild O: Parosmia. Acta Otolaryngol Suppl 360:40–41, 1979.
117. Zuniga JR, Chen N, Miller IJ Jr: Effects of chorda-lingual nerve injury and repair on human taste. Chem Senses 19:657–665, 1994.

PHILIP HARBER, MD, MPH
DAVID DISCHER, MD

OCCUPATIONAL RESPIRATORY FUNCTION TESTING—AN ALGORITHMIC APPROACH

From the University of California
Los Angeles, California (PH)
  and
Private Consulting, Occupational
  and Environmental Medicine
Sunnyvale, California (DD)

Reprint requests to:
Philip Harber, MD, MPH
Professor of Medicine
University of California, Los Angeles
10911 Weyburn Ave., Suite 344
Los Angeles, CA 90024

To many occupational health practitioners, spirometry has become synonymous with pulmonary function testing. This is inaccurate, and this chapter presents an algorithmically-based approach to match tests to the actual purposes of testing. There are several distinct pulmonary functions, and the appropriate tests must be chosen based on the actual function being tested. Selection and performance of the test are only part of occupational pulmonary function testing programs. The interpretation of results on an individual and group basis is equally important.[8]

Details of test performance per se are deemphasized because numerous papers have addressed these topics.[8,27,29,34,62,77] Selection and interpretation of respiratory function tests must be based on an understanding of the precise purpose of testing in a specific situation. This chapter suggests a systematic approach to utilization of testing in occupational medicine practices. Topics include the purposes of testing, specific tests, applications to specific occupational health situations, and algorithms of test selection.

PURPOSES OF TESTING

Components of the Respiratory System

The respiratory system includes several anatomic components (Table 1) that support important bodily functions relevant to functioning in occupational settings. The anatomic components relate to physiologic functions, and these in turn relate to occupational functioning. The upper

TABLE 1. Components of the Respiratory System

Upper respiratory tract	Alveoli
Nose	Pulmonary vasculature
Pharynx	
Ear/eustachian canals	Interstitium
Sinuses	Pulmonary defense systems
Larynx	Respiratory control systems
Major airways	Respiratory coordination system
Small airways	

airway includes the nose, nasopharynx, and larynx. The sinuses and the middle ear are closely linked to these structures.

The intrathoracic large airways, including the trachea, major bronchi, and many branching divisions, conduct air in and out of lungs by bulk flow. The small airways are the terminal divisions that are smaller than 2 mm in diameter. Often, terminal airways are the initial sites of inflammation and airflow obstruction, but symptoms do not develop because there are so many in parallel that effects are minimized.

The alveolar zone is where gas exchange actually occurs. The interstitium, including the supporting tissue and the capillaries bringing blood in close contact with air in the alveoli, is closely associated with the alveolar zone.

The pulmonary circulation is composed of the pulmonary arterial system, bringing blood with depleted oxygen and added carbon dioxide that has come from the body via the right heart; the pulmonary capillaries are the sites at which gas exchange between the alveoli and blood actually occurs; and the pulmonary venous system returns blood to the left heart for distribution to the body. The right ventricle serves as a significant component of the pulmonary circulation, providing the pumping force necessary.

The ventilatory muscles, or thoracic pump, include the diaphragms and the intercostal muscles. The respiratory control system is another major component of the respiratory system. In addition to the central controllers in the brain stem, there are afferent receptors peripherally. These include chemoreceptors for oxygen and carbon dioxide tensions and stretch receptors associated with the chest wall and its musculature. Irritant receptors, located within the lung, can trigger asthmatic responses.

Two other systems that are not directly related to gas exchange per se are the pulmonary defense and the respiratory coordination systems. The respiratory coordination system is responsible for modulating breathing to permit special functions. Detailed adjustments of the respiratory system are necessary to foster the airflow necessary for speaking and eating.

The pulmonary defense system includes immunologic and nonimmunologic components. Impairment or overactivity of components of respiratory defense is directly relevant to occupational medicine. Individuals with macrophage dysfunction (as occurs with silicosis) or immunologic deficits (e.g., due to HIV infection) may be at particular risk of occupational infections. Conversely, individuals with a tendency toward heightened responses may be at increased risk of allergic reactions to high molecular weight workplace antigens. The respiratory defense system not only defends the lungs and nose against inhaled toxins, but it significantly affects systemic uptake, which may have effects at sites distant from the respiratory tract.

Each of these systems has different significance for occupational health, and no single test adequately evaluates the performance of these disparate systems.

TABLE 2. Occupational Functions Supported by the Respiratory System

Support exercise/work
Tolerate irritants
Defend against toxic atmosphere
Support audition and speaking
Maintain alertness

Occupational Pulmonary Functions

Pulmonary physiology describes the internal functioning or malfunctioning of the systems described above. In occupational medicine, however, the focus is generally on the interaction of the pulmonary system with the workplace. In particular, emphasis is often placed on the ability of the distinct respiratory system to support occupational functioning. Therefore, it is useful to define the "occupational respiratory functions"[40] (Table 2). Support of sustained exercise generally has been considered the primary occupational pulmonary function. For example, the use of spirometry or pulmonary exercise testing to determine work ability traditionally rests on the assumption that jobs are associated with particular requirements for sustained average exertion. Peak exertion support differs slightly. Short-term exertion capacity may be most relevant for some occupational settings, in which only brief bursts of heavy exertion are necessary.[47]

Irritant tolerance is another major occupational respiratory function. Many jobs do not require high levels of sustained or peaked exertion but involve exposure to respiratory irritants that may be poorly tolerated by individuals with asthma. Thus, focusing on exertion ability alone would be misleading in assessing occupational effects and occupational ability and disability. Furthermore, if "irritant" is interpreted broadly, respirator use might be considered an irritant, and some disorders may significantly affect this occupational pulmonary function.

The next occupational pulmonary function is vigilance. Some jobs require a high level of alertness. Primary respiratory control disorders, the effect of medication use, or secondary effect of other respiratory disease may lead to hypercapnia with decreased vigilance. Furthermore, a frequent cough may impede the ability to pay constant attention to a critically demanding task such as landing an aircraft or driving in traffic.

Therefore, the relationship of the traditional pulmonary function tests to the actual occupational respiratory functions should be carefully considered. The amount of air expired in the first second following a maximal inspiration (the forced expiratory volume in one second, FEV_1) is not directly related to the workplace.

Context of Occupational Pulmonary Function Testing

The context of testing must be considered. The American Thoracic Society (ATS) has clearly delineated several distinct purposes for testing,[8] and there are additional ones unique for occupational medicine (Table 3).

Clinical diagnostic testing focuses on establishing a diagnosis in an individual patient who is referred because there is suspicion that a particular disorder exists. Surveillance testing is focused on a group rather than an individual. While groups are selected based on an exposure that presumably implies some risk, the subjects are not individually selected for an a priori suspicion of disease. For example, an insulator with a cough may be seen in a clinical diagnostic setting because there is considerable suspicion that a malignancy is present. Intensive testing such as with

TABLE 3. Purposes of Occupational Function Testing

Screening: early detection of disease in individuals with known exposures.
Clinical diagnosis: establishment or refutation of diagnosis of an occupational lung disease when there is an a priori suspicion in a specific individual.
Fitness for duty (work ability): assessment of whether an individual's respiratory system will permit safe and effective work in a particular job.
Impairment: estimation of degree of functional loss, such as for compensation purposes.
Research and surveillance: testing is conducted to collect data for aggregate analysis rather than primarily for the benefit of the individuals being tested.
Functional status improvement: testing for self-monitoring or health promotion to help an individual improve functional status.
Regulatory testing: mandated by law or regulation.

bronchoscopy may be warranted, but such invasive testing is not part of the usual surveillance for asbestos workers.

Screening is a form of surveillance in which members of an at-risk group are tested in an attempt to diagnose disease in an early treatable state in a particular individual. This is a form of secondary prevention. Other forms of surveillance do not necessarily benefit the individual but instead are designed to gain group information likely to help estimate overall risk.

Regulatory testing is mandated by specific regulations, such as those promulgated by the Occupational Safety and Health Administration (OSHA), and may serve other purposes.

Research testing is performed to generate new information. Therefore, in many instances, the testing need not be of documented utility prior to institution.

Testing also may be performed for assessing work ability or for determining disability. While testing of ability and disability theoretically should be the same, in many settings different standards apply. Testing may be conducted for health promotion purposes, and for legal causes such as assessment of tort or workers' compensation liability.

Pulmonary functions may be evaluated to monitor response to treatment, such as the efficacy of bronchodilator medications or change in workplace exposures. Self-monitoring, particularly of peak expiratory flow rates, is another context of testing.

Thus, there are many different purposes for which the respiratory functions are evaluated.

Analytic Framework

Several analytic concepts apply to interpretation of results testing. Concepts of sensitivity and specificity are useful only in a limited number of pulmonary function testing situations. They apply when a diagnosis can be ascertained independent of the test procedure itself. For example, if the presence of occupational asthma is defined by a "gold standard" of a bronchoprovocation test and a simple screening test such as pre/postshift spirometry difference is used, it is meaningful to calculate sensitivity and specificity (sensitivity represents the proportion of the persons with the disease, who are detected as positive by the screening test, and specificity is the proportion of those who do not have the disease, who are identified as negative by the screening test). Even here, sensitivity and specificity cannot be directly calculated. They are dependent on the criterion value selected by changing the definition of how large a pre- to postshift difference is necessary to consider positive. One can trade off sensitivity and specificity. Receiver operating characteristic curves[45,76] can be applied to help select the optimal cut point.

Unfortunately, these concepts cannot be applied to many situations in which occupational pulmonary functions are tested. The diagnosis of obstructive airway disease is generally based on abnormality of spirometry rather than being independent of the test. It is thus not meaningful to state that spirometry has acceptable sensitivity and specificity when its results define the presence of the disease unless there is an external gold standard for reference (e.g., lung biopsy for pneumoconiosis).

In other occupational health situations, the true value cannot be ascertained with certainty. When discussing the relationship between pairs of test procedures such as spirometry and exercise testing, one is actually describing concordance rather than sensitivity and specificity.

Utility, the value associated with a particular outcome, also must be considered. In some situations, the negative utility (cost) of a false positive test may markedly outweigh the potential benefit of a true positive. Harber et al. have conducted formal mathematical analyses in which this concept is applied to the diagnosis of occupational asthma[45] and to assessment of work ability under the Americans with Disabilities Act.[41]

In the current era of budgetary constraints, other considerations are important. Testing of occupational pulmonary functions must consider cost. In a cost-benefit analysis, the total costs of the test, including the indirect costs, are related to the benefit to the individual or more generally to society (when an individual is not expected to benefit in a surveillance setting). For a cost-effective analysis, the increment in value per unit of investment in a testing procedure is considered. Cost-benefit and cost-effectiveness analyses can be conducted based on total or on the marginal costs and benefits of an incremental programmatic change.

Other considerations increasingly affect the choice of modality for testing occupational pulmonary function. In the clinical setting, reimbursement is a major determinant of the feasibility of testing. For surveillance testing, worker population access and availability of professional resources also are fundamental determinants.

Implications

Despite the beliefs of many occupational health professionals, pulmonary function testing is not synonymous with spirometry. The above discussion leads to several implications: what is commonly called "pulmonary" actually refers to a large number of distinct respiratory systems that serve different physiologic purposes (Table 4). The functioning of the respiratory systems within the body is only indirectly related to the worksite pulmonary functions, which are defined in terms relevant to the occupational setting. The purposes for which testing is performed and external constraints also affect test performance and interpretation.

TABLE 4. Physiologic Functions of the Respiratory Systems

Air movement (ventilation)
Gas exchange
Blood distribution
Adjustment to maintain homeostasis
Coordination with other functions such as talking and eating
Resistance to exogenous agents

SPECIFIC TEST PROCEDURES

Measurement of Lung Volumes

Spirometry does not measure actual lung volumes but only describes the air expelled from the mouth. Therefore, it does not describe the total volume of the lung after a maximal inspiratory effort (total lung capacity, TLC), nor does it describe the air left in the lung at the end of normal expiration (functional residual capacity, FRC) or after a maximal expiratory effort (residual volume, RV). For example, the forced vital capacity (FVC) may be reduced because the actual volumes of the lung are reduced due to intrinsic lung disease or external causes such as severe kyphoscoliosis. They also may be reduced because the individual simply cannot inspire and exhale maximally, such as due to neuromuscular disease or severe obstructive lung disease. Generally, lung volume determination is not part of the standard pulmonary functional assessment. It is useful in selected instances:

1. When mixed obstructive and restrictive disease may be present. In the presence of airflow obstruction, the FVC may be reduced. Typically, in asthma and chronic obstructive pulmonary disease (COPD), the true lung volumes are not reduced. During spirometry, air trapping occurs, leading to an increase in the amount of air left in the lung at the end of the forced expiratory maneuver—that is, RV is increased. In addition, the total lung capacity may be increased due to hyperinflation in obstructive disease. The resting position of the lung at the end of the normal tidal breath (FRC) is also increased, meaning that more air remains within the chest. This contrasts with the situation in restrictive lung diseases in which the total lung capacity is reduced.

2. When there are questions about whether complete efforts were made. Occasionally a person may voluntarily perform suboptimally or be unable to effectively complete the expiratory maneuver for spirometry. In some instances, measurement of lung volumes can serve as a useful complement to spirometry per se.

Lung volume determination is commonly accomplished by one of three methods: helium dilution, body plethysmography, and, infrequently, nitrogen washout.[23,32,64]

In the **helium dilution** method, the subject breathes in a circuit including a spirometer in which a known volume of helium or other nonabsorbable inert gas has been placed. The subject then reaches equilibrium with the gas mixture in the circuit. The helium that was present initially in the spirometer is diluted throughout the total volume incorporating the apparatus and the subject. The degree of dilution is therefore related to the volume of the subject. By knowing the amount of helium and the circuit volume, the added volume from the patient can be calculated from the final equilibrium concentration. The method is relatively easy to use, and the equipment is affordable for most large clinical laboratories and pulmonologists' offices.

There are several limitations to the helium dilution method. First, the subject must reach equilibrium with the apparatus. Typically, the subject breathes in and out of the apparatus for about 6 minutes to reach equilibrium. If severe air flow obstruction is present with significant inhomogeneity, 6 minutes may not be sufficient to reach equilibrium, and the measured volume will underestimate the true lung volume. Conversely, if the mouthpiece dislodges slightly during the 6 minutes, helium will leak to the surrounding air and the final concentration will be artificially low, leading to an overestimation of the true lung volume. The method depends on careful timing of the junction of the subject with the apparatus. To measure the functional residual capacity, the technician must turn a valve to connect the subject to the dilution apparatus at the end of the normal breath. Finally, the technician must carefully add enough oxygen to compensate for that absorbed by the patient. If this is not done, volumes will be inaccurate.

The measurements typically made during the helium dilution testing are those of the FRC. The TLC is determined by having the patient take a maximal voluntary inspiration and adding the volume inhaled to the FRC. Similarly, the residual volume (RV) is calculated by having the subject exhale maximally from the FRC position. The TLC and FRC are therefore dependent on the subject making maximal efforts. Unlike the FRC, TLC and RV are not measured directly.

An alternative technique for measuring the lung volumes is **body plethysmography**. The subject pants while seated in a tightly sealed chamber. The method depends on measuring small differences in mouth and ambient (chamber) pressure. Changes of the pressure within the chamber in relation to changes in the airway are related to change in lung volume. Body plethysmography is more complex, and the equipment is more costly than that for helium dilution. Further, it is highly dependent on accurate performance by well-trained technicians. Unlike helium dilution, it provides accurate results even in the presence of airflow obstruction because it does not depend on reaching equilibrium. Unlike helium dilution, body plethysmography-determined volumes include noncommunicating air spaces, such as bullae, which do not communicate with airways.

Airway Hyperresponsiveness Testing

Asthma is a common disorder. Patients with asthma are characterized by hyperresponsiveness of the airways, meaning a tendency of the airways to overrespond to stimuli. In addition, some individuals have asymptomatic airway hyperresponsiveness (AHR). Testing may be needed in the following circumstances:

1. For the diagnosis of asthma. Airway hyperresponsiveness is necessary for the diagnosis of asthma. However, in many instances, it is not necessary to perform formal AHR testing because the diagnosis can be confirmed in other ways. The presence of AHR per se does not establish the diagnosis of asthma in the absence of other findings or symptoms such as wheezing or episodic dyspnea.

2. For assessing disability due to asthma. Studies suggest that the degree of AHR is related to the extent of disability and impairment.[2]

3. For monitoring workers or as a baseline assessment. Theoretically, testing of AHR might represent a sensitive method for the early diagnosis of work-induced asthma. Furthermore, because AHR is common in the general population, baseline testing of individuals who may have potentially relevant exposures may be useful for future reference.

4. First-stage evaluation for occupational asthma with latency. For workers who have had recent exposure to a sensitizing agent, demonstrated absence of AHR significantly decreases the likelihood that asthma is present.[15,87] Absence does not, however, completely rule this out.[65]

Airway hyperresponsiveness represents an exaggerated tendency of airways to respond to external stimuli. There are two major components of airway responsiveness: muscular contraction and inflammation with airway edema. Changes in the former may occur much more rapidly than in the latter.

Three aspects of AHR may be determined: (1) variability of airway function over time, (2) responsiveness to stimuli that increase airflow resistance, and (3) responsiveness to stimuli that decrease airflow resistance. The three types of airway hyperresponsiveness may be related, but they are not necessarily identical. Furthermore, there are several ways to measure each of the phases of airway hyperresponsiveness. AHR is not a constant characteristic but may vary within the same subject over time.[81] Even common respiratory infections such as the common cold may lead to increases in AHR for many weeks after clinical resolution of symptoms.[26]

AHR is not a dichotomous variable, but rather there is a continuous distribution of airway responsiveness. Thus, the habit of describing test results as "positive or negative" should be eschewed in favor of a quantitative measure (just as the FEV_1 is described quantitatively and not by a simple abnormal/normal dichotomy).

Measurement of variability airway function over time is often the easiest to perform. Spirometry may be done repetitively, over days or weeks. Variability may be determined by conducting spirometry before and after a work shift, several times during a week, or over several weeks or months. In interpreting whether variability is greater than that typically associated with normal individuals, three sources of variability must be considered: actual differences in airway function over time, improvement in subject performance due to experience with the testing technique, and error of measurement.

Variability also can be measured with a peak flow meter. Unlike spirometry, this may be done by the worker, which allows more measurements to be acquired. Proper use requires that the subject make maximal efforts and record results accurately. The subject must remember to perform the testing at appropriate times and must be honest about properly recording results. Because of these limitations, the theoretical advantages of peak flow measurements for assessing occupational asthma may not be fully achievable. Studies have found that a relatively small proportion of subjects actually completed recording sufficiently adequately to be useful for diagnosis.[51,79]

Peak expiratory flow meters have less precision than spirometry (i.e., have greater noise of measurement). Therefore, higher levels of variability are needed to indicate excessive variability indicating airway hyperresponsiveness. To interpret peak expiratory flow measurements, variability from day to day and variability within a day should be determined. Optimally, subjects are asked to record their peak expiratory flow rates four times a day. Within-day variability is represented as a difference between the highest and lowest value of the day as a fraction of the highest. Twenty percent diurnal variation is often considered significant.[69] Others emphasize the role of visual inspection of peak flow diaries without a specific percentage.[73]

The second form of AHR measurement is response to agents that decrease airway function (increase airway resistance). Airway function is measured, typically with the FEV_1 but occasionally with direct measurement of airway resistance by body plethysmography. A provocative stimulus is then provided. The response of the subject is measured as a decrement in FEV_1 or increase in airway resistance. If this does not exceed the predetermined value, a larger dose of a provocative stimulus is applied and the lung function measurements are repeated. This continues in an incremental fashion until the dose exceeds a predetermined maximum.

For spirometry, testing usually continues until there has been a 20% drop of FEV_1 from baseline or until the maximal dose of the provocative stimulus has been provided. The actual dose that leads to the 20% drop is the quantitative measure of interest. The data are "censored" because many subjects without AHR will not have a specific value since they do not reach the 20% drop criterion.

The most commonly used provocative agent is methacholine, an analog of the neurotransmitter acetylcholine. This is given by inhalation according to one of several protocols.[14,17,85] Alternatively, histamine may be used, particularly when methacholine is unavailable.[83] Furthermore, inhalation of cold dry air, carbachol, and acid inhalation may be used as provocative stimuli.[80,81,83,86]

A methacholine challenge test is often characterized by the provocative dose to create a 20% drop in FEV_1, symbolized as PD_{20}. For conventional clinical purposes, this is the value that is interpreted. If a 20% drop has not occurred with the maximal dose of 25 mg, the test is considered negative. Conversely, the actual dose that produces the 20% drop is the PD_{20}.

It may be preferable to describe the slope of the dose response relationship rather than the single PD_{20} value. This slope is calculated by comparing the baseline FEV_1 to the FEV_1 at the highest given dose and dividing by the dose—in effect, producing a variable representing the slope of the dose response relationship. The American Thoracic Society has recommended that individuals who respond at a cumulative dose of 8 mg or less be considered to have sufficient AHR to have potential disability.[5]

The third measure of airway responsiveness is response to agents that improve airway function (decrease airway resistance). Short-term responsiveness to an inhaled bronchodilator is usually assessed. After spirometry is performed, a rapidly acting bronchodilator is administered by inhalation, and spirometry is repeated. The proportional increase in the FEV_1 or the FVC is used as a measure of responsiveness to agents increasing airway function. This approach can help differentiate simple chronic obstructive pulmonary disease without a component of AHR from asthma with AHR. By convention, a 12% increase in the FEV_1 or FVC is considered to represent a positive "bronchodilator response."[6] As is the case for response to agents decreasing airway function, a quantitative measure of responsiveness is preferable.

Responsiveness to specific workplace provocative agents can also be determined.[13,22,31]

Some patients have exercise-induced bronchospasm (EIB). A special test is necessary for this diagnosis: spirometry is performed before and after exercise is conducted in a laboratory setting, such as on a treadmill or calibrated bike ergometer).

TIMING OF AHR TESTING

To provide interpretable results, AHR testing must be done at an appropriate time. In general, a patient should not be taking short-term bronchodilators when the testing is performed. Beta agonist medication should be discontinued 12 hours prior to testing. Inhaled or systemic corticosteroid therapy generally is continued, but the interpreter must recognize that this may decrease airway responsiveness. Furthermore, testing should generally not be carried out when there has been an acute respiratory infection, including upper respiratory infections, within 4–6 weeks. Otherwise, the presence of quantitatively significant AHR may be temporary only.

Exercise Testing

Pulmonary exercise testing includes measurement of several parameters that typically are measured at several levels of exercise. Pulmonary exercise testing typically yields a large array of numerical results that may be reduced to several specific parameters to answer relevant questions, as follows:

1. Is there any evidence of objective functional deficit? This determination is useful when a patient has normal spirometry and diffusing capacity yet complains of severe dyspnea. Even if minor abnormalities are seen at maximal exercise, they are not necessarily associated with functional impact that is clinically relevant.

2. What is the maximal exercise level the individual can sustain? The maximal oxygen consumption attained during the exercise test describes this. It is typically expressed as milliliters of oxygen per minute, milliliters of oxygen per kilogram per minute, or mets (weight adjusted). The latter measure is commonly used by cardiologists. The oxygen consumption should be measured directly and not simply estimated from the level of exercise.

For the occupational setting, one is often interested in the actual workload achievable by the individual rather than the oxygen consumption per se. The workload is expressed in terms of watts. Thus, to determine whether an individual can perform a maximal job task, it is the achievable work and not the oxygen consumption that is of interest.[46]

3. What is the level of sustainable exertion of which the subject is capable? Most work demands relate more closely to this measure than to the maximal attainable. Typically, this is answered by taking a fraction of the maximal attainable exercise. Usually, it is assumed that an individual can maintain 40–50% of the maximal for a full workday.

4. What factor limits exercise ability? Here, the exercise test is used diagnostically. Normally, exercise is limited by cardiovascular performance rather than by pulmonary factors. Thus, when the subject has achieved his or her maximal exertion level in the exercise test, there should be evidence of reaching cardiovascular limitation but with pulmonary reserve. In abnormal conditions, there may be limitations due to pulmonary ventilation/gas exchange, deconditioning, voluntary exercise limitation, or muscular limitations.

Typically, when the exercise is terminated, the subject has a heart rate close to the predicted maximal based on age. In addition, the person should have crossed the anaerobic threshold, meaning that oxygen delivery to the exercising muscle has become limited. Crossing the anaerobic threshold is indicated by the increase in the respiratory exchange ratio (carbon dioxide excretion to oxygen uptake ratio) to more than 1 and similar measures.

When exercise is limited by cardiovascular factors, there is generally sufficient reserve in the pulmonary system at maximal exercise. This is typically measured by comparing the ventilation at maximal exercise (in liters per minute) to the individual's predicted maximum (generally calculated at 35–40 times the FEV_1). If there is adequate reserve—greater than 25%—it is unlikely that limitation is due to pulmonary factors. Conversely, if there is no pulmonary reserve at maximal exercise, it is likely that pulmonary disease limits exercise.

In addition, the oxygen tension is ascertained—either by direct measurement of arterial blood gas tensions or by the use of an oxygen saturation meter that is placed on a fingertip or earlobe and does not require arterial punctures. Normally, oxygen concentration does not drop with maximal exercise. However, in certain pulmonary diseases, particularly if there is limitation of pulmonary vasculature as occurs in emphysema or restrictive interstitial disease such as severe asbestosis, the oxygen concentration may decrease with exercise.

In some individuals, neither cardiac nor pulmonary systems are functioning at their maximal level at the time of exercise limitation. In such circumstances, exercise may be limited by deconditioning, neurologic or musculoskeletal factors, or voluntary limitation.

Exercise testing can help differentiate limitation due to pulmonary disease, cardiac disease, and deconditioning. For disability assessments, this is important if disability must be assessed and apportioned to specific origins. However, it is unimportant when the origin is not relevant, as in Social Security disability assessment.

5. Is the pulmonary response to increasing exercise normal? Under normal circumstances, the pulmonary system has sufficient reserve to continue functioning efficiently as the exercise level increases. The dead space ratio (proportion of tidal volume that does not bring air in contact with the alveoli) normally remains the same or decreases with exercise. However, with severe lung disease, the proportion of wasted ventilation increases with exercise. Similarly, if arterial blood gas tensions are determined, the alveolar-arterial oxygen gradient normally does not increase significantly with exercise.

6. Did the patient make a valid effort during the exercise test? Exercise testing is subject to legitimate efforts on the patient's part. If the cardiovascular system or the pulmonary system has reached its functional limit, such as by achieving the maximal predicted heart rate or maximal predicted ventilation, it is likely that the effort has been valid. Consistency of effort also can be assessed by the linearity of the relationship between exercise level (watts) and oxygen consumption or ventilation.

7. Has the patient's exercise capacity been reduced by a particular disease or injury? This is the most difficult question to answer. Simply comparing the patient's maximal attained oxygen consumption to a "predicted value" may be misleading. Predicted values are typically those of healthy, fit individuals, and a specific subject may have had less exercise ability prior to the illness due to a sedentary lifestyle. Conversely, an individual who exercises regularly may have had greater than typical maximal exercise ability, and simply matching the predicted value would underestimate the degree of loss.

Also, oxygen consumption is affected by body weight. This can lead to interpretive difficulty, particularly if peak oxygen consumption is weight-adjusted, that is, expressed as milliliters of oxygen consumption per kilogram per minute or as mets.

8. Can the patient meet the demands of a particular job? Exercise testing alone is incapable of answering this question. Only if the job demands are well characterized can the exercise test results be interpreted for this specific question. Furthermore, specific job demands such as use of respirators may add significant burdens. In borderline cases, the exercise test should be performed with the respiratory protective equipment in place.

9. Is exercise-induced bronchospasm present? Some asthmatics have bronchospasm after they exercise.

Spirometry and Peak Expiratory Flow Testing

Spirometry testing has evolved considerably. Spirometry is particularly useful in occupational health for several reasons:

1. It is sensitive to many of the lung disorders that may be induced by occupational exposures.
2. Testing can be done at a reasonable cost.
3. Standards are available to ensure consistent testing methods.
4. Testing can be done at worksites.
5. There are reasonably well defined normal reference standards.

Spirometry may be used as a test itself or as part of a more complex procedure such as determination of airway hyperresponsiveness, antigen bronchoprovocation testing, or serial measurements to reflect variability of lung function.

There have been several detailed reviews of this technique.[24] This section discusses the use of spirometry as the test itself.

Spirometry testing involves several steps: (1) determination of whether spirometry is necessary and sufficient, (2) selection of equipment and training of personnel,

(3) timing of testing, (4) testing performance, (5) interpretation of individual results, (6) aggregate interpretation, and (7) longitudinal analysis for one individual and for groups.

APPROPRIATE USE OF SPIROMETRY

Spirometry is extremely useful on an individual (clinical) and on a population basis.[6,8,58,77] It is useful for early detection and for assessment of severity of advanced disease. However, radiography may be more sensitive for the early detection of pneumoconiosis. Furthermore, spirometry is diagnostically nonspecific. While it is effective in demonstrating the presence of abnormality, it does not describe the cause. Spirometry also may be time-specific. For disorders such as asthma that have considerable day-to-day variability, a single spirometry session may overestimate or underestimate the likelihood or magnitude of the disorder.

Spirometry is not particularly useful for several major classes of respiratory disorders, including pulmonary vascular disease, early interstitial disease, and respiratory control disorders such as sleep apnea. For these purposes, other tests are requisite.

EQUIPMENT AND PERSONNEL

Most modern spirometers are automated, eliminating the need for hand calculations. There are two general categories of spirometers: those that measure volume and those that measure flow. Volume measurements were often preferred in occupational settings, but both types are now widely used.

The American Thoracic Society, which is instrumental in setting the de facto community standards for spirometry practice, has recently revised its recommendations for spirometry equipment and methodology.[8] This has significant implications for occupational medicine purposes.[43] One major change relates to the BTPS factor. This factor is multiplied by the air volume measured at the spirometer temperature to determine the volume of air that actually was expelled from the subject (at body temperature, pressure, and water saturation). For flow measuring devices in particular, the temperature of air reaching the sensor is typically between ambient temperature and body temperature, and use of a room temperature-derived BTPS factor would lead to overestimation of true spirometric volumes.[18,35,36,37,54,63,66,72,75] Current recommendations for spirometer manufacturers require that the instrument be accurate when the design is tested under varying temperature and saturation conditions, whereas prior recommendations by ATS did not require this. In effect, this suggests that each manufacturer should specify how BTPS is adjusted for the particular model of spirometer. The results of this change may be significant.[44]

Several factors should determine the selection of a spirometer.[33] Volume-measuring devices are typically easier to calibrate but are larger and therefore more difficult to move from place to place. Many flow-sensing spirometers allow rapid throughput of subjects being tested and therefore may be preferable during routine surveillance of relatively healthy populations. The reputation of the manufacturer and availability of repair service are other factors to be considered. The quality of the prompting the spirometer system provides should be assessed. Extensive prompting may interfere with the productivity of experienced technicians, whereas it may be particularly important for individuals conducting such testing on an intermittent basis.[11] The graphic display during spirometry maneuvers varies among instruments. Generally, online observation of results as the subject is exhaling can help both the subject and the technician. When testing is part of a corporate program, compatibility with the overall data system is necessary. Finally, the purchaser must decide whether the spirometer operates with a free-standing personal computer or the processor is built into the spirometer itself.

Personnel should be adequately trained.[30,52] A limited number of OSHA standards set specific requirements for technician training, which generally consists of completion of a brief NIOSH-approved spirometry course. Periodic retraining has been recommended.

TEST PERFORMANCE

Accurate results are dependent on proper test technique.[52] The subject must be adequately instructed in advance. The testing is performed several times in each testing session, and the best values for each subject are selected as being representative. This differs from other clinical testing procedures, in which the average of replications is used. An adequate number of spirometric efforts for each patient is necessary. In general, this requires at least three adequate efforts for each patient. Up to eight could be needed if the technician feels the methodology or effort is inadequate or the repeatability criteria are not met. In the past, adequate consistency was ascertained by having the results of the two best efforts be within 5% of each other. Under the newer ATS recommendations, this percentage approach has been supplanted by an absolute value requiring that the best results be within 200 ml.[8] Use of proportion criteria has been shown to introduce potential biases.[8] Unfortunately, many spirometry systems still use the 5% difference rule, and many spirometry technicians have been trained in the 5% approach. Therefore, gradual transition to the upgraded repeatability technique is permitted.[8]

Use of test results when data do not meet the repeatability criteria has received considerable attention. Several studies have demonstrated that persons who do not meet repeatability criteria are more likely to have lung disease than those who do meet such criteria.[12,25,53,55,69,88] Hence, excluding their data may bias any surveillance or study analysis by preferentially excluding individuals with disease. However, including the inaccurate data with more accurate data also would be misleading. Therefore, it is probably useful to conduct analyses with and without the subjects with less repeatability. Whether the specific type of respiratory disorder is associated with inadequate repeatability is moot. Some, but not all, investigators feel that asthma is particularly common in the nonrepeatability group.

It is important for the technician to be allowed the option of designating the test result as being poorly repeatable.

TEST INTERPRETATION

Measurement of the values is only the first step in interpretation. Test interpretation is done in two ways: clinical and aggregate. For clinical purposes, three questions are answered:
- Are the test results normal?
- If abnormal, how abnormal are they?
- What disease process is most likely?

The values must be compared to those of a reference population. However, the reference population value set mandated in several OSHA standards[57] is not generally accepted now. In most instances, the equations of Crapo,[21] Morris,[67] or the newer Knudson[56] equations are preferred in the United States except where mandated by OSHA regulations. The reference equations in common use have been derived from populations of healthy, white, non-Hispanics and thus are not directly applicable to African American, Asian American, and other individuals.

For African Americans, it is common to apply a proportioning factor, reducing the predicted values based on the population. No such method is commonly applicable to Asians within the United States. White, Hispanic populations have been shown in several studies to have different results, but they are not sufficiently consistent to recommend adjustment for this factor.[19,20,78] Some studies are specifically based on blue-collar working populations.[74]

Classification of an abnormal/normal category is generally done on a statistical basis rather than by comparison to an external diagnostic standard. Two theoretical bases may be applied: (1) Are the individual subject's results lower than those of an arbitrary fraction (usually 95%) of the reference population? (2) From a statistical sampling perspective, is it less than 5% likely that the subject's results are from the same population from which the reference population was sampled? The former, arbitrary approach is most commonly used. Although there has been a strong tradition of dependence on using the percentage of predicted value as the metric for comparing results of an individual subject to a reference population, confidence intervals (depending on the magnitude of difference rather than the ratio) are increasingly being used. This approach is embodied in the ATS's and the American Medical Association's guidelines for disability assessment.[1,3] For statistical reasons, it is more consistent with the homoscedascasity of lung function distribution.[49]

Spirometry data represent a description of the subject's physiologic state rather than establish a cause, but they are relevant in establishing diagnoses. The role of spirometry results and integration with other testing are described later in this chapter.

Aggregate Analysis

Spirometry is commonly used in epidemiologic health surveillance as well as on an individual clinical basis. Particular emphasis is needed to assure rigid quality control when data will be aggregated over a large number of subjects. Differences that might not be considered clinically significant may become relevant when they are found consistently in a population. Differences in instrumentation, performance of the technician, and subject selection/exclusion criteria can have major effects in aggregate analysis. Special efforts are needed to assure consistency of the technician's performance, including application of computer monitoring of test performance and periodic reevaluation and retraining of the technician.[28]

Longitudinal Analysis of Spirometry Data

Longitudinal analysis, the comparison of results over time, may be performed on a clinical or an aggregate/surveillance basis. In a clinical application, a subject's values in one year are compared to results from prior years. A sudden drop in spirometry results suggests that an adverse effect—whether due to disease or exposure—may have occurred. Thus, disease can be detected even if the recent results are technically within the normal limits as defined by comparison to an external reference population. This is based on the concept of tracking. While some individuals have larger lungs than others even after adjustment for height and other body size parameters, any individual tends to maintain the same position in reference to the larger population. That is, individuals with an FEV_1 of 85% of the predicted value should maintain this position over a period of years, just as an individual with an FEV_1 of 110% of the predicted value should continue to be above average.

While clinical longitudinal data analysis is theoretically attractive, several practical factors constrain its use. The normal rate of decline in lung function is relatively small when assessed on a year-to-year basis. For this reason, small errors in measurement or random variability might be overinterpreted as representing accelerated decline. It is difficult to have workers tested with exactly the same equipment and technician over a period of years, thereby introducing possible temporal extraneous variability. Furthermore, patients often change health care providers or employers relatively frequently, thereby making consistent data collection for clinical purposes difficult.

Longitudinal analysis of spirometry data holds great promise as surveillance or epidemiologic tools. A consistent pattern of increased rates of decline may be the earliest indicator that disease has developed, and it might be more sensitive on a short-term basis than comparing results of an exposed to that of an unexposed population.

Rigid quality control is necessary when spirometry is conducted on a longitudinal basis.[59] Change in technique may produce significant systematic artifacts.

There is still incomplete consensus about the appropriate statistical models for longitudinal data analysis.[4] Generally, the rate of decline of each subject should be ascertained and then averaged over the group, rather than the group average being compared over time. In other words, the data for each subject should be used for an individual regression to find the temporal coefficient, and the subject-derived regression coefficients should be combined to represent the group. This contrasts with simply taking the average lung function of the overall group in each year and comparing it over time to measure longitudinal change.

SUMMARY

Spirometry has been the mainstay of physiologic testing in the worksite, but it is only one of many available techniques. Spirometry is only an indirect indicator of the true goal of testing in the worksite. To be useful, spirometry must be done properly. The sources of variance of spirometry results should be carefully considered and controlled wherever possible. Whether a source of variance is signal or noise depends on the situation. For example, short-term variability of FEV_1 may be considered noise in a study of pneumoconiosis but it is the primary signal in determining whether a particular patient has asthma. One source of variability—measurement error—is always noise and should be minimized by scrupulous attention to technical detail.[27,28]

SOFTWARE

A wide array of computerized spirometry equipment, which often includes packaged interpretative software, is available. If one chooses to use such software, the underlying logic should be adaptable to the situation at hand. For example, some vendors provide screening prompts to help the technician determine prior to administering the test whether the subject has tight clothing, loose dentures, cold or other URI, or has smoked or taken a relevant medication recently.

Software can facilitate spirometry programs in several ways:

1. It may support quality control. It can monitor technician performance by summarizing the performance of each technician, indicate the frequency of tests without at least three acceptable trials, indicate tests without reproducibility of the two best FEV_1s or FVCs, and allow physicians' comments on individual test quality.

2. Software can support physician review of testing. Overreaders frequently discard a trial that contains an artifact not detected by the software as unacceptable based on an inspection of the spirometry curves. The direct visual comparison of these curves without referring to the reproducibility of calculations can be helpful in assessing the issue of submaximal efforts on the successive forced expiratory trials.

The overreader looks at prior spirograms, checks for questionnaire responses, reviews other examination findings that would help explain the abnormality, and reviews the worker's recent exposures on the job if the abnormality appears to be a new finding.

3. Statistical software can be helpful in making calculations for group comparisons or longitudinal trends in data. These analyses may be complicated by the use of different equipment and software. Interpretation can be difficult when the retrospective data come from multiple sources and are without graphic displays. Documentation is needed for calibration or quality checks. Variances in sitting versus standing during testing also may confound comparisons.

4. It may foster overreading of data from bronchodilator effect testing or spirometry performed under controlled or worksite provocation. Some vendors provide modules for entering free text on clinical observations and even brief questionnaire routines.

5. Software is commercially available and provides preliminary test interpretations. General interpretation algorithms involve selecting appropriate prediction equations; the best FEV_1, FVC, and FEV_1/FVC ratios are the three most common ventilatory parameters used to categorize abnormalities. An overreader will observe the quality rating and often add an interpretive statement such as follows: "Trials 3, 4, and 6 are acceptable and the best trial (6) and the second best trial (4) are within the reproducibility criteria for both FEV_1 and FVC. The test interpretation is that of borderline obstruction." This is based on the criterion of "borderline obstruction" meaning that the best trial ratio observed value is below 75%.

6. Commercial software can help plant-level epidemiologic analyses. By focusing on operations within or between departments and displaying the aggregated data, one might identify a hazard not previously observed. This approach, using the data from an annual medical surveillance program, was used in a corporate research and development facility of a resin manufacturer and helped identify unrecognized health risks from recurrent exothermic releases.[68]

7. Peak flow meters are often recommended for use by workers. Computer software can greatly facilitate interpretation. The usual analytic approach to peak flow data is to calculate the daily average variability, comparing variability on the exposure day to nonexposure days. The spirometry observed peak flow can be compared to the values obtained in the clinic using the dispensed peak flow device to calibrate the device. Moreover, one can focus on the evening after work data—for example, for egg protein aerosol-exposed workers on the day shift because of the typical delayed asthmatic reaction with this sensitizer.[84] Thus, the low peak flows may be consistently noted after work.

Asthmatic patients often are given a diary and a peak flow device and asked to record symptoms and peak flows during the day for a week while starting a new medication or job. The occupational physician will have a choice between cross shift testing using technician-administered spirometry versus worker-administered and -recorded peak flow measurements. Sometimes the best approach will be a combination of both, so as to retrain the worker on the peak flow technique during the shift while obtaining cross shift spirometry and to use the peak flow after the shift when clinic hours are over. The usual instruction of peak flow is to record only the highest of three puffs. With new electronic peak flow devices one can store all puffs, and no data entry by hand is required; one can even download the peak flows daily or weekly by telephonic transmission.

Diffusing Capacity for Carbon Monoxide Testing

The diffusing capacity of the lung for carbon monoxide (DLCO) is a gas transfer test rather than a ventilatory test. It has general application to occupational conditions such as pneumoconioses rather than asthma. In silicosis, for example, the interstitial lung pathology involves a reduced alveolar surface area and membrane thickening with reduced efficiency or transport.

The single breath technique has been most standardized.[7] It involves inhaling a mixture of gas with a small concentration of carbon monoxide (typically, about 0.3%) in about 10% helium gas and air, and holding the breath for 10 seconds. An alveolar sample is obtained by discarding the initial portion of the forced expired air. The helium concentration is a function of the lung volume, while the carbon monoxide concentration is a function of both the lung volume and the amount absorbed across the alveolar membrane. The typical computer package calculates alveolar lung volume and the diffusing capacity, the latter based on the carbon monoxide absorbed in 10 seconds, for example. Since with silicosis the efficiency of transport of carbon monoxide or any absorbed gas is reduced, the diffusing capacity is lowered. Because diffusing capacity standardization is not as widely used as spirometry standardization, comparisons between testing facilities can be difficult. A steady state diffusing capacity test is also performed occasionally. The diffusing capacity test is somewhat nonspecific, however, and is reduced in a variety of pulmonary conditions. Many of the comments about overread and trend analysis stated above for spirometry and peak flow testing also apply to this test.

APPLICATION TO SPECIFIC OCCUPATIONAL HEALTH SITUATIONS

Occupational Asthma

Pulmonary function testing is an essential part of the evaluation and prevention of occupational and other forms of asthma. Periodic pulmonary function testing and an asthma symptom questionnaire can be effectively used to detect asthma and assess exposure risk. Questionnaires should be tailored to elicit job tasks and exposure conditions specific to the workplace, and they can be administered by a spirometry technician or other allied health professional. While immunologic or skin tests are occasionally available, they typically have the inherent problem of interpreting the significance of positive results in an asymptomatic worker.

Respiratory function testing is useful in the following situations:

1. To provide objective evaluation in an individual with symptoms. When respiratory symptoms are present, spirometry is likely to be abnormal if the symptoms are due to airflow obstruction such as asthma. In this setting, therefore, it is important for the timing of the spirometry to coincide with symptoms.

2. To identify asthma that is intermittent and variable in course. In such cases, the results of spirometry can be normal even when disease is present. Therefore, if asthma is strongly suspected in a symptomatic patient, additional testing such as with a methacholine challenge is indicated. Normal spirometry does not rule out asthma.

3. To express the severity of asthma. The severity of asthma ranges from minimal to life-threatening. The impact on occupational functional, necessary work accommodation, and preclusion measures depend on severity of illness. The use of spirometry and other respiratory function tests for assessment of severity is discussed later in this chapter. Objective assessment of severity, rather than reliance on symptoms alone, is feasible.

4. To evaluate the response to therapy. Asthma is very responsive to a proper therapeutic program. In addition to the proper selection of medications, patient compliance is often an issue. Periodic lung function testing can assess the efficacy of drug selection and patient compliance.

5. To evaluate the response to environmental modification. Many asthmatics are allergically sensitive to specific workplace or home antigens. Elimination of exposures (such as by changing job location) or accommodation (such as institution of local exhaust ventilation or personal respiratory protection) can be evaluated by responses to lung function testing.

6. To confirm the diagnosis of allergic sensitization asthma (occupational asthma with latency) when used in conjunction with a bronchoprovocation test. In this testing, lung function is measured typically with spirometry or airway resistance before and after exposure to a putative agent. The exposure may be in a laboratory setting or in the worksite as naturally occurs. A significant change in results with the exposure agents but not with the control exposure strongly suggests specific sensitization.

7. To conduct surveillance on populations exposed to chemical and biologic agents that may be allergic sensitizers or otherwise cause airway responses. For example, spirometry is mandated before and after a shift in populations exposed to cotton dust.[70]

8. For research studies involving the detection of degree of hazard associated with new chemicals and processes.

The diagnosis and management of occupational asthma is discussed by Chan-Yeung.[15] Lung function testing should be integrated with other measures.

Pneumoconioses

The pneumoconioses are dust diseases of the lung produced by exposures to inorganic dust. In many instances, a dust exposure also can lead to nonpneumoconiotic effects. For example, coal dust produces pneumoconiosis but also produces significant chronic bronchitis, and it may produce obstructive and emphysema effects.[9] This discussion, however, focuses on the pneumoconiotic effect.

Screening and Surveillance

Radiography, not pulmonary function testing, has traditionally been the primary means of detecting pneumoconioses in individual cases. However, pulmonary physiology testing is essential for assessing the impact of pneumoconioses for an individual. Such testing is particularly useful in describing the degree to which symptoms can reasonably correlate with radiographic or pathologic findings. While radiographic methods may be particularly sensitive for detection in individuals, lung function methods provide excellent surveillance tools for populations. Thus, when considering aggregates of data as opposed to individual worker data, changes in average pulmonary function data can be very sensitive.

For screening purposes, in which the goal is to detect early cases, pulmonary function testing should be secondary to radiographic testing. For detecting the nonpneumoconiotic effects such as obstructive lung disease, spirometry is extremely useful.

The forced vital capacity may be reduced because of restrictive lung disease, such as progressive massive fibrosis or asbestosis, but it also may be reduced due to obstructive lung disease such as that due to cigarette smoking. Therefore, a reduced FVC per se does not necessarily indicate a pneumoconiosis is present. It is helpful to interpret the FVC in conjunction with the FEV_1/FVC ratio. The ratio will be significantly reduced if airflow obstruction is present. Lung volume determination also can be helpful.

In theory, the DLCO may be a useful screening tool for pneumoconiosis. It is particularly sensitive for pneumoconioses such as asbestosis. Even with automated instrumentation, DLCO is more expensive and requires greater technical expertise than spirometry. For that reason, there has not been widespread utilization of DLCO on a screening basis.

DIAGNOSTIC ASSESSMENT

A different approach may be used with diagnostic assessment. Such efforts are focused on a single individual for whom there is an a priori likelihood of disease. In these circumstances, both diffusing capacity and spirometry should be used. Furthermore, lung volume determination such as with plethysmography or helium dilution can be important if air flow obstruction (reduced FEV_1/FVC ratio) is present. Furthermore, the spirometry may be repeated after bronchodilator administration if the baseline spirometry is abnormal.

In most instances, lung volume measurements may not be necessary. However, in the presence of obstructive airway disease, they may play a significant role. Individuals with emphysema may have reduction of the FVC and diffusing capacity for carbon monoxide; these are the same phenomena seen in restrictive lung disease such as pneumoconioses. However, the effect on lung volume is opposite: because of air trapping, the functional residual capacity is increased with COPD/emphysema, but this does not occur to a comparable degree with pneumoconioses. The pressure-volume relationship is not linear. Thus, with pulmonary fibrosis, the effect is most markedly seen at high lung volumes (near total lung capacity). An individual with "stiff lungs" is particularly affected at high lung volumes, and therefore the total lung capacity is a particularly good differentiator.[48]

Lung volume measurements also can serve as a complement to radiographic techniques. Emphysema decreases the radiodensity of the lung and CT occasionally can differentiate emphysema from pneumoconioses. A recent analysis, however, showed that CT's incremental benefit for finding asbestosis was limited.[50]

The pressure volume curve, commonly summarized by a single measure of lung compliance, has been suggested. This determines the "stiffness" of the lung. Lung compliance measurements are of relatively limited utility, and because the testing requires passage of an esophageal catheter orally, rarely necessary.

Other tests occasionally may be abnormal in individuals with pneumoconioses. For example, as with many forms of interstitial lung disease, there may be a decrease in the arterial oxygen tension as the exercise level increases. Furthermore, exercise testing may show other typical abnormalities such as inadequate volume recruitment. However, the results are nonspecific and do not serve a diagnostic role, except in limited cases of assessing the physiologic impact.

ABILITY AND DISABILITY ASSESSMENT

For the pneumoconioses, lung function tests are extremely useful for assessing the physiologic impact and the consequent disability. Their utility in this setting is greater than in most other disease groups.

The impact may be measured by spirometry and diffusing capacity. In borderline cases, it may be useful to measure total oxygen consumption in a pulmonary exercise test. Generally, the exercise testing should be done only if there is a need for the information to classify the individual properly. The exercise test is unnecessary when the severity of the functional abnormalities shown by the more basic tests is great.

There is one circumstance in which physiologic tests may not directly relate to disability: many workers may have radiographic findings of pneumoconiosis but do not have associated physiologic abnormalities until the radiographic findings are relatively advanced. Thus, the individual may be physically able to do the job because of the absence of any impairing physiologic effect. However, if pneumoconiosis is present radiographically, disability may be present if the radiographic findings per se constitute a reason to change jobs. For example, simple coal workers' pneumoconiosis (CWP) is not typically associated with any physiologic effect of clinical importance. However, miners with simple CWP should be removed from further exposure because their risk of developing progressive massive fibrosis (PMF) is much greater than for other comparably exposed miners without simple CWP. In this situation, there may be disability in the absence of physiologic impact.[16,61,82]

Work Ability and Disability Assessment

Physiologic testing forms the cornerstone of ability and disability assessment of lung disease.[1,2,3,5] Properly applied, lung function testing can make assessment of the individual's status virtually independent of subjective factors. Unfortunately, this high degree of objectivity in patient assessment is not matched by the precision of determining workplace demands. Thus, if the focus of the disability assessment is classifying individuals into one of several arbitrary groups, such as those defined in the AMA's *Guides to the Evaluation of Permanent Impairment*,[1] there may be high precision. Conversely, if the question is ability to do a particular job or to work effectively in the labor force, uncertainty is introduced because of limited knowledge of the job demands.

Physical demands differ considerably among different jobs and even among individuals doing the same job. Furthermore, there are temporal shifts in the overall arduousness of work, yet many disability programs rely on outdated work surveys. Even for a single worker, there is difference in the job demands over the course of a day since workers rarely do exactly the same task continuously. The limited number of studies that have measured oxygen consumption indirectly throughout the workday describe oxygen consumption as a distribution of work levels as a cumulative probability or time function.[47] Even such a cumulative distribution function may not fully account for the temporal distribution.[46] Working at a high level of exertion 60 minutes a day is tolerated much better if the work is broken into 12 five-minute segments than if performed continuously for an hour.

Physiologic testing in respiratory disability assessment has traditionally emphasized lung mechanics and oxygen consumption. The central dogma has been that lung function tests estimate maximal attainable oxygen consumption, which is related to the sustainable oxygen consumption achievable by an individual. This, in turn, is assumed to be related in a linear fashion to the oxygen consumption demand of the job. Reliance on the central dogma is suspect for several reasons. First, oxygen delivery is only one of the respiratory system's functions. Disability may exist when another function is significantly impaired. Second, job demands are not homogeneously distributed. Third, the proportion of the maximal attainable oxygen consumption which may be sustained throughout a workday has been estimated to be 40–60%; however, this has not been demonstrated to be valid for all disease groups.

The two major categories for physiologic assessment for disability and work ability determination are ventilation/oxygen consumption and irritant sensitivity. The former has been the traditional focus of disability and impairment assessment. However, asthma is extremely common regardless of whether it was caused by work.

Assessment of Ventilatory Mechanics and Gas Exchange

Spirometry and diffusing capacity testing are the primary physiologic tests used to assess ventilatory mechanics and gas exchange. FEV_1, FVC, and their ratio is of the most importance. Measures such as the midflow rate (such as the forced expiratory flow from 25–75% of the vital capacity ($FEF_{25-75\%}$) do not in themselves limit exertion.[42]

Spirometry is dependent on effort. It is therefore particularly important in disability assessment that the test is adequately performed. In some instances, it may not be possible to obtain adequate results. Physicians interpreting spirometry should examine the tracings themselves and not rely on printed numerical results alone. The morphology and consistency of tracings can provide information about the degree of effort.

The diffusing capacity test may be particularly helpful in disability assessment if vascular limitation is of concern.

Exercise testing has an important but limited role in disability and impairment assessment.[71] It is particularly useful when the spirometry and diffusing capacity tests are intermediate: neither completely normal nor sufficiently severely abnormal to automatically imply total disability.

Pulmonary exercise tests collect a great deal of information, the most important of which includes (1) maximal oxygen consumption, attained at the highest exercise level, (2) ventilatory reserve, and (3) cardiac-related parameters.

The appropriate exercise protocol should be chosen to meet the needs, but, unfortunately, some laboratories use the same protocol regardless of the purpose of the test. Testing may be done with rapidly changed exercise levels or with more prolonged exercise at fewer levels. The former approach is useful from the pulmonary diagnostic standpoint. However, when the exercise levels are changed rapidly, results of any level may be subject to a phase lag and not truly reflect the individual's ability to sustain that level of exertion. Similarly, if ability to work with personal respiratory protective equipment or protective clothing is the question, routine pulmonary exercise testing has limits and should be modified.

In contrast to formal pulmonary exercise tests, whose role is limited, informal exercise testing can be implemented easily in disability assessment. A great deal can be learned by accompanying a patient as he or she ascends one or two flights of stairs. Disparity between objective and subjective responses may be evident.

Airway Hyperresponsiveness and Irritant Sensitivity

Asthma, both due to work and other situations, is increasing in frequency. The usual approach to disability assessment may be inadequate for the following reasons[38]:

- The disorder is highly variable from day to day, and results on one examination may not reflect those at other times.

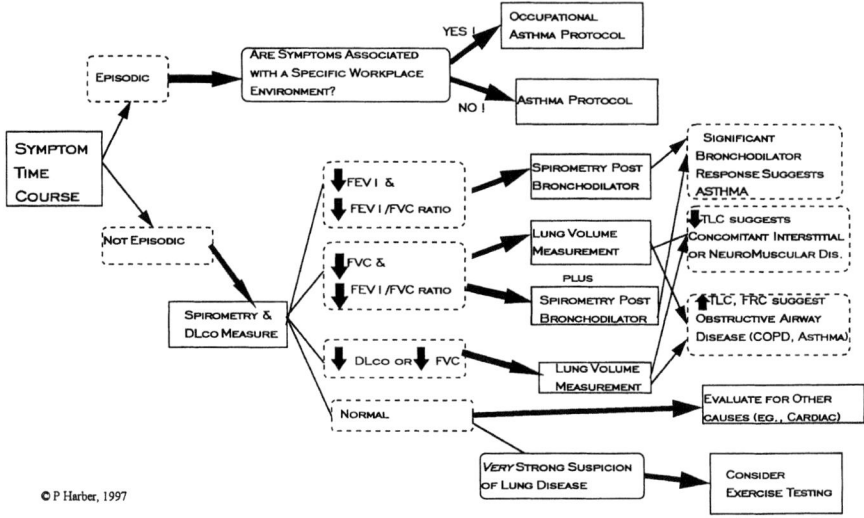

FIGURE 1. Sequence of test selection for evaluation of a dyspneic patient.

- Asthma is responsive to therapy. Thus, the degree of impairment depends on the appropriateness of treatment and on patient compliance with the appropriate treatment.
- In instances of occupational asthma due to allergic sensitization to a specific chemical, even minimal exposures may trigger severe attacks, and the disability therefore may be specific to a single job.
- Testing in a clean medical office may not reflect lung function when the patient is working in an atmosphere with moderate levels of nonspecific irritants.

The American Thoracic Society's guideline for assessment of impairment[5] is based upon the sum of impairment on three separate scales: (1) baseline lung function, before bronchodilator administration, (2) degree of airway hyperresponsiveness, and (3) medication needs. These scales allow one to deal with complex situations. For example, impairment is considered to be present even if nearly normal lung function is achieved at the cost of extensive and potentially dangerous medication use. Respiratory function testing is applied in two ways: spirometry is used for the assessment of the baseline lung function, and airway hyperresponsiveness is measured. Testing includes peak expiratory flow measurement at the worksite, worksite spirometry such as cross shift change, and "ambulatory spirometry" at the worksite.

SUMMARY

Overall, assessment of pulmonary impairment in disability is critically dependent on the use of objective lung function tests. However, they should not be applied by rote. They must be interpreted for the individual case with regard to the other clinical factors and the specific function being assessed. Reliance on older protocols, emphasizing fixed airway obstruction such as due to chronic obstructive pulmonary disease, and emphasizing interstitial disease such as asbestosis may be complemented by different protocols for assessing asthma-related conditions. Special testing is necessary for impairment assessment for respiratory control disorders and other classes of pulmonary disease.

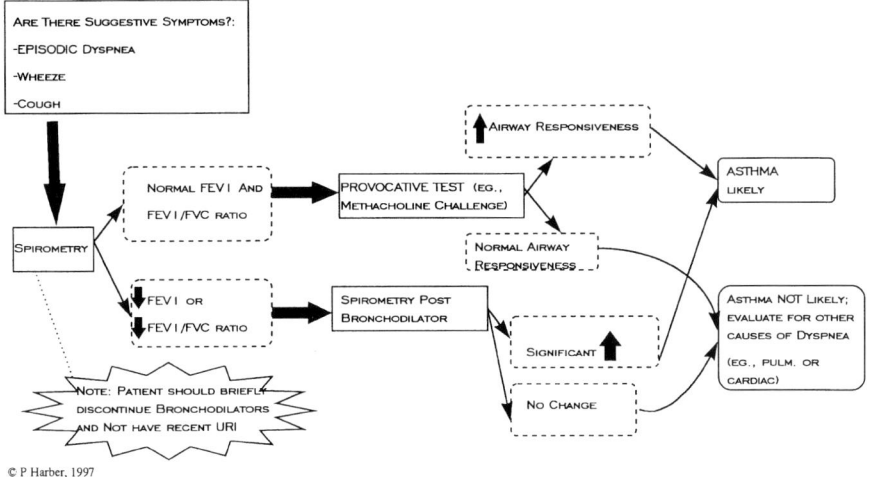

FIGURE 2. Sequence of testing for the diagnosis of asthma.

ALGORITHMS FOR TEST SELECTION

Methods for selecting and using pulmonary function testing in the workplace are described below. Although protocols are presented, individual judgment must be used. The protocols serve two purposes. First, although individualization to the specific patient or workplace situation is requisite, the protocols should provide guidance. Second, these protocols suggest that a systematic logical approach should be used.

Protocols for Test Use

Pulmonary function testing can be extremely cost-effective. The high sensitivity and specificity of many tests make their use advisable in appropriate situations. Although there are significant differences in the costs of different tests, cost is only

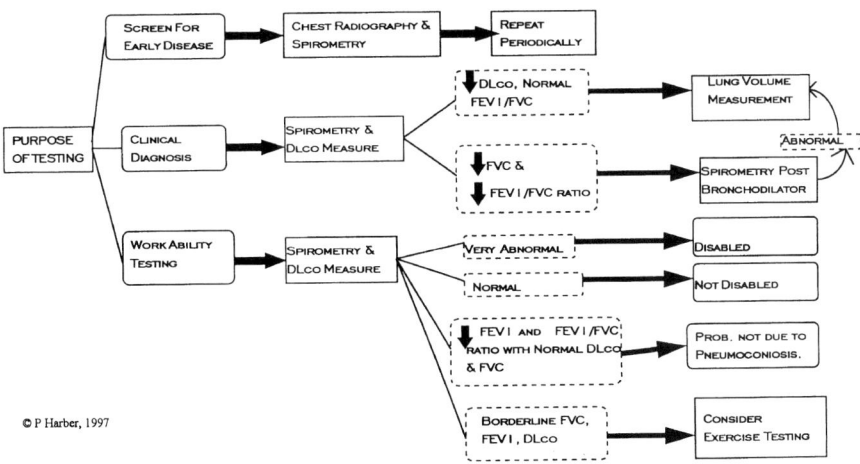

FIGURE 3. Test selection algorithm for pneumoconioses.

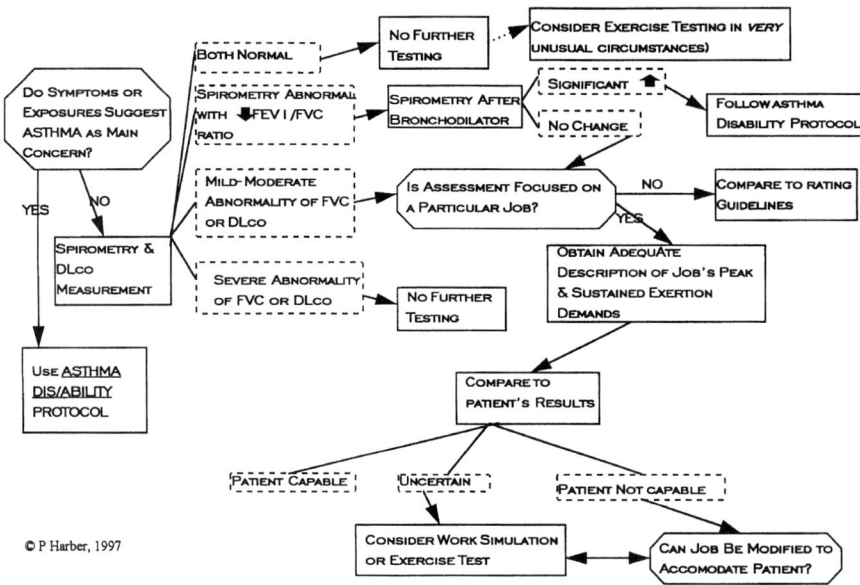

FIGURE 4. Testing sequence for ability and disability evaluation.

one consideration. Programmatic operation expenses for worksite screening programs, recordkeeping, communication and interpretation of results for workers, and administration may cost more than the actual test itself.[10,39] Use of highly sensitive but nonspecific tests can add significant costs by requiring subsequent more detailed testing, confirmatory testing, and clinical evaluations.

Testing should generally be done in a stepwise fashion. The protocols described in Figures 1–5 progress from simple to more complicated testing and include the following: test selection protocol for patients complaining of dyspnea, testing for

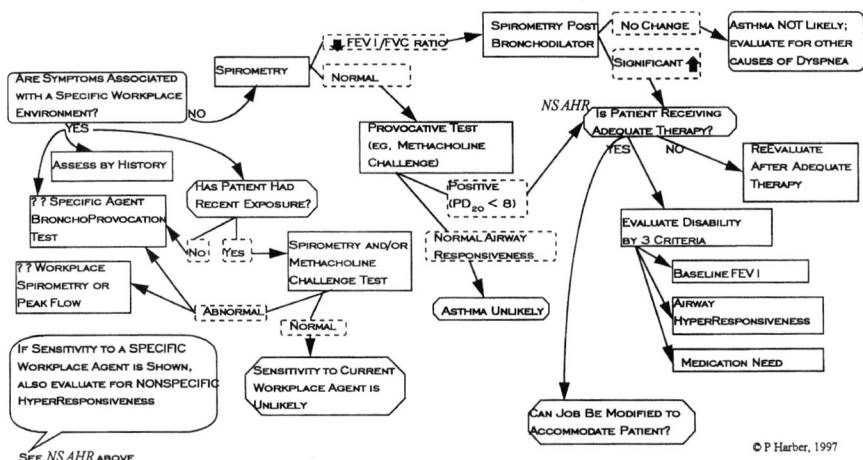

FIGURE 5. Testing sequence for asthma ability and disability evaluation.

evaluation of asthma, testing for evaluation of pneumoconioses, testing for occupational asthma, and testing for assessment of ability and disability.

These protocols are derived by the authors from published literature and experience. They focus on the use of respiratory function testing and therefore do not include many other appropriate forms of testing. In addition, they focus on the most common respiratory functions that are tested: exercise ability, ventilatory mechanics, and gas exchange. They do not address the muscular components of the respiratory system, the pulmonary defense components, upper airway aspects, the respiratory control system, or other important functions.

SUMMARY

Pulmonary function testing is an essential component of many occupational respiratory programs. Testing is performed for several different reasons. Proper selection of tests depends on whether they are used for screening a healthy population, establishment of a clinical diagnosis in a specific individual, or determination of work ability or disability.

There are many pulmonary conditions and relevant exposures. The appropriate tests should be chosen based on the specific situation.

ACKNOWLEDGMENT

The authors thank Weiling Chen for her extensive work in preparing this manuscript.

REFERENCES

1. American Medical Association: Guides to the Evaluation of Permanent Impairment, 4th ed. Chicago, American Medical Association, 1993.
2. American Thoracic Society: Evaluation of impairment/disability secondary to respiratory disease. Am Rev Respir Dis 126:945–951, 1982.
3. American Thoracic Society: Evaluation of impairment/disability secondary to respiratory disorders. Am Rev Respir Dis 133:1205–1209, 1986.
4. American Thoracic Society: European Respiratory Society Longitudinal Data Analysis Workshop. Am J Respir Crit Care Med 154:S207–S284, 1996.
5. American Thoracic Society: Guidelines for the evaluation of impairment/disability in patients with asthma. Am Rev Respir Dis 147:1056–1061, 1993.
6. American Thoracic Society: Lung function testing: Selection of reference values and interpretative strategies. Am Rev Respir Dis 144:1202–1218, 1991.
7. American Thoracic Society: Single-breath carbon monoxide diffusing capacity (transfer factor): Recommendations for a standard technique—1995 update. Am J Respir Crit Care Med 152: 285–298, 1995.
8. American Thoracic Society: Standardization of spirometry: 1994 update. Am J Resp Crit Care Med 152:1107–1136, 1995.
9. Attfield MD, Hodous TK: Pulmonary function of U.S. coal miners related to dust exposure estimates. Am Rev Respir Dis 145:605–609, 1992.
10. Balmes JR: Medical surveillance for pulmonary endpoints. Occup Med State Art Rev 5:499–513, 1990.
11. Banks DE, Wang ML, McCabe L, et al: Improvement in lung function measurement using a flow spirometer that emphasizes computer assessment of test quality. J Occup Environ Med 38:279–283, 1996.
12. Becklake MR: Epidemiology of spirometric test failure. Br J Ind Med 47:73–74, 1990.
13. Bernstein IL, Chan-Yeung M, Malo JL, Bernstein DI (eds): Asthma in the Workplace. New York, Marcel Dekker, 1993.
14. Chai H, Farr RS, Froelich LA, et al: Standardization of bronchial inhalation challenge procedures. J Allergy Clin Immunol 56:323–327, 1975.
15. Chan-Yeung M: Assessment of asthma in the workplace. Chest 108:1084–1117, 1995.
16. Cochrane AL, Moore F, Thomas J: The radiographic progression of progressive massive fibrosis. Tubercle 42:72, 1961.
17. Cockeroft DW, Killian DN, Mellon JJA, Hargreave FE: Bronchial reactivity to inhaled histamine: A method and clinical review. Clin Allergy 7:235–243, 1977.

18. Cole P: Recordings of respiratory air temperature. J Laryngol 68:295–307, 1954.
19. Coultas DB, Howard CA, Skipper BJ, Samet JM: Spirometric prediction equations for Hispanic children and adults in New Mexico. Am Rev Respir Dis 138:1386–1392, 1988.
20. Crapo RO, Jensen RL, Lockey JE, et al: Normal spirometric values in healthy Hispanic Americans. Chest 98:1435–1439, 1990.
21. Crapo RO, Morris AH, Gardner RM: Reference spirometric values using techniques and equipment that meet ATS recommendations. Am Rev Respir Dis 123:659–664, 1981.
22. Dimich HD, Sterling TD: Ventilatory function changes over a workshift. Br J Ind Med 38:152–155, 1981.
23. DuBois AB, Botelho SY, Bedell GN: A rapid plethysmographic method for measuring thoracic gas volume: A comparison with a nitrogen washout method for measuring functional residual capacity in normal subjects. J Clin Invest 35:322–335, 1956.
24. Eisen EA (ed): Spirometry. Occup Med State Art Rev 8:241–414, 1993.
25. Eisen EA, Dockery DW, Speizer FE, et al: The association between health status and the performance of excessively variable spirometry tests in a population based study in six US cities. Am Rev Respir Dis 136:1371–1376, 1987.
26. Empey DW, Laitinen LA, Jacobs L, et al: Mechanisms of bronchial hyperreactivity in normal subjects after upper respiratory tract infection. Am Rev Respir Dis 113:131–139, 1976.
27. Enright PL: Surveillance for lung disease: Quality assurance using computers and a team approach. Occup Med State Art Rev 7:209–225, 1992.
28. Enright PL, Connett JE, Kanner RE Jr, Lee WW: Spirometry in the lung health study: II. Determinants of short-term intraindividual variability. Am J Respir Crit Care Med 151:406–411, 1995.
29. Ferris BG: Epidemiology standardization project: Recommended standardized procedures for pulmonary function testing. Am Rev Respir Dis 118:1–120, 1978.
30. Gardner RM, Clausen JL, Crapo RO, et al: Quality assurance in pulmonary function laboratories. Am Rev Respir Dis 134:626–627, 1986.
31. Ghio AJ, Castellan RM, Kinsley KB, Hankinson JL: Changes in forced expiratory volume in one second and peak expiratory flow rate across a work shift among unexposed blue collar workers. Am Rev Respir Dis 146:1231–1234, 1991.
32. Goldman HI, Becklake MR: Respiratory function tests. Normal values at median altitudes and the prediction of normal results. Am Rev Tuberc 79:457–467, 1959.
33. Hankinson JL: Instrumentation for spirometry. Occup Med 8:397–407, 1993.
34. Hankinson JL: Pulmonary function testing in the screening of workers: Guidelines for instrumentation, performance and interpretation. J Occup Med 28:1081–1092, 1986.
35. Hankinson JL, Castellan RM, Kinsley KB, Keimig DG: Effects of spirometer temperature in FEV_1 shift changes. J Occup Med 28:1222–1225, 1986.
36. Hankinson JL, Viola JO: Dynamic BTPS correction factors for spirometric data. J Appl Physiol 44:1354–1360, 1983.
37. Hankinson JL, Viola JO, Petsonk EL, Ebeling TR: BTPS correction for ceramic flow sensors. Chest 105:1481–1486, 1994.
38. Harber P: Assessing occupational disability from asthma. J Occup Med 34:120–128, 1992.
39. Harber P: Pulmonary prevention: Programmatic characterization. Occup Med State Art Rev 6:133–143, 1991.
40. Harber P, Hsu P, Chen W: An "atomic" approach to dis/ability assessment. J Occup Environ Med 38:359–366, 1996.
41. Harber P, Hsu P, Fedoruk J: Personal risk assessment under the Americans with Disabilities Act: A decision analysis approach. J Occup Med 35:1000–1010, 1993.
42. Harber P, Kanter R, Tashkin DP, Rask-Andersen A: Functional impact of small airway dysfunction. Am Rev Respir Dis 139:A390, 1989.
43. Harber P, Peterson K: Spirometry update. OEM Reporter 10:49–51, 1996.
44. Harber P, Peterson K, Lehman A: Change in spirometer: Impact on longitudinal data. Am J Resp Crit Care Med 153:A97, 1996.
45. Harber P, Rappaport S: Clinical decision analysis in occupational medicine: Choosing the optimal FEV_1 criterion for diagnosing occupational asthma. J Occup Med 27:651–658, 1985.
46. Harber P, Rothenberg LS: Controversial aspects of respiratory disability determination. Semin Respir Med 7:257–269, 1986.
47. Harber P, Tamimie J, Emory J: Estimation of the exertion requirements of coal mining work. Chest 85:226–231, 1984.
48. Harber P, Tashkin DP, Lew M, Simmons M: Physiologic characterization of asbestos-exposed workers. Chest 92:494–499, 1987.

49. Harber P, Tockman M: Defining "disease" in epidemiologic studies of pulmonary function: Percent of predicted or difference from predicted? Bull Eur Physiopath Respir 18:819–828, 1982.
50. Harkin TJ, McGuiness G, Goldring R, et al: Differentiation of the ILO boundary chest x-ray (01-1/0) in asbestosis by high resolution CT scan, alveolitis, and respiratory impairment. J Occup Environ Med 38:46–52, 1996.
51. Henneberger PK, Stanbury MJ, Trimbath LS, Kipen HM: The use of portable peak flow meters in the surveillance of occupational asthma. Chest 100:1515–1521, 1991.
52. Horvath EP Jr (ed): Manual of Spirometry in Occupational Medicine. Cincinnati, National Institutes for Occupational Safety and Health, 1981.
53. Humerfelt S, Eide GE, Kvale G, Gulsvik A: Predictors of spirometric test failure: A comparison of the 1983 and 1993 acceptability criteria from the European community for coal and steel. Occup Environ Med 52:547–553, 1995.
54. Johnson LR, Enright PL, Voelker HT, Tashkin DP: Volume spirometers need automated internal temperature sensors. Am J Respir Crit Care Med 150:1575–1580, 1994.
55. Kellie SE, Attfield MD, Hankinson JL, Castellan RM: The ATS spirometry variability criteria: Associations with morbidity and mortality in an occupational cohort of coal miners. Am J Epidemiol 125:437–444, 1987.
56. Knudson RJ, Lebowitz MD, Holberg CJ, Burrows B: Changes in the normal maximal expiratory flow-volume curve with growth and aging. Am Rev Respir Dis 127:725–734, 1983.
57. Knudson RJ, Slatin RC, Lebowitz MD, Burrows B: The maximal expiratory flow-volume curve. Normal standards variability and effects of age. Am Rev Respir Dis 113:587–600, 1976.
58. Lewinsohn HC, Bresnitz EA, Gould KG Jr, et al: Spirometry in the occupational setting: Notes for guidance. J Occup Med 34:559–561, 1992.
59. Linn WS, Solomon JC, Gong H Jr, et al: Standardization of multiple spirometers at widely separated times and places. Am J Respir Crit Care Med 153:1309–1313, 1996.
60. Liss GM, Tarlo SM: Peak expiratory flow rates in possible occupational asthma. Chest 100:63–69, 1991.
61. Lyons JP, Campbell H: Relation between progressive massive fibrosis, emphysema, and pulmonary dysfunction in coal workers' pneumoconiosis. Br J Ind Med 38:125–129, 1981.
62. McKay RT, Lockey JE: Pulmonary function testing: Guidelines for medical surveillance and epidemiological studies. Occup Med State Art Rev 6:43–57, 1991.
63. Madan I, Bright P, Miller MR: Expired air temperature at the mouth during a maximal forced expiratory maneuver. Eur Respir J 6:1556–1562, 1993.
64. Meneely GR, Ball CT, Kory RC, et al: A simplified closed circuit helium dilution method for the determination of residual volume of the lungs. Am J Med 28:824–831, 1960.
65. Merget R, Dierkes A, Rueckmann A, et al: Absence of relationship between degree of nonspecific and specific bronchial responsiveness in occupational asthma due to platinum salts. Eur Respir J 9:211–216, 1996.
66. Miller MR, Pincock AC: Linearity and temperature control of the Fleisch pneumotachometer. J Appl Physiol 60:710–715, 1986.
67. Morris JF, Koski A, Johnson LC: Spirometric standards for healthy nonsmoking adults. Am Rev Respir Dis 103:57–67, 1971.
68. National Institute for Occupational Safety and Health: Hexcel Corporation, Dublin, California: Health Hazard Evaluation. AETA 85-131-1731. Cincinnati, NIOSH, Division of Surveillance, Hazard Evaluations, and Field Studies, 1986.
69. Ng'Ang'a LW, Ernst P, Jaakkola MS, et al: Spirometric lung function distribution and determinants of test failure in a young adult population. Am Rev Respir Dis 145:48–52, 1992.
70. Occupational Safety and Health Administration: Pulmonary function standards for cotton dust: CFR 1910. 1043 Cotton Dust, Appendix D:808–32; 1980.
71. Oren A, Sue DY, Hansen JE, et al: The role of exercise testing in the impairment evaluation. Am Rev Respir Dis 135:230–235, 1987.
72. Perks WH, Sopwith T, Brown D, et al: Effects of temperature on vitalograph spirometer readings. Thorax 38:592–594, 1983.
73. Perrin B, Lagier F, L'Archeveque J, et al: Occupational asthma: Validity of monitoring of peak expiratory flow rates and non-allergic bronchial responsiveness as compared to specific inhalation challenge. Eur Respir J 5:40–48, 1992.
74. Petersen M, Hankinson J: Spirometry reference values for nonexposed blue-collar workers. J Occup Med 27:644–650, 1985.
75. Pincock AC, Miller MR: The effect of temperature on recording spirograms. Am Rev Respir Dis 128:894–898, 1983.
76. Post WK, Steyerberg E, Burdorf A, et al: Choosing optimal values of FEV_1 and FEV_1/FVC for surveillance for respiratory disorders in occupational populations. J Occup Environ Med 38:673–680, 1996.

77. Quanjer PH, Tammeling GJ, Cotes JE, et al: Lung volumes and forced ventilatory flows: Report of working party, standardization of lung function tests. European Community for Steel and Coal—official statement of the European Respiratory Society. Eur Respir J 6:5–40, 1993.
78. Quintero C, Bodin L, Andersson K: Reference spirometric values in healthy Nicaraguan male workers. Am J Ind Med 29:41–48, 1996.
79. Quirce S, Contreras G, Dybuncio A, Chan-Yeung M: Peak expiratory flow monitoring is not a reliable method for establishing the diagnosis of occupational asthma. Am J Respir Crit Care Med 152:1100–1102, 1995.
80. Rabone SJ, Phoon WO, Anderson SD, et al: Hypertonic saline challenge in an adult epidemiological survey. Occup Med 46:177–185, 1996.
81. Redline S, Tager IB, Speizer FE, et al: Longitudinal variability in airway responsiveness in a population-based sample of children and young adults. Intrinsic and extrinsic contributing factors. Am Rev Respir Dis 140:172–178, 1989.
82. Reisner MTR: Results of epidemiologic studies on the progression of coal workers' pneumoconiosis. Chest 78:406–407, 1980.
83. Ryan G, Latimer KM, Dolovich J, Hargreave FE: Bronchial responsiveness to histamine: Relationship to diurnal variation of peak flow rate, improvement after bronchodilator, and airway calibre. Thorax 37:423–429, 1982.
84. Smith AB, Bernstein DI, London MA, et al: Evaluation of occupational asthma from airborne egg protein exposure in multiple settings. Chest 98:398–404, 1990.
85. Spector S: Bronchial inhalation challenge procedures with allergens and other bronchoconstrictor substances. Allerg Immunol 28:112, 115–118, 1996.
86. Tager IB, Weiss ST, Muñoz A, et al: Determinants of response to eucapneic hyperventilation with cold air in a population-based study. Am Rev Respir Dis 134:502–508, 1986.
87. Tarlo SM, Broder I: Outcome of assessments for occupational asthma. Chest 100:329–335, 1991.
88. Venables KM, Graneek BJ, Taylor AJ: Bronchial responsiveness and the reproducibility of forced expiratory volume in one second. Scand J Work Environ Health 19:342–345, 1993.

TIMOTHY A. SHAPIRO, MD
PAUL M. COADY, MD

DIAGNOSTIC TESTING OF CARDIAC FUNCTION

From the Hospital of the University
of Pennsylvania (TAS)
and
Thomas Jefferson University
Hospital (PMC)
Philadelphia, Pennsylvania
and
Lankenau Hospital and Medical
Research Center (TAS, PMC)
Wynnewood, Pennsylvania

Reprint requests to:
Timothy A. Shapiro, MD
Lankenau Hospital
3320 Lankenau Medical Science
Building
Wynnewood, PA 19096

Disorders of the cardiovascular system are among the most common problems encountered by physicians. New or continuing cardiac diseases and conditions prompt individuals to seek health care. Evaluations of these conditions range from quick, simple, and relatively inexpensive tests to highly sophisticated, complex, and expensive techniques to assess and manage cardiovascular disease. This chapter discusses various cardiac testing procedures with emphasis on patient selection, sensitivity and specificity, predictive value, and reliability.

THE ELECTROCARDIOGRAM

The electrocardiogram (ECG) is among the most commonly performed tests in medicine. The clinical ECG is a record of the changing potentials of the electrical field of the heart. Although the ECG provides only an approximation of the actual voltage generated by the heart, its usefulness as a diagnostic tool is a result of innumerable studies correlating the ECG to clinical and laboratory findings; with basic electrophysiologic properties of the heart; and with anatomic, pathologic, and experimental observations.[13,17] Thus, over time, the ECG has evolved into a useful tool for identifying hemodynamic, metabolic, anatomic, and ionic changes and is often an independent marker of cardiac disease.[11] In any patient with complaints referable to the cardiovascular system (chest pain, shortness of breath, syncope, edema) or examination findings suggesting a cardiovascular disorder, such as elevated blood pressure, irregular pulse, edema, bruits, and rales, an electrocardiogram should be performed as part of the evaluation. An ECG is the gold standard for the diagnosis of arrhythmia, and no other technique is as sensitive and specific.[14] Although dysrhythmias most frequently reflect disorders of specialized conduction tissue of the heart, the ECG reflects the electrical activity of the most complex rhythm disturbances.

While echocardiography is rapidly becoming a widely used tool in cardiovascular disease management, the ECG continues to provide readily available, inexpensive, and reliable information about cardiac chamber size, hypertrophy, and other disorders of myocardial and valvular structure and function.

Atrial Abnormalities

A terminal portion of the P wave in the lead V1, one box in depth (1.0 mm) and one box in duration (0.04 seconds) is found in 2.5% of the normal population and 70–90% of patients with left-sided valvular disease and left atrial enlargement.[22] On the other hand, a P wave with a height of 2.5 mm or more with a P wave of normal duration in leads II, III, and AVF is characteristic of P. pulmonale but is found in only 20–40% of patients with chronic lung disease.[4]

Ventricular Hypertrophy

The ECG diagnosis of left ventricular hypertrophy is based mainly on an increasing QRS voltage. Many clinical and anatomic studies have been conducted to determine the accuracy of various ECG criteria. In general, high voltage in the precordial leads was the most sensitive criteria but also was most frequently responsible for false positive diagnoses. Criteria requiring lower voltage were more sensitive but less specific. Romhilt and associates performed one of the most extensive anatomic correlation studies. The sensitivity and specificity of the most frequently used criteria for the diagnosis of left ventricular hypertrophy were evaluated in older patients.[25] Patients younger than 35, particularly men, can have higher QRS voltages that are normal. The ability of the ECG to predict *right* ventricular hypertrophy is not as good. An anatomic correlation study by Flowers and Horan showed the best criteria to have a sensitivity of 28%, specificity of 24%, and correctness of 76%.[12] Correctness is calculated by dividing the true positives and true negatives by the total group.

Myocardial Ischemia, Injury, and Infarction

The electrocardiogram is a reliable test that can be performed serially and is a cornerstone of the diagnosis and treatment of acute ischemic syndromes. In patients with clinical complaints of chest pain characteristic or suspicious for angina, the initial ECG is diagnostic of acute myocardial infarction in 50% of patients, abnormal but not diagnostic in about 40% of patients, and normal in 10% of patients. Serial tracings increase the sensitivity to nearly 95%.[10] The classic evolutionary pattern of infarction—T wave elevation and/or prolongation followed by ST (sinus tachycardia) segment elevation followed by T wave inversion with ST segment return to the baseline and formation of Q waves—is seen in a half to two thirds of patients with acute infarction. The other patients develop ST segment shifts or T wave changes only or reflect a non Q wave pattern on the ECG. Blanke et al. studied 152 patients arteriographically to correlate ECG patterns with the site of obstruction.[2] The sensitivity, specificity, and positive predictive value for anterior myocardial infarction and occlusion of the left anterior descending coronary artery was 90%, 95%, and 96%, respectively; for inferior myocardial infarction and right coronary artery occlusion, 56%, 97%, and 80%, respectively; and posterior or lateral infarction and circumflex occlusion, 24%, 98%, and 75%, respectively.

The diagnosis of transmural and nontransmural infarction, when based on the presence or absence of Q waves on the ECG, shows poor clinical correlation with autopsy findings. Perhaps as many as half of nontransmural myocardial infarctions have Q waves on the surface electrocardiogram. Thus, the term *Q wave* and *non Q wave* myocardial infarction should replace *transmural* and *nontransmural* for the electrocardiographic diagnosis of myocardial infarction. Factors confounding the ECG diagnosis of acute infarction include previous myocardial infarction, bundle branch block patterns, left ventricular hypertrophy, paced rhythms, pericardial disease, and electrolyte imbalances.

Nondiagnostic ST Segment and T Wave Changes

Nondiagnostic ST segment and T wave changes are the most common ECG abnormalities, accounting for 80% of the abnormal tracings in a general hospital population and 2–4% of all ECGs. Because the T wave is highly sensitive to a variety of changes, T wave abnormalities are least likely to suggest a specific condition or problem. Some causes of nondiagnostic or nonspecific ST segment and T wave changes include position, temperature, tachycardia, psychotropic drugs, cerebrovascular accident, anemia, electrolyte imbalance, endocrine disorder, ischemia, and dilated and infiltrative cardiomyopathy.

AMBULATORY MONITORING

Prolonged electrocardiographic monitoring, whether constant (Holter) or intermittent (transient event detection) while patients are involved in routine daily activities, is the most useful noninvasive approach to the diagnosis and treatment of complex cardiac arrhythmias. Newer, more sophisticated systems also provide information regarding T wave changes and ST segment shifts as well as alterations of the QRS morphology. Indications for such testing include chest pain, dizziness, syncope and near syncope, and palpitations.

The traditional Holter monitor takes a continuous 24-hour recording of two channels of the electrocardiogram. Most recordings are computer-scanned and provide accurate information with regard to irregularities of the cardiac rhythm. About 25–50% of patients will report a symptom during the 24-hour period of recording, and 2–15% of symptoms are related to dysrhythmia. Importantly, in young people, marked sinus bradycardia, Wenckebach phenomena (especially during sleep), up to 3-second pauses, junctional complexes, atrial premature complexes, or ventricular premature complexes are all normal Holter findings in young, healthy patients. Holter monitoring has shown that the long-term prognosis for asymptomatic healthy persons with frequent and complex ventricular premature complexes resembles that of the healthy population, without increased risk of sudden cardiac death.[31] Holter monitoring also is used in testing drug efficacy and in one study led to predictions of antiarrhythmic drug efficacy more often than did electrophysiologic testing in patients with sustained ventricular tachycardia, with no difference in the success as selected by the two methods.[21]

Patient complaints often are episodic and fail to be documented by a single 24-hour continuous recording. Transient event detection systems are patient-activated devices that record the cardiac rhythm during the course of an event and transtelephonically transmit the recording for analysis. This is a helpful means of detecting dysrhythmias, but it depends on the patient's ability to quickly recognize symptoms and activate the device. The dysrhythmia must be of sufficient duration to be recorded, and access to a phone for transmission of the recording is necessary at all times.

EXERCISE STRESS TESTING

The association of exercise-induced ST segment and T wave changes in patients with ischemic heart disease was recognized as early as 1923.[9] Since then, a large body of research has helped define the usefulness and limitations of this procedure, allowing exercise stress testing to evolve into an important diagnostic and prognostic tool in the assessment of patients with ischemic heart disease.

Physiology

The anticipation of exercise frequently results in an increase of cardiac output in normal subjects at rest. Early in exercise, cardiac output is raised by augmentation of stroke volume through the Frank-Starling mechanism and heart rate. In later phases of exercise, an increase in ventricular rate is primarily responsible for increased cardiac output. During strenuous exercise, vasoconstriction occurs to all arterial beds except exercising muscle and coronary and cerebral circulation. As skeletal muscle blood flow is increased, oxygen extraction also increases by as much as threefold. Systemic, mean arterial, and pulse pressure usually increase. Diastolic blood pressure response is variable. The pulmonary circuit can accommodate a four- to sixfold increase in cardiac output with only modest increases in pulmonary artery and pulmonary capillary wedge pressure. Maximum heart rate and cardiac output all decrease in older individuals. Hemodynamics return to baseline within minutes of termination of exercise.

Exercise Protocols

Exercise can be dynamic or static. The most common dynamic exercises include arm or bicycle ergometry and treadmill exercise. Protocols for treadmill exercise are standardized, and the Bruce protocol is the most popular. Variations of the Bruce protocol or other protocols are available for elderly patients or those with limited exercise capacity due to cardiac, pulmonary, or orthopedic limitations. All exercise protocols are designed to assess myocardial oxygen consumption through an increase in heart rate and systolic blood pressure.

Exercise Electrocardiograms

Lead placement for an exercise ECG is modified to reduce motion artifact. This will result in a rightward shift of the QRS axis and increased voltage in the inferior leads, potentially masking inferior Q waves.

In normal subjects, the P-R, QRS, and Q-T intervals shorten as the heart rate increases. Depression of the J point is a normal finding. Myocardial ischemia results in horizontal or downsloping ST segment depression. ST segment depression must exceed 1 mm in three consecutive leads 80 msec after the J point to be considered an abnormal response. Patients with resting ST segment depression must depress the ST segments an additional 1 mm to be considered abnormal. In patients with resting ST segment elevation due to early repolarization, a return to baseline with exercise is a normal finding. ST depression does not localize the site of ischemia and does not indicate which coronary artery is involved.

ST segment elevation with exercise of greater than 1 mm that occurs 80 msec after the J point is abnormal and is relatively specific for the territory and coronary artery involved. ST segment elevation in an infarct territory with abnormal Q waves on a resting electrocardiogram is a marker for more severe left ventricle wall motion abnormalities and adverse prognosis. T wave changes are dependent on body position, respiration, and hyperventilation. Pseudonormalization of abnormal resting T wave changes is a nondiagnostic finding.

Diagnostic Use of Exercise Testing

The most common use of stress testing is for the diagnosis of coronary artery disease and determination of functional capacity and prognosis. The test should not be used to screen low-risk asymptomatic individuals because the test has limited diagnostic and prognostic (low positive predictive) value in this group, due to the low prevalence of disease. The sensitivity of exercise electrocardiography for single-vessel coronary artery disease ranges from 25–71%, with exercise-induced ST segment displacement most common with left anterior descending coronary disease. An overview of 147 consecutive reports involving more than 24,000 patients who had exercise testing and concomitant coronary angiography revealed a mean sensitivity of 68% and specificity of 77%. In patients with multivessel coronary artery disease, the sensitivity rose to 81% with a specificity of 66%.

The early onset of symptoms and an ischemic ST segment response with a concomitant fall in the blood pressure at low work loads are important exercise parameters associated with severe coronary disease and adverse prognosis.

According to Bayes' theorem, the diagnostic power of the exercise test is maximal when the pretest probability of coronary artery disease is intermediate.

Prognostic Use of Stress Testing

An abnormal electrocardiographic response may occur in 5–12% of asymptomatic middle-age men. While the risk of developing a cardiac event is nine times greater in patients with a positive stress test, over 5 years only one of four men with a positive stress test will experience an event, most commonly the development of angina.

Patients with established coronary disease have an excellent prognosis when able to exercise to 10 METS (metabolic equivalents of oxygen consumption) or greater. Patients with known coronary disease able to exercise past the third stage of a Bruce protocol with a normal ECG response have an annual mortality that is less than 1% per year over 4 years.

Postmyocardial infarction stress testing provides valuable information about functional capacity, hemodynamic response, and arrhythmias. The ability to complete 5–6 METS of exercise or 80% of maximum predicted heart rate in the absence of an abnormal electrocardiogram or blood pressure response is associated with a 1–2% mortality over the first year post myocardial infarction. Poor functional capacity, ST segment depression, or a decrease in blood pressure are associated with an increased risk of postmyocardial infarction events.

In other circumstances, such as prior myocardial infarction, rhythms other than sinus, and bundle branch block patterns, the electrocardiogram is unreliable for interpretation during a stress test. For this reason, means of assessing myocardial flow or assessing myocardial function have become important adjuncts to exercise testing. Additionally, when patients are unable to exercise, pharmacologic stress testing (adenosine, dipyridamole, dobutamine) has evolved as an alternative means of evaluation for myocardial ischemia.

Myocardial Perfusion Imaging

Radiopharmaceuticals that accumulate in the myocardium proportional to blood flow were first studied in 1964.[5] Exercise studies were first performed in

1973.[29] Currently, the two most commonly used compounds are thallium 201 and technetium 99m labeled compounds.

For the diagnosis of ischemic heart disease, the imaging agents are injected in conjunction with exercise ECG evaluation during rest and during exercise. Image acquisition is performed with standard views. Single photon emission computed tomography (SPECT) imaging has replaced planar imaging as the dominant means of image assessment. SPECT is designed to acquire multiple planar images and reconstruct them into a three-dimensional object. Patient position and preparation are extremely important. Motion of the patient is a common cause of artifact. An imaging arc of 180° is used with thallium 201, and a 360° arc can be used with technetium 99m.

To be considered a true abnormality, a SPECT perfusion defect should be seen on at least three consecutive slices. Slightly less inferoseptal uptake can be noted in males as a normal variant. In females, basal short axis slices usually show a septal defect, a normal finding representing the membranous portion of the septum. Defects present on both rest and exercise scans usually represent scar from infarction. A defect present on a stress scan and no longer present or present to a lesser degree on the rest scan is a reversible defect that indicates myocardial ischemia. The phenomena of reverse distribution occurs only with thallium 201. This is the finding of stress images that are normal or with a defect, and rest images show a new defect or a more intensive defect. This finding was frequently observed in patients who have received thrombolytic therapy or angioplasty and is felt to represent an initial excess of tracer in the reperfused area with a mixture of scar and viable tissue.

Uptake of tracer in the lungs or enlargement of the ventricle after exercise compared to rest can sometimes be seen and represents exercise-induced left ventricular dysfunction.

Each year 2.5 million patients undergo stress myocardial perfusion imaging in the United States. About 60–70% of these studies are performed in conjunction with physical exercise, and 30% take place with pharmacologic stress. The clinical usefulness of this technique has been well established in the detection of coronary artery disease. Prognostically, patients with evidence of ischemia have a higher incidence of future cardiac events than those with fixed defects. The number and extent of myocardial perfusion defects and the degree of reversibility also are predictive of events during follow-up after uncomplicated myocardial infarction.[15]

An important clinical application of myocardial perfusion is preoperative evaluation of patients undergoing a noncardiac surgery, particularly aortic and peripheral vascular surgery. Studies demonstrate that patients can be stratified appropriately based on clinical variables alone; however, most patients fall into an intermediate risk group and can further be categorized quite effectively by perfusion imaging.[8]

Echocardiography

Exercise echocardiography has rapidly progressed to the point where it is a reliable adjunct to bicycle or treadmill exercise for detection and assessment of ischemic heart disease. Abnormal wall motion is the first event to occur with ischemia and the last to recover. The mean sensitivity and specificity of exercise echocardiography for the detection of coronary artery disease are 84% and 87%, respectively. Prognosis for individuals with a normal exercise echo is good, but a large amount of data on the importance of an abnormal study for detection of coronary artery disease or postmyocardial infarction is not yet available.[23]

Echocardiography also can be combined with pharmacologic stimulation, particularly with dobutamine, in patients who cannot exercise. Dobutamine echocardiography

ASSESSMENT OF RESTING CARDIAC FUNCTION

may provide a means of assessing myocardial viability in the region of the ventricle where angiography reveals compromised coronary blood flow.[24]

Echocardiography has become an instrumental part of the clinical evaluation of patients with cardiovascular disease or complaints potentially related to the cardiovascular system. Routine transthoracic echocardiographic evaluation includes M-mode examination, two-dimensional echocardiography, and Doppler echocardiography. Transesophageal echocardiography also can be used to provide echocardiographic information about the heart.

M-mode Images

M-mode images of the heart are "ice-pick" views of the heart that give one-dimensional imaging of cardiac chambers and structures in real time. One can garner information about the size and function of the left ventricle, aortic root, left atrium, right ventricle, and pericardium. One also can define certain valvular abnormalities of the mitral, aortic, and pulmonic valves. With advancements in imaging techniques, the information obtained from M-mode echocardiography has been largely supplanted by two-dimensional and Doppler echocardiography.

Two-Dimensional Echocardiography

Two-dimensional echocardiography displays pie-shaped slices of the heart that are imaged in real time, usually at a rate of 30 slices per second. These images are easily displayed on a monitor and recorded on videotape for detailed review. The two-dimensional echocardiographic examination has become an integral component of the work-up of patients with suspected cardiac pathology. The size and shape of the aortic root is easily defined. The aortic valve can be imaged for function or the presence of vegetations. Detailed information is obtained regarding left ventricular size and regional and global myocardial function. The mitral valve and its apparatus are relatively easily viewed. Left atrial size is obtained. Right ventricular and right atrial size can be evaluated. In addition, pericardial effusions are clearly defined. Because so much information may be obtained about the structure and function of cardiac chambers and valves, the two-dimensional echocardiogram is an indispensable tool.

Doppler Echocardiography

M-mode and two-dimensional echocardiography create images of the heart, but the principles of the Doppler effect are used in Doppler echocardiography to map blood flow. Information about blood flow can be displayed on a monitor in what is called a spectral Doppler. Doppler information also can be interpreted with an audio component, which can be helpful in distinguishing various types of flow. Finally, the Doppler flow information can be displayed and superimposed directly onto the two-dimensional echocardiographic image. This is performed by using a color scheme to define flow toward and away from the transducer. Color Doppler has greatly enhanced the ability to evaluate valvular lesions and intracardiac shunts as well as other cardiac pathophysiologic states with altered flow characteristics, such as hypertrophic obstructive cardiomyopathy.

Transesophageal Echocardiography

The information obtained from transthoracic echocardiography, including M-mode, two-dimensional, and Doppler evaluation, is enormous and often sufficient.

However, the transthoracic echocardiographic technique has limitations. On occasion, image quality can be poor, often due to a patient's body habitus. Transthoracic echocardiography often gives limited information about certain cardiac structures, such as the intra-atrial septum, the aorta, prosthetic valves, valvular vegetations, the left atrial appendage, and intracardiac masses. Echocardiography can be performed via the esophagus by placement of an ultrasonic probe on an adapted endoscope. This technique, transesophageal echocardiography, now has been widely applied to further investigate the heart when the transthoracic examination cannot supply enough information.[26] Therefore, transesophageal echocardiography is commonly employed when endocarditis is suspected and one wants to rule out a valvular vegetation.[19] In addition, it is used to image the aorta to exclude dissections and other aortic pathology,[6] to evaluate patients with prosthetic valves,[7] and in patients with atrial fibrillation to image the left atrial appendage to evaluate for the presence of thrombus prior to attempting electrical cardioversion.[20]

Application of Transthoracic Echocardiography

Transthoracic echocardiography often is useful in patients who present with symptoms that have a potential cardiac etiology. A careful history and physical examination often will point the clinician in a particular direction and define the likelihood of significant cardiac pathology. However, it is often useful to obtain confirmatory information about the structure and resting function of the heart that can be supplied by a transthoracic echocardiographic examination. For instance, patients who present with dyspnea and have a normal examination and normal resting electrocardiogram have a low likelihood of a cardiac cause for their symptoms. Nevertheless, a normal transthoracic echocardiogram including a Doppler study further helps to exclude any potential cardiac etiology. Definitively excluding cardiac pathology is reassuring for many patients.

For young patients with chest pain, a resting echocardiogram often is used to exclude cardiac pathology or to detect mitral valve prolapse, which may have a relationship to their clinical syndrome. For patients with palpitations secondary to dysrhythmias, it is helpful to exclude structural heart disease such as mitral valve prolapse, atrial septal aneurysms, and other structural cardiac problems that can be associated with arrhythmias. For patients with murmurs, transthoracic echocardiography with a Doppler examination has been a wonderful adjunct to our diagnostic aptitude.

Even when the physical examination is classic for a particular valvular lesion, echocardiography helps to confirm the degree of pathology along with defining cardiac chamber size and function, which may likely affect further evaluation and treatment. In patients with mitral valve prolapse and a murmur, an echocardiogram can help to define the degree of pathology of the mitral valve and the extent of mitral regurgitation as estimated by Doppler examination.[27] For patients with aortic stenosis, echocardiography with Doppler is valuable in defining the type of aortic valve pathology (i.e., bicuspid valve or calcific degenerative valve), the degree of valvular stenosis, and the status of left ventricular function.[28] In patients with a suspected benign flow murmur, a normal echocardiographic and Doppler examination can be reassuring and limit the unnecessary use of prophylactic antibiotics for dental procedures.

Other Cardiac Imaging Techniques

Echocardiography is the principal clinical tool for evaluating resting cardiac function. However, when the information it yields is limited and when an invasive procedure (transesophageal echocardiography or cardiac catheterization) is not called for, cardiac function can be assessed by other techniques. Nuclear medicine techniques such as equilibrium radionuclide angiography (formerly called MUGA scans) are frequently employed. In this technique the blood pool is labeled with technetium 99m, and electrocardiographic-gated imaging is performed over the heart. Left ventricular regional or global function can be analyzed with this technique.[3]

Cardiac magnetic resonance imaging can also be performed when more detailed structural information is required. The clinical use of cardiac magnetic resonance imaging is predominantly limited to evaluating intracardiac masses, pericardial processes, right ventricular pathology, and congenital heart disease.[16]

VASCULAR DIAGNOSIS

History and Physical Examination

Like other areas in medicine, the history and physical examination are extremely helpful when evaluating patients with suspected vascular disease. In chronic arterial occlusive disease, pain that is reproducibly experienced at a certain level of exercise and is promptly relieved by rest is a symptom of intermittent claudication. Claudication does not occur at rest. Claudication in the calf is generally caused by obstructive disease in the superficial femoral artery, while pain that extends to the thigh and buttocks generally applies to disease of the aortoiliac segments. This type of pain needs to be distinguished from osteoarthritis of the hip, lumbar disc disease with radiculopathy, spinal stenosis, and peripheral neuropathy. Physical examination of patients with arterial vascular disease predominantly focuses on examination of pulses and identification of bruits. Pulses that are easily palpable in the feet exclude arterial disease as the cause of lower extremity pain. Bruits are generally detected in the femoral area when disease of the iliofemoral region is present. However, sometimes there may be lack of bruits when there is significant proximal obstructive disease and the distal vessel is filled predominantly by collaterals. Other signs that are sometimes considered to be indicative of diminished flow to an extremity, including lack of hair growth, toenail thickening, and delayed capillary refill, are less specific signs of arterial occlusive disease. Obstructive disease in the carotid system leads to symptoms of amaurosis fugax, transient ischemic attacks, reversible ischemic neurologic deficits, or stroke. Physical examination of the neck is suggestive of carotid disease when a bruit is present. This sometimes can be difficult to distinguish from a transmitted murmur of aortic stenosis if a systolic murmur exists. Examination of the eye grounds may demonstrate cholesterol emboli in the branches of the retinal artery, which is highly suggestive of carotid bifurcation disease.

Evaluation of a Patient with Peripheral Vascular Disease

Evaluation of a patient with suspected lower extremity occlusive disease is indicated if the patient has symptomatic claudication that significantly limits his or her lifestyle. In addition, the presence of nonhealing infections of the lower extremity often indicates further evaluation of suspected vascular disease. Initial laboratory tests obtained in patients with vascular disease include ankle/brachial pressure indices and ultrasound and Doppler findings. Ankle/brachial pressure indices are indicative of the severity of obstructive arterial disease. They generally are reflected as a ratio of lower limb to brachial pressures. An ankle/brachial index of less than 0.60 usually is reflective of significant and severe disease that may require further evaluation and treatment.[18]

Vascular ultrasound imaging is commonly described as Duplex scanning that combines B-mode ultrasound imaging of arterial segments with information from Doppler flow velocities. Duplex scanning allows rapid location of sites of stenosis by the presence of lumen narrowing and an acceleration of velocities. Changes in peak systolic and end diastolic velocities can be used to further measure stenosis severity. A greater than 70% stenosis generally is present if the peak systolic velocity is greater than 160 cm/sec and there is an increase in peak systolic velocity of 100% with respect to the more proximal arterial segment.[1]

Color Doppler imaging also is added to Duplex scanning to further improve diagnostic yield. Color-coded flow acceleration often helps identify areas of most severe disease.[30] If disease is suspected based on symptoms or physical exam and is confirmed by abnormal ankle/brachial indices and Duplex imaging with color flow scanning, definitive study with arteriography is indicated to confirm the site and severity of the disease. Therapeutic options then include continued medical therapy versus percutaneous intervention with angioplasty or stenting versus surgical correction.

Carotid Disease

Suspected carotid disease is evaluated by Duplex scanning, whose results have been considered to be almost as accurate as arteriography. If the patient has symptoms and a carotid stenosis of 70% or greater, most clinicians would consider surgical treatment. In an asymptomatic patient with a bruit, surgery is sometimes entertained for patients with a stenosis of greater than 80%. Some surgeons feel that Duplex scanning is adequate for assessing the severity and location of carotid stenosis, but many require additional imaging with arteriography or magnetic resonance imaging.

REFERENCES

1. Blair JK, Bandyk DF: Real-time color Doppler in arterial imaging. In Yao JST, Pearce LO (eds): Technologies in Vascular Surgery. Philadelphia, WB Saunders, 1992, pp 129–149.
2. Blanke H, Cohen M, Schlicter GV, et al: Electrocardiographic and coronary arteriographic correlation during acute myocardial infarction. Am J Cardiol 54:249–255, 1984.
3. Burow RD, Strauss HW, Singleton R, et al: Analysis of left ventricular function from multiple gated acquisition cardiac blood pool imaging: Comparison to contrast angiography. Circulation 56:1024–1028, 1977.
4. Calatayud JB, Abod JM, Khan NB, et al: P-wave changes in chronic obstructive pulmonary disease. Am Heart J 75:444–453, 1970.
5. Carr EA, Gleason G, Shaw J, et al: The direct diagnosis of myocardial infarction by photo scanning after administration of cesium-131. Am Heart J 68:627–636, 1964.
6. Chirillo F, Cavallini C, Longhini C, et al: Comparative diagnostic value of transesophageal echocardiography and retrograde aortography in the evaluation of thoracic aortic dissection. Am J Cardiol 74:590–595, 1994.
7. Daniel WG, Mugge A, Grote J, et al: Comparison of transthoracic and transesophageal echocardiography for detection of abnormalities of prosthetic and bioprosthetic valves in the mitral and aortic positions. Am J Cardiol 71:210–215, 1993.
8. Eagle KA, Singer DE, Brewster DC, et al: Dipyridamole thallium scanning in patients undergoing vascular surgery. Optimizing preoperative evaluation of cardiac risk. JAMA 257:2185–2189, 1987.
9. Feil H, Siegel ML: Electrocardiographic changes during attacks of angina pectoris. Am J Med Sci 175:255–260, 1928.
10. Fisch C: Electrocardiography. In Braunwald E (ed): Heart Disease. A Textbook of Cardiovascular Medicine. 5th ed. Philadelphia, WB Saunders, 1997, pp 108–152.
11. Fisch C: Electrocardiography of Arrhythmias. Philadelphia, Lea & Febiger, 1989.
12. Flowers NC, Horan IG: LV hypertrophy and infarction: Subtle signs of RV enlargement and their relative importance. In Schlant R, Hurst JW (eds): Advances in Electrocardiography. New York, Grune & Stratton, 1972, pp 297–308.

13. Fye WB: A history of the origin, evolution and impact of electrocardiography. Am J Cardiol 73:937–949, 1994.
14. Fye WB: Disorders of the heartbeat: A historical overview from antiquity to mid 20th century. Am J Cardiol 72:1055–1070, 1993.
15. Gibson RS, Watson DD, Craddock GB, et al: Prediction of cardiac events after uncomplicated myocardial infarction: A prospective study comparing pre-discharge exercise thallium-201 scintigraphy and coronary angiography. Circulation 68:321–326, 1983.
16. Higgins CB, Byrd BF, Farmer DW, et al: Magnetic resonance imaging in patients with congenital heart disease. Circulation 70:851–860, 1984.
17. Horan LG: Manifest orientation: The theoretical link between the anatomy of the heart and the clinical electrocardiogram. J Am Coll Cardiol 9:1049–1056, 1987.
18. Lennihan R Jr, Mackereth MA: Ankle blood pressures as a practical aid in vascular practice. Angiology 26:211–224, 1975.
19. Lowry RW, Zoghbi WA, Baker WB, et al: Clinical impact of transesophageal echocardiography in the diagnosis and management of infective endocarditis. Am J Cardiol 73:1089–1091, 1994.
20. Manning WJ, Silverman DI, Gordon SP: Cardioversion from atrial fibrillation without prolonged anticoagulation with use of transesophageal echocardiography to exclude the presence of atrial thrombi. N Engl J Med 328:750–755, 1993.
21. Mason JW: A comparison of electrophysiologic testing with Holter monitoring to predict anti-arrhythmic drug efficacy for ventricular tachyrhythmia. Electrophysiologic study versus electrocardiographic monitoring. N Engl J Med 329:445–451, 1993.
22. Morris JJ Jr, Estes EH Jr, Whalen RF, et al: P-wave analysis in valvular heart disease. Circulation 29:242–252, 1964.
23. Presti CF, Armstrong WF, Feigenbaum H: Comparison of echocardiography at peak exercise and after bicycle exercise in evaluation of patients with known or suspected coronary artery disease. J Am Soc Echocardiol 1:119–126, 1988.
24. Roger VL, Pellikka PA, Oh JK, et al: Stress echocardiography. Part I: Exercise echocardiography: Techniques, implementation, clinical application and correlation. Mayo Clin Proc 70:5–15, 1995.
25. Romhilt DW, Estes EH Jr: Point score systems for the ECG diagnosis of left ventricular hypertrophy. Am Heart J 75:752–758, 1968.
26. Schiller NB, Maurer G, Ritter SB, et al: Transesophageal echocardiography. J Am Soc Echocardiol 2:354–357, 1989.
27. Shah PM: Echocardiographic diagnosis of mitral valve prolapse. J Am Soc Echocardiol 7:286–293, 1994.
28. Taylor R: Evolution of the continuity equation in the Doppler echocardiographic assessment of the severity of valvular aortic stenosis. J Am Soc Echocardiol 3:326–330, 1990.
29. Zaret BL, Strauss HW, Martin NR, et al: Non-invasive regional myocardial perfusion with radioactive potassium. N Engl J Med 288:809–812, 1973.
30. Zierler RE: Duplex and color-flow imaging of the lower extremity arterial circulation. Semin Ultrasound CT MR 11:168–179, 1990.
31. Zipes D: Genesis of cardiac arrhythmias: Electrophysiological considerations. In Braunwald E (ed): Heart Disease. A Textbook of Cardiovascular Medicine. 5th ed. Philadelphia, WB Saunders, 1997, pp 548–592.

JOHN KRAUS, MD

THE INDEPENDENT MEDICAL EXAMINATION AND THE FUNCTIONAL CAPACITY EVALUATION

From the Bryn Mawr Rehabilitation Hospital
Malvern, Pennsylvania

Reprint requests to:
John Kraus, MD
Bryn Mawr Rehabilitation Hospital
414 Paoli Pike
Malvern, PA 19355

THE INDEPENDENT MEDICAL EXAMINATION

An independent medical examination (IME) is an evaluation performed by a health care professional to furnish information requested by a third party. The third party is usually an insurer, an attorney, or a judge who is seeking answers to a series of questions that have been provided in advance. The information that is requested generally pertains to the health status of an individual. Some of the frequent reasons for requesting an IME include (1) to confirm the presence or absence of a particular diagnosis, (2) to evaluate whether additional testing is needed, (3) to evaluate whether additional treatment is needed, (4) to determine functional limitations in daily activities, (5) to determine job limitations and precautions, (6) to evaluate the degree of an impairment, (7) to document causality, and (8) to determine whether maximal medical improvement has occurred.

An IME requires an objective assessment and is therefore performed by someone who has not previously treated the individual. Because an IME is not requested by the individual, the results of the evaluation are provided to the referral source and not to the individual. For the same reason, the IME is paid for by the referral source. No patient-doctor relationship is established in an IME because no continuing follow-up care is expected. Therefore, the term *patient* is not used in this chapter. An IME is generally performed by a physician, but a psychologist, physical therapist, or other health care professional may perform a specialized assessment. The physician or other health care professional who agrees to perform an evaluation is expected to have sufficient knowledge and clinical skill to answer the questions that are asked. This chapter uses the word *physician* generically to refer to the examining health care professional.

The results of an IME may become a crucial part of the evidence presented in a court of law. The physician must avoid personal prejudice when drawing conclusions about the person, the injury or disease process, or any other litigants or events pertaining to the case. The physician should, in advance of the examination, inform the referring party of any known prior professional or personal contact with the individual. Although it is natural to feel loyalty to an insurer or attorney who has requested and is paying for the service, the physician must avoid persuasion from the payer to draw conclusions that conflict with the medical facts.

An IME is performed once. The IME physician does not have the advantage of examining a person on multiple occasions and comparing findings, as does a primary treating physician. The evaluation may occur on a day when the person is feeling better or worse than average. Pain, especially if chronic, often fluctuates. Sudden changes in weather, a sleepless night, or heightened anxiety about the examination can change symptoms. An individual who arrives for an IME following a physical therapy session of hot packs may respond differently to the physician's palpating fingers than one who arose from bed an hour earlier or arrived after a 90-minute car ride. A person may consciously or unconsciously exaggerate his symptoms to persuade the examining physician in his favor. The physician can help to allay a person's concerns by explaining that the physical examination is one part of the IME and that the reports from other health care providers and prior test results also will be used to render a total picture of his current status. Because the IME is performed on one occasion, the physician must carefully interpret his findings in relation to what other physicians have documented. For example, when a person with a diagnosis of reflex sympathetic dystrophy (RSD) demonstrates minimal physical findings on the examination, the physician must decide not only whether he agrees with the diagnosis of RSD but whether he believes the person's symptoms are episodic, which explains the variability in the examination on that day. Prior records from other physicians that document episodic findings may support such a conclusion.

All of the comforts and rights to privacy that are given to a physician's patients in the routine daily practice setting should be provided to the person undergoing an IME. The physician must maintain a neutral demeanor and avoid confrontation if the person is uncooperative. Confrontation decreases compliance, and a poor interaction will almost certainly be communicated by the individual to his attorney who may use this information to discredit the IME.

Some of the common medical conditions for which the occupational medicine physician performs IMEs include neck, back, or limb pain due to an accident or to repetitive motion; head injury; occupational lung disease; the effects of exposure to pollutants or toxins; and the complications of infectious disease. Exposure to physical or chemical hazards may lead to multi-organ complaints involving the central nervous system, cardiopulmonary system, hematologic system, endocrine system, gastrointestinal system, genitourinary system, or skin. Nonwork-related illness such as cardiovascular disease, diabetes, or seizure disorder may lead to a dispute regarding a person's fitness to return to work and require an IME. The occupational medicine physician who performs IMEs is called upon to address a wide variety of physical complaints.

This chapter focuses on the IME for assessing musculoskeletal disease. How many IMEs are performed annually and the frequency of the various medical conditions for which they are ordered are unknown, but many are requested to assess pain and the consequences of work-related injuries. Musculoskeletal problems and, in particular, neck and back injuries constitute a large volume of such problems. The Bureau of Labor Statistics reported that, in 1993, 47% of work-related injuries occurred in the neck/head, back, or trunk.[35] In a survey of the Boeing Company, 19% of all workers' compensation claims and 41% of the total injury costs were for back injuries.[30] Such high-cost injuries are more likely to become chronic and lead to a request for an IME. Litigation issues resulting from motor vehicle accidents are another source of IMEs. Many of these injuries also are musculoskeletal in nature. Although this chapter focuses on the musculoskeletal system, it also illustrates points that have universal applicability. Summaries that review the assessment of nonmusculoskeletal occupation-related illnesses are available elsewhere.[10,27]

In general, the parts of an IME are similar to those of any other comprehensive medical evaluation. The parts, which are described below, include reviewing the medical records, meeting and obtaining a history from the individual, performing an examination, formulating conclusions and responding to the questions, and writing the report.

Medical Records Review

It is the responsibility of the referral source to provide all available medical records and the responsibility of the physician to review them all. The physician examines the records to identify key facts that will help to answer the questions being asked. Although many physicians prefer to review the records at the time of the scheduled IME, others review them sufficiently in advance in the event that more information or clarification of questions is needed prior to the examination. The thoroughness of record review depends on the complexity of the questions. The physician must remember, however, that information that is not reviewed is useless. Even seemingly unrelated reports may contain important details. For example, a notation from a primary care doctor during an office visit for cold symptoms may uncover an entry about back pain that the person denies having experienced prior to an alleged work-related back injury.

A questionnaire completed by the individual and submitted in advance or on the day of the office visit provides important supplemental information. The questionnaire allows the individual to state the history and the nature of the problem in his own words. The questionnaire also provides the physician with a statement about the person's key concerns and the emphasis he places on various details of his medical history. It may reveal inconsistencies between the individual's statements and information from other medical records. The physician should develop his or her own questionnaire (Fig. 1) to meet particular needs for length and detail. Having the individual complete a pain diagram (Fig. 2) is useful when a predominant symptom is pain.

Whenever possible, it is best for the physician to personally examine copies of relevant radiologic studies and not solely rely on reports. If radiographs were performed in a private physician's or chiropractor's office and no official radiologic interpretation obtained, one should consider requesting both viewing them personally and having them reviewed by a radiologist to render an official interpretation. In reporting the results of such studies in the IME, the doctor should document whether the interpretation came from a specialist (i.e., radiologist) in an official report, from another doctor, or from himself.

```
Name_____      Age_____ Date_____
Address_____      Phone No. (Home)_____
        _____      Phone No. (Work)_____
                                           Referred by_____
List names of all current physicians_____
_____

Marital Status:_____      No. of Children:_____
Education: Last grade completed_____    Occupation:_____
Date Last Worked:_____       # of Yrs. Worked At Last Job:_____
List current medications and number of tablets taken each day:_____
_____
_____
_____

Allergies:_____
Check if you have had any of the following problems:

        Heart disease          _____     Thyroid disease         _____
        Heart attack           _____     Arthritis               _____
        Hypertension           _____     Fractures               _____
        Pacemaker insertion    _____     Cancer                  _____
        Asthma                 _____     Fainting or dizziness   _____
        Bronchitis/emphysema   _____     Falling                 _____
        Diabetes               _____     Neurological problems   _____

        If you have checked any of the above, describe in more detail with
        dates:
        _____
        _____

List all prior hospitalizations:_____
_____

List all prior operations:_____
_____
```

FIGURE 1. Questionnaire to assist with the medical records review by the physician.
(Figure continued on opposite page.)

THE INITIAL ENCOUNTER

When meeting the individual, begin by stating the reason for the visit, the name of the referring company or person requesting the IME, and the names of the persons who will receive the report. Explain that the purpose of the examination is to perform an objective assessment of the person's status and to answer questions that have been asked by the referral source. State that there will be no physician-patient relationship established from this office visit and the reason.

During the initial dialogue, look for signs that demonstrate the individual's level of cooperation. In some instances cooperation is poor because he or she feels

INDEPENDENT MEDICAL EXAMINATION/FUNCTIONAL CAPACITY EVALUATION   529

Where is the pain located? _____

When did the pain begin? _____

Describe what event or activity you think caused the pain: _____
_____

What makes the pain worse? _____
_____

What makes the pain better? _____
_____

How many hours must you spend lying down or sitting during the daytime hours because of the pain? _____

Do you need help to dress or bathe, or to perform ordinary household activities? _____ If yes, describe: _____
_____

What treatments (PT, chiropractic, psychology, etc.) have you received for the pain, for how long, and where were they obtained? _____
_____
_____

If you have had any other pain problems in the past, describe _____
_____
_____

If anyone in your family has ever had long-standing pain problems, describe? _____
_____
_____

Are you receiving workers' compensation benefits?

    Yes _____   No _____

Are you represented by an attorney for your pain problem?

    Yes _____   No _____

***FIGURE 1** (continued).*   Questionnaire to assist with the medical records review by the physician.

coerced into having the examination and enduring another privacy intrusion. The individual knows that the purpose of the examination is not to relieve his symptoms but to gather information for someone else's use. He may have undergone evaluations in the past by physicians who have not made him better. This leads to anger toward the health care system. He may offer cynical or negative comments about other health care professionals he has visited. He may state that he is in too much pain to perform some of the tasks requested during the examination or that he is certain he will experience more pain for several days after the examination.

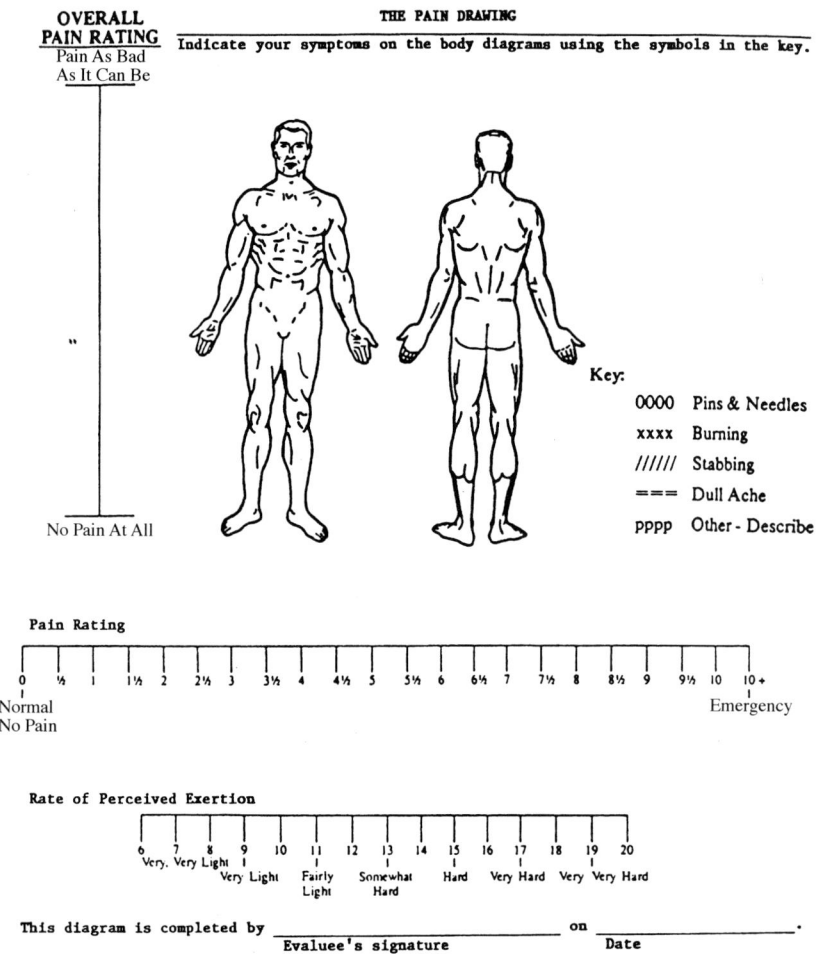

FIGURE 2. Form with which the individual describes his or her pain.

Never force or intimidate him into undergoing any part of the examination he opposes or to answering any questions he does not wish to answer. If he refuses to comply with any part of the IME, document in the report what was not performed or answered.

The individual may insist that another person remain in the exam room during the history-taking and the physical examination. The physician decides whether this is acceptable and, in doing so, uses the same criteria that she uses when examining patients in her routine practice. When an attorney, paralegal, or other professional wants to remain in attendance, the physician must decide whether she feels that an objective evaluation can be performed. In such circumstances, the person may feel a need to "perform" for the observer. At the same time, the physician should not respond defensively or with trepidation when an attorney or other observer is present. The physician's knowledge and skill exceed that of the others in the exam room. At times the person will change his mind when he realizes he must remain disrobed during the examination in view of the observer. A call to the referral source to discuss the person's/observer's request may resolve whether to comply with the demand or to cancel the evaluation. Always document in the report the presence of an observer during any part of the IME and any pertinent comments made by the observer.

It is unfortunate when a person informs his primary treating physician following an IME that "the insurance company made me see one of its doctors and all he asked was where does it hurt, spent 5 minutes examining me, and walked away without saying another word." When the individual communicates this opinion to his own physician or attorney, the confrontation level between them and the opposing side escalates. As a result, the IME may be devalued in the judicial system and the physician who performed the examination gains a poor reputation among his colleagues and referral sources in the community.

Obtaining the History

Taking pertinent information from the prior medical records and the person's written answers to the questionnaire, the physician should verbally review relevant facts to verify that the person agrees. Any conflicting statements among sources are clarified with the person and documented in the report. Depending on the nature of the problem, the following are some of the questions that should be asked.

First, thoroughly review the circumstances surrounding the injury or the start of the illness. What happened? What does he feel were the causal factors? If an accident occurred, what events immediately preceded the accident? What happened right after the accident? When did the symptoms begin in relation to the precipitating event? What were the initial symptoms? When was the first medical encounter? Who saw him? What tests were ordered? At some point during the interview, the relevant diagnostic tests in the medical records are reviewed with the person and confirmation obtained regarding whether any other tests were performed, especially recently. How have the symptoms changed over time? What are the current symptoms? When do they occur? What is their location, frequency, and intensity? What treatments have been received throughout the course of the illness, including all therapies, operations, and injections? Who performed the treatments, and what were the results? Has he received any treatments not recorded in the medical records? What about alternative therapies? Individuals often do not volunteer information about acupuncture, manipulation, and similar treatments unless specifically asked. Even psychological or psychiatric care may not be reported unless directly asked. What medications have been used in the past for the symptoms, and what is taken currently? If medications are used on an as-needed basis, what is the average number of pills taken daily? If he cannot estimate this because use is variable, how many pills are taken weekly or monthly? Prescription records, if available, should be compared with the individual's report of the number of pills taken. What else does he do to relieve his symptoms? What activities or positions increase his symptoms?

What does he believe is his diagnosis? It is natural for persons to seek a name to explain their symptoms, particularly when the symptoms are chronic.[15] "Labeling" a collection of symptoms with a medical diagnosis may be done by a doctor or, more dangerously, by the individual himself, often after misunderstanding what he has heard. A disc bulge becomes a herniated disc. Tension headaches become migraine headaches. When a person is given a diagnosis, sick role behavior may increase.[20] It is therefore important to evaluate whether the diagnosis is correct. Is the diagnosis the person is using truly reflective of that disease process and confirmed by other physicians and test results?

General health history is obtained next. Past medical history includes questions about acute and chronic disease, prior hospitalizations and surgery, other current medications, and drug allergies. Completion of a questionnaire that includes a general health survey helps to expedite this part of the interview. Ask whether he ever sustained similar pain in the past. If so, how long did it last, and how was it treated? What about past history of other injuries? Some individuals report a history of multiple work-related or motor vehicle accidents. Even if the injury was not work-related, has he ever missed periods of employment because of poor health? Ask about the use of alcohol, illicit drugs, or smoking. Alcohol abusers have an increased risk of disability.[18] If he denies a history of alcoholism or illicit drug use and is later found to have an abuse history, his entire credibility may be questioned. What is his current weight? Height and weight are obtained during the physical examination. In addition, however, ask the person to estimate his weight in the questionnaire. Often the estimate is significantly lower than the actual weight. Has he gained weight since the injury? Obesity can play a role in the etiology of injury and in its recovery. Document family history of related illness or injury. For example, has any family member ever experienced a significant back problem that required surgery or extended time out of work or that resulted in disability? Answering yes to this question may signify that the individual has been influenced by another "role model" in dealing with his symptoms.

What is his current ability to perform daily activities? This includes the degree of independence in self-care such as bathing and dressing; tolerance for walking, sitting, standing, lifting, and carrying; and performance in routine activities such as household activities, grocery shopping, lawn care, and driving an automobile. What is the average amount of time spent lying down or resting during the daylight hours each day? If he requires assistance for self-care or household activities, who provides that assistance? Does the family help to perform basic needs?

How long has he worked with his current employer? How long has he worked at his current job? What were his prior jobs, and who were his employers? Why did he leave his prior jobs? The etiology of back pain after lifting a 20-pound sack in a new job is more easily explained when one learns that the person's previous job of 5 years required repetitive lifting of 100-pound weights. Did he work at more than one job at the time of the injury? This is not an unusual occurrence and may suggest that fatigue played a role in the injury. Describe a typical workday just prior to the accident. If pertinent, ask him to describe any current or past exposure to noise or chemical pollutants, dust, physical hazards, vibrations, or repetitive motions. Following the injury, how much work time was lost? If he continued to work, was he placed on any job restrictions? How does he feel about his employer? His job? If not currently working, does he want to return to his prior job? How reasonable is it for him to return to his prior job in view of the time missed from work, the physical demands of the job, and his pain complaints? What is his education history? What are his career goals? Are they realistic for his level of education and training? Is he receiving disability benefits? When did they start? Is he applying for long term-disability, such as Social Security benefits?

Answers to questions about compensation, litigation, and attorney representation may provide clues about an individual's primary goals in the recovery process. Although most individuals want their symptoms to resolve, except perhaps malingerers or those with severe psychiatric disease or personality disorders, the literature has demonstrated that litigation and workers' compensation issues influence the success of treatment. Studies have shown the presence of litigation or attorney representation results in less functional improvement and a slower rate of recovery,[34] higher dropout rates in work hardening programs,[29] less likelihood of returning to work,[29] and persistent abnormalities on the Minnesota Multiphasic Personality Inventory (MMPI).[34] Financial incentives result in greater disability even in individuals who have less severe injury.[6] Individuals receiving compensation or involved in litigation have reported greater disruptions in life.[9,32] Beals summarized the paradox of compensation laws: financial compensation discourages return to work; the appeals process increases disability; open claims inhibit return to work; and recovering individuals often are unable to return to work because employers are inflexible about light duty and restricted hours.[4]

The Examination

PHYSICAL ASSESSMENT

Observe the general appearance and movements of the person during the history-taking and the examination. Are there inconsistencies between the person's report of dependence in self-care activities and what is observed? What are his posture and movement patterns? Are they guarded, as one would expect in the presence of severe low back pain? If observed, how much effort does he use to remove his socks or to rise on and off the exam table? Are movement patterns consistent with his verbal reports?

The components of the physical examination depend on the medical condition being assessed. Many IMEs require only a regional examination. For example, it is generally unnecessary to perform a fundoscopic examination on a person who has back pain. Strength testing may not be relevant when assessing someone with abdominal pain. Strength testing may be essential, however, when evaluating the functional status of an individual who states he is deconditioned because of occupationally-induced asthma. Should a rectal examination be performed on an older man with persistent low back pain? The physician who performs a thorough assessment and uncovers a previously missed diagnosis will have served all sides in the case. If the physician believes that further examination or diagnosis of a body system is necessary but is outside the scope of his specialty or experience, he should recommend in his report another consultation by the appropriate specialist.

The physician should be thoroughly familiar with generally acceptable examination principles and report the findings using correct terminology. "The straight leg raising test is positive" should be described. What was positive—back pain or leg radiation? The elements of a thorough physical or psychological/psychiatric examination for an IME are beyond the scope of this chapter; if necessary, the physician can review general textbooks on physical examination or specialty texts for regional examination.[12,24]

After the person has left the office, no physician wants to remember that she forgot to perform some aspect of the examination. One method to remember all necessary parts of the examination is to use a structured format from a written outline or check-off sheet. An example of a musculoskeletal/neurologic exam outline is shown in Figure 3. The best outline is one developed by the physician to meet her own needs for her patient population.

Just as a medical student is taught the skills of auscultation of the heart and the nomenclature for describing murmurs, the physician who evaluates the neurologic or musculoskeletal systems must understand how to perform a manual muscle test (MMT) and a joint range of motion (ROM) test and how to describe the findings

```
                    Orthopedic/Neurologic IME
Name_____     Date_____
Temp_____ Pulse_____ BP_____ Resp_____ Wgt._____ Hgt_____
General Appearance: _____
_____
Mental Status: _____
_____
CN's: _____
Posture, Body Movements: _____
Palpation Neck, Back: _____
_____

ROM: Neck (N)   Flexion    N ___    Rt. Rot.   N ___   Rt. Bend   N ___
     Back (B)              B ___               B ___              B ___

                Extension  N ___    Lt. Rot.   N ___   Lt. Bend   N ___
                           B ___               B ___              B ___


Spinal Curvatures: _____
Limbs:      ROM            _____
                           _____
            Atrophy        _____
            Circumferences _____
            Leg Lengths    _____
            Pulses         _____
            Palpation      _____
            SLR            _____
            Other Tests    _____
                           _____
```

FIGURE 3. An independent medical examination outline or checklist of the essential components of the exam. CN = cranial nerves; ROM = range of motion; SLR = straight leg raise. *(Figure continued on opposite page.)*

accurately. Many texts describe the principles of manual muscle testing[11,17,23] and joint range of motion.[11,17,23] Several important principles should be emphasized.

ROM testing for an IME requires precision in measurement. Estimating ROM is unacceptable because it lacks reproducibility. The simplest measurement tool for evaluating limb ROM is a goniometer. Hellebrandt found the variability on repeated measurements with a goniometer was less than 5°.[21] More experienced clinicians obtained smaller variabilities. For measuring spinal movement, either two mechanical inclinometers or one computerized inclinometer is recommended.[1] It is essential

Strength:

	Rt	Lt
Sh flex		
Elb flex		
Elb ext		
Wrist flex		
Wrist ext		
Fing flex		
Fing ext		
Intrinsics		
Grip		
Other		

	Rt	Lt
Hip flex		
Hip ext		
Hip abd		
Hip add		
Knee ext		
Knee flex		
Ank dorsi		
Ank plantar		
Ank eversion		
Toe ext		
Other		

Sensation: _____

DTR's   Rt   Lt

Other Reflexes: _____

Gait: _____

FIGURE 3 (continued). An independent medical examination outline or checklist of the essential components of the exam. DTR = deep tendon reflex.

for the physician who tests ROM to understand the principles of measurement, including the landmarks that are used for placing the goniometer, the movement being tested, and the normal ranges for that particular movement. Because the degree of spinal motion is highly dependent on a person's flexibility at any given moment, at least three separate trials are taken for each movement tested, and the average of the three trials becomes the true reading. It also is necessary to obtain more than one measurement when testing any limb joint whose range is significantly limited by stiffness, pain, or contracture. When repeated measures show a variability of more than 10° or more than 10% for ranges greater than 50°,[1] consider the presence of a technical error or poor patient cooperation. When a physician who performs IMEs works regularly with therapists who perform functional capacity evaluations, both should consider using the same goniometers/inclinometers to minimize measurement variability due to instrumentation differences.

Manual muscle testing is highly subjective and variable;[12,24] terminology used for an MMT is shown in Table 1. An MMT does not take into account age and sex

TABLE 1. Gradings Used in Manual Muscle Testing

Grade	Description
5/5 = Normal	Muscle accepts normal resistance through full joint range of motion (ROM).
4/5 = Good	Muscle accepts some resistance through full joint ROM.
3/5 = Fair	Muscle moves through full joint ROM against gravity but cannot accept resistance.
2/5 = Poor	Muscle moves through full joint ROM with gravity eliminated.
1/5 = Trace	Muscle has palpable contraction but no movement.
0/5 = Zero	Muscle has no palpable contraction.
+ or –	The muscle strength falls between two grades. For example, 3+/5 means the muscle can accept some resistance against gravity but through less than 50% of the joint ROM. 4–/5 means the muscle can accept some resistance against gravity for more than 50% but less than 100% of the joint ROM.

differences and the effects of a person's preexisting strength. A body builder may have neurologic weakness, but the examiner is unable to appreciate the weakness because his strength is not great enough to overcome that of the body builder. Strength in an ill person may vary from day to day because of pain or fatigue. Just as in testing ROM, it is necessary to use a standardized technique when performing an MMT to reduce variability as much as possible. For example, the examiner must consider the variable effects of applying his own lever arm at different distances from the joint fulcrum. He should make the person initiate the movement starting at the same joint angle each time. Kendall provides a description of manual muscle testing that is widely used.[23]

When testing muscle strength, the physician must prevent muscle substitution. Muscle substitution occurs when an individual uses a muscle or muscle group to assist or substitute for a weaker muscle or muscle group during the test. For example, a person may externally rotate the thigh and use the hip adductors to assist a weak iliopsoas to flex the hip. When testing elbow flexion, the medial deltoid can assist the biceps if the arm is permitted to abduct and internally rotate at the same time that the elbow is flexed. While such substitutions do demonstrate the amount of functional strength in a particular movement, substitution patterns are not reliably reproduced and do not isolate the muscle of interest. Muscle substitution therefore does not provide an accurate measure of strength on an MMT.

PSYCHOLOGICAL ASSESSMENT

Depression is frequent in the general population of the United States,[16] with a lifetime prevalence of 15% in men and 24% in women.[22] Despite its high prevalence, a recent consensus conference highlighted the fact that depression is seriously undertreated.[22] Depression commonly accompanies chronic pain. Disruption of lifestyle such as job loss is another causal factor. It is therefore not surprising that depressive disorders are present in many people who undergo an IME. Depression is also associated with somatic symptoms, which adds further complexity to identifying a physical cause for a person's symptoms. The diagnosis of depression may be uncovered merely by asking an individual if he or she is depressed. Prior medical records may reveal evidence of depression. Observe him during the IME for a depressed mood. More sophisticated assessment is obtained by incorporating a paper and pencil test. Although the MMPI is a well-known tool, it takes a long time to administer, and its interpretation requires expertise. Shorter assessment tools are available, such as the Beck Depression Inventory.[5] Once depression is diagnosed, third-party payers may not recognize it as a disorder that requires treatment under workers' compensation.[22] Many argue that personal and family emotional strife have no bearing on an individual's ability to work. There is, however, a well-established relationship between depression, chronic pain, and disability. One study found a 4$\frac{1}{2}$ times greater risk of disability in individuals with major depression compared to a nondepressed population.[8] When the question of maximal medical improvement is asked and the individual appears depressed, the physician should evaluate whether the depression has been adequately treated, just as he evaluates whether the physical treatment has been adequate.

When significant depression or anxiety is found or unusual behavior identified and there is a history of trauma such as a fall or motor vehicle accident, ask the person if he sustained any loss of consciousness. Mild traumatic brain injury can result in such symptoms, and further cognitive testing is indicated.

Another diagnosis is somatoform disorder, which occurs when one or more physical symptoms suggest a physical disorder for which there are no demonstrable organic findings or known physiologic causes. Psychological factors appear to dominate. Somatization is increasing in our culture; individuals are more often seeking a diagnosis for their symptoms, and physicians are accommodating these requests by ordering multiple tests and giving the symptoms names, regardless of whether objective pathologic findings are present. At the same time, the trend by insurers to reduce medical utilization by limiting diagnostic testing and specialty physician visits clashes with patient wishes and exacerbates the problem of somatitization.[3]

Another term used to describe nonphysiologic disease is symptom magnification. A symptom magnifier exaggerates symptoms in the history or during the examination. This may be an unconscious effort on the part of the individual to solicit sympathy about his pain. Symptom magnification is difficult to recognize with one encounter, and the physician often must rely on historic records to support this diagnosis. Symptom magnification is suspected when a person demonstrates inconsistencies and atypical symptoms, or overreacts to parts of the physical examination. For example, a supine straight leg raising test, a seated straight leg raising test, and a standing bend-forward-and-touch-toes test generally should produce the same response. Furthermore, when a supine straight leg raising test causes neck pain or when back pain worsens upon flexing both the hip and knee while lying supine—both nonpathologic reactions—suspect nonsomatic pain or symptom magnification. Waddell described a group of tests for low back pain whose responses have no organic basis.[37] A functional capacity evaluation also may help to identify inconsistent responses that suggest symptom magnification.

A diagnosis of symptom magnification or somatoform disorder does not indicate the cause. A symptom magnifier, for example, may respond in an excessive manner because of a low pain threshold, fear or apprehension, other underlying psychological distress, or a desire to overtly demonstrate his pain. These diagnoses are different from malingering. Malingering is a premeditated and conscious attempt to deceive or falsify. Malingering is more difficult to diagnose and often requires information from sources outside the health care system, such as surveillance videotapes or eyewitness accounts of behavior that is counter to the person's statements.

Forming a Diagnosis

When questioning a diagnosis, the physician must use care in drawing a conclusion outside the scope of his training. Just as the individual must be educated about improperly labeling his own symptoms, the physician must be reasonably certain of the accuracy of any label that he applies. For example, "This person is bipolar" is a psychiatric diagnosis. In a legal setting, a nonpsychiatrist who makes this diagnosis will be held to the same standard of knowledge as a psychiatrist. An alternative statement is: "This person demonstrates symptoms that suggest a bipolar disorder. A psychiatric evaluation should be considered." These sentences suggest the diagnosis but also recommend further confirmation. By using this approach, confrontation with the opposing side about one's credentials when offering a new diagnosis outside of one's specialty is avoided, and the risk that the opposing side will refute the validity of the entire report is reduced.

Also use care in inferring a nonmedical cause for a person's symptoms. As already discussed, although the influence of compensation and litigation on recovery is well described in the literature, the physician should have clear evidence before concluding that the person has a somatoform disorder or is embellishing symptoms because of pending litigation or compensation disputes.

IMPAIRMENT RATING

Physicians and nonphysicians often use the terms *impairment*, *disability*, and *handicap* interchangeably. To the IME physician, these words have specific meanings and differences. The American Medical Association defines an impairment as an alteration of an individual's health status.[1] Impairment is assessed medically. A functional definition for impairment is the inability to complete a specific task in activities of daily living because of insufficient physical, psychological, or intellectual skills or because of anatomic variation.

A disability is a medical impairment or incapacity that restricts or prevents someone from performing an activity such as employment in a normal manner. A disability affects a person's ability to fulfill personal, social, or occupational needs or to meet regulatory or statutory requirements.[1]

A handicap is an impairment that substantially limits one or more life activities or roles expected of a person of a particular age and sex.[1]

An impaired person is not necessarily disabled. Disability involves factors that cannot be easily measured by a medical assessment alone. Behavioral, social, attitudinal, and economic factors contribute to a disability. An often-used example is that of a person who sustained a partial amputation of the small finger of the nondominant hand. An impairment has occurred. If the person is a general internal medicine physician, little or no disability has resulted because he can continue to fulfill essentially all of his job and personal life functions. For a concert pianist, the amputation results in a major disability in carrying out his profession.

An IME often is requested for the purpose of calculating an impairment rating or percentage. An impairment percentage is a measure of the loss in the capacity of the individual to carry out his activities of daily living. The most frequently used impairment rating system is the American Medical Association's *Guides to the Evaluation of Permanent Impairment*.[1] The guides are mandated or recommended for workers' compensation cases in 40 of the 53 jurisdictions in the United States. Even in the 13 jurisdictions that do not use the guides, the physician who performs IMEs should be familiar with the rating system because it provides a systematic approach for evaluating impairment. The guides contain a collection of specific instructions and tables that allow the physician to calculate an impairment percentage for all of the principal organ systems of the body.

The AMA's Guides are not a perfect measurement system. They were developed by teams of specialists, each team evaluating an organ system. Some of the rating scales are more subjective than others. The ratings are based on the assumption that a person has achieved a level of permanent impairment. This is often not the case for certain disorders, such as chronic back pain. Age and sex differences are not accounted for, which is important for some tables, such as range of motion of the spine. The physician also is given leeway in the percentage rating he assigns to many of the impairments. Despite its flaws, the Guides are an immense reference intended to gather multiple symptoms and findings and objectify and categorize them into a system that provides a numerical and comparative rating scale.

Disability rating systems, such as Social Security Disability, evaluate a person's ability to earn wages in the presence of an impairment due to a work-related injury. The physician is asked to assess an impairment, and a compensation panel uses the physician's report to determine whether a disability is present in a given individual. In addition to the federal Social Security Disability program, each state has a compensation board and legislates its own workers' compensation laws. The IME physician must become familiar with the workers' compensation regulations in his state. Demeter provides an excellent reference regarding disability evaluations.[13]

CAUSALITY

The workers' compensation system varies by state but in general is a no-fault system based on the premise that an injury is work-related and compensable if it occurs both during the course of employment and as a result of employment.[19] The determination of whether an injury is compensable often requires a physician evaluation that addresses the question of causality. To form an opinion about causality, the physician should try to understand the precise mechanism of the injury or illness that the person feels led to his current condition. When a hand is amputated in the course of using machinery on the job, the cause of the amputation is reasonably clear. A claim of back pain that becomes chronic after lifting a 10-pound carton may raise doubt about whether the injury resulted only from that one event. As already described, it is important to gather as much information as possible about the event and the pertinent prior history to draw an informed conclusion. In the case of a motor vehicle accident, were others injured and to what extent? Obtaining the cost of the vehicular damage may indicate the force involved in the accident and provide some evidence about the severity of an injury. The physician may express the view that she feels the mechanism of injury as described could not produce the injury claimed by the individual.

The causality of an injury becomes more difficult in the case of a cumulative stress disorder. In that situation, the nature of the job must be carefully analyzed by the frequency and type of movements involved. Neck pain in a cashier who must turn his head multiple times each day may be a legitimate cause of a work-related injury. What is his work history? Even in the absence of prior work-related injury, performing the same job over many years for different employers, called "job roulette," may lead to cumulative trauma and explain the cause of injury from a trivial event early in the course of a new job. A history of working at two different jobs when the injury occurred may suggest that fatigue or overuse played a causal role. Inquire about hobbies or avocational interests that require repetitive activity such as woodworking, yard work, sewing, or sports. These kinds of activities may actually cause or at least contribute to symptoms first felt on the job.

Lack of fitness,[18] obesity, or chronic disease such as diabetes complicate the question of causality. A previous injury that has not fully healed raises the question of proportional causality. Risk-taking in certain jobs, especially jobs that pay in proportion to the amount of work produced, results in injury due to fatigue and neglect of basic safety precautions. Is the employer or the employee to blame? For the physician, this determination often is made from a legal and not from a medical perspective. For work-related injuries in most states, the workers' compensation system is a no-fault system that gives employees the benefit of the doubt. Even after meticulous review of records and a thorough examination, however, the physician may still have reasonable doubt regarding causality. When this occurs, the only honest response is to state that "the claimant says that the injury occurred as a result of . . ."

Predicting Return to Work

Can the person return to work? To answer this question, many issues require consideration. First, the person should be asked whether he feels he can return to work. If the answer is no, what part of his job can he not perform? Sometimes the person will say he is unable to perform only one or two aspects of the job, which, with modification, will allow him to resume working. If that is not so, does he feel he can work at any other job in his company? He may say other jobs are available but he thinks he will not be chosen because of seniority or education. Past history may be a good indicator of ability to return to work. After the injury, did he try to return several times in the past, was unsuccessful, and had to stop again for long periods? The longer an individual is out of work, the more difficult it is to return, even following a physical rehabilitation program. Studies suggest that fewer than 50% of persons with a back injury return to work if they have been out for more than 6 months.[25,26] Attitude toward the employer and insurer has a significant impact on return to work. Is he angry? Does he believe his employer is not interested in helping him? He may say he was originally injured because of a dangerous work environment demand. He may state that the insurer or case manager has been confrontational and has prevented him from receiving necessary rehabilitation services. Regardless of whether these perceptions are correct, a person who identifies the employer or insurer as an antagonist has less desire to cooperate and less motivation to return to his job.

Another predictor of return to work comes from assessing the physical demands of the job. For example, an individual whose job requires loading trucks with 150-pound crates has a low probability of return to work following a significant back injury. The answer is often not as clear for many less physically challenging jobs; in such cases a functional capacity evaluation is helpful in identifying the person's restrictions for returning to his job. The Americans with Disabilities Act in certain cases requires an employer to modify the job or provide comparable work to a person who is unable to return to his prior job. When factors such as age and education appear to interfere with return to work, even when physical recovery has occurred, the physician may wish to note these impediments in his report but not base a return-to-work opinion on them. A vocational specialist is responsible for determining whether a person's skills, subject to the physician's restrictions, match the job opportunities in the current labor market.

Maximal Medical Improvement

One of the most subjective decisions a physician is asked to make is whether an individual has achieved maximal medical improvement (MMI). In responding to this question, physicians recognize that predicting the outcome of an illness is an inexact process. The legal system expects the physician only to respond to such questions with a 51% degree of certainty. MMI implies that permanency has occurred. How is permanency predicted even at a 51% level? Certain disorders lead to easier predictions than other disorders. For example, an individual with a below-knee amputation who ambulates independently with a prosthesis, is pain-free, and is functional in daily life skills has most likely reached MMI. Occupational asthma attains a steady state about two years after onset if the person is using appropriate medication. At that stage of the disease, MMI has occurred. In many other disorders, however, MMI is not as easy to predict.

The essential question is whether the person has achieved optimal treatment for a reasonable period without resolution of symptoms. "Optimal treatment" refers to all reasonable care currently available and prescribed by knowledgeable physicians to treat the condition. Using an experimental drug, experimental procedure, or unconventional therapy may be appropriate for some diagnoses but not necessary to receive before concluding MMI is achieved. What is unconventional today may have been state of the art in the past. An example is chymopapain injections for low back pain,[14] a treatment that was common in the 1980s but is no longer performed. Another question is whether the treatment was provided in a reputable facility and by a skilled practitioner. The physician can best answer this through awareness of the quality of various health care resources in his community. Is the physical therapy facility where the person was treated known to provide excellent care? Was comprehensive treatment documented in the therapy notes? Should rehabilitation be recommended again in another facility that is better known for its success rate before concluding that MMI has occurred? Does the individual have another diagnosis that has not yet been optimally treated? For example, if he is depressed and the depression is contributing to symptomatology, has he received any psychological or psychiatric services? Has a comprehensive physical rehabilitation program been provided? If surgery was suggested but the individual refused surgery, if the risks of surgery outweigh the benefits, or the potential for recovery is uncertain, the person has reached MMI.

The strong effects of litigation and the workers' compensation system on recovery from illness have already been described. Use care when concluding that MMI has occurred in someone who appears consumed by the litigation process. Further recovery is known to occur following settlement. In such circumstances, the physician can report that the individual has plateaued and MMI may have occurred but that future "spontaneous" recovery remains possible.

Prolonged bedrest causes well-known changes in physical capacity, including cardiovascular deconditioning, muscle atrophy, and decrease in bone density.[7] An individual who spends a significant portion of the day resting in bed has not achieved MMI unless a previous attempt at a physical rehabilitation program failed. If the reason for bedrest is pain, has the person received a reasonable amount of analgesic medication to allow a trial of physical rehabilitation to commence? Without a trial of rehabilitation, it is difficult to state that MMI has occurred.

If additional testing or treatment is recommended, maximal medical improvement has not occurred. In some persons, although maintenance therapy may help to manage symptoms even after MMI is achieved, a recommendation for further treatment to try to improve a condition generally is not consistent with a conclusion of MMI.

The Report

WHAT TO TELL THE INDIVIDUAL

Many physicians dictate a narrative of the history in the presence of the individual prior to the physical examination. This allows the individual an opportunity to disagree with the information as understood by the physician, providing additional verification of the history. It also indicates to the person that the physician respects his opinion and may increase his cooperation during the physical examination. When using this technique, one should document in the report that it was performed.

The physician should refrain from summarizing his findings and conclusions to the examined individual or any observer. Recommend that he request a copy of the report from the referring party. If he persists about obtaining an immediate opinion, the physician may say that he must review all of the data in more detail before drawing any final conclusions. By not sharing conclusions immediately, confrontation and disagreement are avoided in the office. In addition, the referring party may later refuse to accept the physician's report. For example, the referrer may request a verbal summary from the physician prior to receiving the formal written report. Based on the discussion, the referrer may choose not to receive a written report, particularly if the conclusions are different from what the referrer desired. The referrer does have a legal right to reject the physician's conclusions. An awkward situation would result if the physician shared his findings with the individual and later learned that the referring party did not want a formal report. An exception to this recommendation is the rare instance when a written report is refused and the physician has uncovered an important medical finding or recommendation that he believes can help the individual. He then has an ethical obligation to inform the person directly or the person's treating physician. Even when a written report is accepted, occasions may arise when the severity of a diagnosis requires that the physician inform the person immediately to seek further medical advice.

COMMUNICATING TO THE REFERRAL SOURCE

A written report summarizes to the referral source the record review, the interview, the examination and the conclusions, and answers to questions. When preparing the report, it is important to remember the high probability of its circulation through the judicial system. Unambiguous terminology understandable to nonphysician readers, liberal use of definitions, and accurate descriptions are essential. Avoid abbreviations. Include headings. Use short paragraphs and simple sentences. Regarding content, the report should reflect the time and effort the physician put into the evaluation. Include the essential information obtained in the review of old records and the person's narrative of the history. Report pertinent negatives (i.e., "He denies any current or past history of numbness"). Document sources of information by writing "He states . . ." or "Dr. Smith concluded. . . ." Maintain a balance between repeating everything stated in old records versus highlighting the pertinent and essential information. Although it may seem that a long report will appear more authoritative and justify a higher fee, it is not necessary to repeat all of the past medical history from physicians and tests but rather to summarize key data that demonstrate all material was reviewed. One method that suggests to the reader that a thorough review was performed is to begin the report by itemizing all of the records that were received, including the names of physicians, hospitals, other health care providers, pertinent diagnostic tests, and inclusive dates. Finally, always proofread the report, preferably twice.

Conclusion

The physician who agrees to perform an independent medical examination has a responsibility both to the individual he examines and to the referring source to provide an unbiased and thorough assessment. The physician is considered an expert in the IME process and must possess the knowledge and skill to provide an expert report for those who are placing their trust in his judgment. It is hoped that this section illustrates that a good independent medical examination requires a commitment of time and effort by the physician in order to perform a reliable evaluation, drawing conclusions that are based on factual information and examination findings. Only when a physician is willing to provide this commitment of time and effort should he agree to participate in the IME process.

FUNCTIONAL CAPACITY EVALUATION

The functional capacity evaluation (FCE) is a systematic assessment of an individual's ability to perform a series of tasks safely. An FCE is indicated (1) to obtain baseline measures of a person's current functional abilities, (2) to quantify the degree of impairment as it pertains to functional skills, (3) to match a person's current capacity to his job demands, (4) to match a person's current capacity to the demands of his occupation, (5) to measure the amount of work a particular job task requires, and (6) to provide information on what accommodations are needed to perform a particular job.

Insurers and other third parties are increasingly requesting FCEs. There are several reasons for this heightened interest. Some work-related disorders, such as repetitive motion injuries, are more common. The workforce is aging, and older workers may have an increased risk of developing acute and chronic injury. More persons with chronic medical disease such as spinal cord injury or cardiopulmonary dysfunction are living longer and more productive lives and want to work. At the same time, insurers and case managers are demanding more precision from doctors when requesting return-to-work estimates. An FCE provides information that cannot be predicted through an IME or a simple examination alone.

Purpose

The FCE presents a snapshot of a person's functional abilities at any one point in time. Functional abilities are purposeful activities that an individual must carry out in daily life. Basic self-care needs such as bathing, dressing, and toileting are functional activities but are generally not tested in an FCE. If these activities require testing, they are more often evaluated by a general physical therapy or occupational therapy assessment. In an FCE, the functional abilities most often tested are more advanced household activities or general job functions. Such abilities may include lifting, carrying, pushing, pulling, bending, sitting, and standing tolerances; housekeeping tasks; and tolerances for walking distances on level surfaces and walking on stairs.

When the physician must answer questions in an IME pertaining to return to work and achieving maximal medical improvement, an FCE will provide him with more objective information for responding. The FCE may simply verify what the physician found on the physical examination. On the other hand, it also may demonstrate findings that were not seen on the IME. For example, a person may feel more comfortable in a large open therapy space than in a small examination room under the constant and close surveillance of a physician; he may "let down his guard" during a 4-hour FCE. During an FCE, the therapist may observe the person perform an activity or assume a posture that the person had told the physician he could not do because it caused pain. A symptom magnifier may not exaggerate all of his pain complaints as consistently during the FCE as he did during the IME.

Case managers of IMEs frequently ask the physician to *estimate* a person's current functional capacities (Fig. 4). One of the most subjective decisions in medicine occurs when a physician completes a functional capacities form on the basis of the

```
Name:_____    Patient No.:_____
Diagnosis:_____    Date of Injury:_____
```

Patient can work as follows (circle full capacity for each):

```
        Total No. of Hours at Once        Total No. of Hours in an 8-Hour Day
Sit     1  2  3  4  5  6  7  8        Sit    1  2  3  4  5  6  7  8
Stand   1  2  3  4  5  6  7  8        Stand  1  2  3  4  5  6  7  8
Walk    1  2  3  4  5  6  7  8        Walk   1  2  3  4  5  6  7  8
```

Patient can lift/carry (please check as appropriate):

```
            Never         Occasionally    Frequently
lbs.     Lift  Carry    Lift  Carry     Lift  Carry          Comments
0-10
11-20     ___   ___      ___   ___       ___   ___      _____
21-50     ___   ___      ___   ___       ___   ___      _____
51-100    ___   ___      ___   ___       ___   ___      _____
100+      ___   ___      ___   ___       ___   ___      _____
```

Patient can use hand repetitively (please check as appropriate):

```
         Simple Grasping    Fine Manipulation    Pushing & Pulling
         Yes      No        Yes        No        Yes        No
Right    ___     ___        ___       ___        ___       ___
Left     ___     ___        ___       ___        ___       ___
```

Patient can use feet for repetitive movement such as foot controls (please check as appropriate):

Right ____ Yes ____ No   Left ____ Yes ____ No

Patient is able to (please check as appropriate):

```
         Not At All    Occasionally    Frequently    No Restrictions
Bend       ___            ___            ___             ___
Climb      ___            ___            ___             ___
Kneel      ___            ___            ___             ___
Squat      ___            ___            ___             ___
Reach      ___            ___            ___             ___
```

FIGURE 4. A form for estimating an individual's current functional capacities.
(Figure continued on opposite page.)

physical examination alone. It truly becomes an estimate of function and often a poor estimate. Many times the physician relies solely on the person's self-report of his tolerances. A better method is to obtain a functional capacity *evaluation* that can test these capacities, allowing the physician to provide an estimate based on objective evidence. When completing an estimated functional capacities form, it is generally wise for the physician or the therapist to review the recommendations with the person, which allows an opportunity for discussion and disagreement.

```
Is patient restricted by environmental factors, such as heat/cold, dust,
dampness, height, etc.?

____    No Restriction
____    Yes - Please explain:_____
        _____


As a result of this evaluation, patient could perform (please check as
appropriate):
                                                        Part-   Full-
                                               No Work  Time    Time
Sedentary Work -
(10 lbs. maximum lifting; carrying 10 lb. articles
frequently; walking/standing on occasion)       ___     ___     ___

Light Work -
(20 lbs. maximum lifting; carrying 10 lb. articles
frequently; walking/standing on occasion)       ___     ___     ___

Medium Work -
(50 lbs. maximum lifting with frequent lifting/
carrying of up to 25 lbs.; frequent walking/
standing)                                       ___     ___     ___

Heavy Work -
(100 lbs. maximum lifting with frequent lifting/
carrying of up to 50 lbs. or more; frequent
walking/standing)                               ___     ___     ___

Very Heavy Work -
(lifting objects over 100 lbs. and frequent
lifting/carrying of 50 lbs. or more;
frequent walking/standing)                      ___     ___     ___


Comments:_____
_____
_____
_____
_____



                              _____
                              Signature & Credentials

                              _____
                              Date
```

FIGURE 4 (continued). A form for estimating an individual's current functional capacities.

The FCE is useful in establishing or setting goals in a physical rehabilitation program by identifying areas of weakness. It also can monitor progress in meeting treatment goals if repeated at intervals through the course of the program.

When the question is whether the person can hold any job, the FCE assesses general functional tasks and identifies the limits of safe performance. Once the limits are determined, they are matched to a variety of job descriptions. The job descriptions often are provided by the person's current or potential employer. When this information is not available, the therapist may refer to the Directory of Occupational Titles, a compendium from the U.S. Department of Labor that describes work duties for numerous jobs, including professional positions, clerical work, agricultural jobs, service occupations, and industrial work.[36]

Test Options

An FCE examines general functional performance at one point in time. The evaluation typically lasts 2–6 hours. It does not assess sustained activity or many activities specific to a particular job. Despite these limitations, it frequently is used to make return-to-work recommendations. To test more specific activities, a specialized type of FCE is obtained, a work capacity evaluation (WCE). In contrast to an FCE, a WCE tests a person's ability to safely understand and perform specific job duties. Job duties might include climbing a ladder, building a cement wall, or repairing small appliances. A WCE may require use of specialized equipment appropriate to the person's job. If the supplies and tools are not available on the site of the WCE test facility, the WCE may be performed at the individual's place of employment. Unlike the FCE, the WCE can test a person's endurance for repeated work. Because a WCE is more comprehensive, it lasts from half a day to several days.

Other phrases often encountered in functional testing include *job capacity evaluation*, *work tolerance screen*, and *work sample*. These evaluations are distinguished principally by the degree in which they evaluate specific vs. general job tasks. Some functional tests are standardized assessments that have norms to allow comparisons with large populations.[31]

Components of the FCE

The format of the FCE can vary depending on the person who is performing the test and the information that is requested. A sample FCE is shown in the Appendix.

The therapist should first obtain some history and preferably will have medical records, particularly medical records from the physician who has ordered the test. A history also is obtained from the individual, focusing on the problem being evaluated. When return to work is under consideration, detailed information is obtained about job history and career interests and goals.

Musculoskeletal and neurologic evaluations are first performed to assess range of motion of the limbs and trunk, strength of limbs, presence of deformity, location of painful areas, fine and gross motor coordination, balance, posture, and mobility.

Endurance is measured by ambulating on a treadmill when possible. Alternatives are available for limited or nonambulatory individuals, such as a stationary bicycle or an arm ergometer.

The functional assessment portion of the test may involve many different general and job-specific activities depending on the questions being asked. The general activities tested in most FCEs include lifting, pushing, pulling, carrying, crawling, kneeling, crouching, and squatting. Lifting from floor to waist, waist to eye, and above eye level are tested separately. Lifting or carrying objects with the person's torso in various sitting or rotational positions also may require testing.

When the therapist also must evaluate specific job functions, he should request a job description in advance of the FCE to simulate the functional tasks as closely to the job requirements as possible.

The summary section includes not only numerical information on capacities but also observations on the person's level of cooperation and any pertinent comments regarding physical distress or reactions to the test itself. The test report concludes with a description of the person's abilities and restrictions. Answers to specific questions from the referring source and recommendations for further treatment are provided when appropriate.

Strength Assessment

An FCE can evaluate strength using several methods. One common technique is isokinetic testing. The theory of isokinetic testing and strengthening is well described.[28,33] In contrast to a manual muscle test, isokinetic testing provides a more objective and reproducible method to assess strength. It can quantify strength. It measures subtle changes and therefore can identify weakness in a strong individual. However, isokinetic testing has limitations. The equipment is expensive. Therapists must learn to perform and interpret a complex test. An important concern when performing isokinetic testing for a WCE is that muscles or muscle groups are usually tested in a certain position[2] with the limb often fixed by straps. The therapist, however, may need to test a movement pattern required for a particular job that is different from the movement patterns allowed by the instrumentation. Free weights are much more versatile in testing certain movement patterns and therefore may be more informative for some work capacity tests. Another difficulty with isokinetic testing is that it cannot be used to estimate impairment when using the AMA's *Guides to the Evaluation of Permanent Impairment*.[1]

There are many types of isokinetic instrumentation. No one device has a clear advantage over another. Perrin has summarized various equipment options.[28]

Numerous studies have evaluated the retest reliability of isokinetic testing. Perrin also reviewed that data.[28] When performing analysis with a Pearson product moment or intraclass correlation coefficient, most authors have generally obtained correlations of greater than 0.85 for upper extremity testing and even higher values for most lower extremity joint testing and trunk muscle testing.

Maximum Effort

During the FCE, the therapist must decide when to stop various parts of the test. There are several options. The individual himself reports he cannot continue because of pain, weakness, shortness of breath, or other distress. Alternatively, the therapist recognizes the person is performing the test with increasing difficulty and risking possible injury. For example, as a person lifts heavier objects, his body mechanics change as he approaches his limits, struggling to recruit additional muscle groups to help perform the tasks. Posture may worsen. In the case of endurance testing, blood pressure and heart rate parameters may reach unsafe levels. A maximal effort is defined as one in which the person continues to work until he is stopped for one of the above reasons.

A third reason for stopping any part of the test is that the individual has achieved preestablished goals or the achieved level has provided sufficient information to answer questions that were asked by the referral source. An example is stopping a lift capacity test when a person achieves 30 pounds of floor to waist lift and the person is returning to a light duty occupation that will require maximum lifts of 20 pounds.

Interpretation of Results

In making a determination about return to work, the physician must consider all of the factors needed for a person to successfully resume a job, including factors that are not tested routinely on the FCE. What is his ability to drive to and from work? Will the additional time sitting in a car affect his job performance? An individual who has a spinal cord injury may require one to two hours each morning merely to dress and perform personal hygiene activities. This additional time must be included in the estimate of the person's daily work capabilities. Another consideration is the person's initial endurance and recovery time. Can he return immediately to work 8 hours each day, 5 days each week, or should he resume at a part-time schedule of half days every other day? In some circumstances, consider extending a WCE over multiple consecutive days to assess the person's endurance for a 40-hour work week. The FCE and WCE record a person's capability at one point in time and do not guarantee he will not fail in a job. A person's performance also depends on general physical and psychological health status, motivation to return to work, and social factors involving coworkers and supervisors. Despite their flaws, these evaluation tools are the best methods for determining return-to-work capabilities at present.

Special Populations

Modification of the evaluation protocol is possible for the purpose of performing an IME on special populations. Individuals who have physical or mental disabilities or the elderly can undergo a modified FCE. For example, when a person's endurance cannot be assessed by treadmill walking because of a prior stroke or amputation, arm pedaling of a bicycle ergometer is a substitute. Special precautions must always be considered. Monitoring cardiac status by checking heart rate and blood pressure regularly and extending the warm-up time before requiring the individual to make a full effort reduce the potential for unexpected complications. Extending a 1-day test over 2 days is another common strategy.

Medicolegal Considerations

A therapist should consider performing an FCE only under the prescription of a physician. It is the physician's obligation to identify any precautions the therapist should take when performing an FCE. Are there any restrictions for lifting or carrying weight? Should cardiac precautions be followed? Are any orthopedic injuries present that require the test to be modified? If the therapist identifies medical concerns such as an excessively elevated blood pressure or a complaint of increased pain, the therapist must refer the individual to a physician of record to further assess the problem. When an FCE is ordered by a non-physician, such as a case manager or insurer, the results may not receive a medical interpretation. For example, an individual may demonstrate the ability to climb a ladder on the FCE, but a thorough physician review of his medical history may lead to a decision that climbing is not safe because he has episodic vertigo. Such information may not be known to the therapist performing and interpreting the FCE or to the non-physician report receiver.

When performing an FCE, the therapist should describe each stage of the evaluation process to the person. If the person is tested on a piece of complex equipment, the therapist first demonstrates the equipment and the test protocol and then allows the person to try the equipment using minimal resistance before beginning the test. The therapist should remain in close contact with the person at all times in the event that equipment failure or patient fatigue forces the test to end prematurely. Providing reasonable precautions usually results in a safe and uncomplicated test.

We live in a highly litigious society. Any increased pain during or after the FCE may lead to a complaint that the test was unsafe or was poorly supervised. It is strongly recommended that prior to the FCE, the person sign an informed consent that outlines the risks of the test and his obligation to immediately inform the staff of any pain or discomfort during the examination. Although an informed consent does not release the therapist, doctor, or facility from all liability, it does provide some modest protection by documenting that the person was made aware of the potential risks in advance of consenting to the FCE.

Conclusion

The functional capacity evaluation is an important adjunct to the physical examination in measuring a person's functional ability. When performed by a knowledgeable staff and a willing participant, an FCE records objective and reliable information for both the referral source and the individual.

REFERENCES

1. American Medical Association: Guides to the Evaluation of Permanent Impairment. 4th ed. Chicago, American Medical Association, 1993.
2. Balogun JA, Akomolafe CT, Amusa LO: Grip strength: Effects of testing posture and elbow position. Arch Phys Med Rehabil 72:280–283, 1991.
3. Barsky AJ, Borus JF: Somatization and medicaligation in the era of managed care. JAMA 274:1931–1934, 1995.
4. Beals RK: Compensation and recovery from injury. West J Med 140:233–237, 1984.
5. Beck AT, Ward CH, Mendelson M, et al; An inventory for measuring depression. Arch Gen Psychiatry 4:561–571, 1961.
6. Binder LM, Rohling ML: Money matters: A meta-analytic review of the effects of financial incentives on recovery after closed head injury. Am J Psychiatry 153:7–10, 1996.
7. Bloomfield SA: Changes in musculoskeletal structure and function with prolonged bed rest. Med Sci Sports Exerc 29:197–206, 1997.
8. Broadhead WE, Blazer DG, George LK, et al: Depression, disability days, and days lost from work in a prospective epidemiologic survey. JAMA 264:2524–2528, 1990.
9. Carron H, DeGood DE, Tait R: A comparison of low back pain patients in the United States and New Zealand: Psychosocial and economic factors affecting severity of disability. Pain 21:77–89, 1985.
10. Chan-Yeung M, Malo JL: Occupational asthma. N Engl J Med 333:107–112, 1995.
11. Cole TM, Barry DT, Tobis JS: Measurement of musculoskeletal function. In Kottke FJ, Lehmann JF (eds): Krusen's Handbook of Physical Medicine and Rehabilitation. 4th ed. Philadelphia, WB Saunders, 1990, pp 20–71.
12. DeLisa J, Gans B (eds): Rehabilitation Medicine Principles and Practices. 2nd ed. Philadelphia, JB Lippincott, 1993.
13. Demeter S, Andersson GBJ, Smith GM (eds): Disability Evaluation. St. Louis, Mosby, 1996.
14. Deyo RA: Fads in the treatment of low back pain. N Engl J Med 325:1039–1040, 1994.
15. Deyo RA: The role of the primary care physician in reducing work absenteeism and costs due to back pain. Spine State Art Rev 2:17–30, 1987.
16. Eisenberg L: Treating depression and anxiety in primary care. N Engl J Med 326:1080–1083, 1992.
17. Erickson RP, McPhee MC: Clinical evaluation. In DeLisa J, Gans B (eds): Rehabilitation Medicine Principles and Practice. 2nd ed. Philadelphia, JB Lippincott, 1993, pp 25–65.
18. Frymoyer JW, Cats-Baril W: Predictors of low back pain disability. Clin Orthop 221:89–98, 1987.
19. Hadler NM: Occupational illness: The issue of causality. J Occup Med 26:587–593, 1984.
20. Haynes RB, Sackett DL, Taylor DW, et al: Increased absenteeism from work after detection and labeling of hypertensive patients. N Engl J Med 299:741–744, 1978.
21. Hellebrandt FA, Duvall EN, Moore ML: The measurement of joint motion, part III: Reliability of goniometry. Phys Ther Rev 29:302–310, 1949.
22. Hirschfield RMA, Keller MB, Panico S: The National Depressive and Manic-Depressive Association consensus statement on the undertreatment of depression. JAMA 277:333–340, 1997.
23. Kendall FP, McCreary EK, Provance PG: Muscles Testing and Function. Baltimore, Williams & Wilkins, 1993.
24. Kottke FJ, Lehmann JF (eds): Kursen's Handbook of Physical Medicine and Rehabilitation. 4th ed. Philadelphia, WB Saunders, 1990.
25. Kramer J, Yelin E, Epstein W: Social and economic impacts of four musculoskeletal conditions. Arthritis Rheum 26:551–556, 1983.

26. Liang M: Costs and outcomes in rheumatoid arthritis and osteoarthritis. Arthritis Rheum 27:210–220, 1984.
27. Newman LS: Occupational illness. N Engl J Med 333:1128–1134, 1995.
28. Perrin DH: Isokinetic Exercise and Assessment. Champaign, IL, Human Kinetics, 1993.
29. Petersen M: Nonphysical factors that affect work hardening success: A retrospective study. J Occup Sports Phys Ther 22:238–246, 1995.
30. Spengler DM, Bigos SJ, Martin NA, et al: Back injuries in industry: A retrospective study. 1. Overview and cost analysis. Spine 11:241–245, 1986.
31. Stolov WC, Hooks DL: Prevocational evaluation. In Kottke FJ, Lehmann JF (eds): Krusen's Handbook of Physical Medicine and Rehabilitation. 4th ed. Philadelphia, WB Saunders, 1990, pp 206–214.
32. Tait RC, Margolis RB, Krause SJ, et al: Compensation status and symptoms reported by patients with chronic pain. Arch Phys Med Rehabil 69:1027–1029, 1988.
33. Thistle HG, Hislop HJ, Moffroid M, et al: Isokinetic contraction: A new concept of resistive exercise. Arch Phys Med Rehabil 48:279–282, 1967.
34. Trief PT, Stein N: Pending litigation and rehabilitation outcome of chronic back pain. Arch Phys Med Rehabil 66:95–99, 1985.
35. U.S. Department of Labor, Bureau of Labor Statistics: Occupational injuries and illnesses: Counts, rates and characteristics, 1993. Washington, DC, BLS, 1996.
36. U.S. Department of Labor, Employment and Training Administration: Directory of occupational titles. 4th ed. Washington, DC, ETA, 1991.
37. Waddell G, McCulloch JA, Kummel E: Nonorganic physical signs in low-back pain. Spine 5:117–125, 1980.

APPENDIX
Functional Capacity Evaluation

DATE:

NAME: AGE: 49   ONSET:

DIAGNOSIS: Guillain-Barré syndrome

REASON FOR REFERRAL: Functional Capacity Evaluation to determine abilities/limitations

CURRENT SYMPTOMS: "Below ankles and above neck 'troubles'; the rest of my body is at least 90%."

MEDICATIONS: None noted at time of evaluation

MEDICAL PRECAUTIONS: None noted (Dr. Kraus) at time of evaluation

FUNCTIONAL RESTRICTIONS (DR.): None noted (Dr. Kraus) at time of evaluation

EDUCATIONAL LEVEL: High school graduate

MEDICAL HISTORY/PREVIOUS TREATMENT: Refer to Dr. Kraus' evaluations/follow-ups.

WORK HISTORY: Mr. _____ worked in maintenance for _____ (foil division) full time for 24 years up until his injury.

CLIENT GOALS/PLAN FOR RETURN TO WORK: "Return to work, gradually."

Pain Diagram: Correlates with reported symptoms.

Pain Intensity Rating: Pre-evalaution pain rating = 3 with a 30-day range of 3 to 5 out of a possible 10+. He reported a post-evaluation pain rating of 3½ with increased foot pain. He is presently collecting unemployment compensation; however, he would like to return to work at least on a part-time basis.

THE PAIN DRAWING

OVERALL PAIN RATING

Pain As Bad As It Can Be

No Pain At All

Indicate your symptoms on the body diagrams using the symbols in the key.

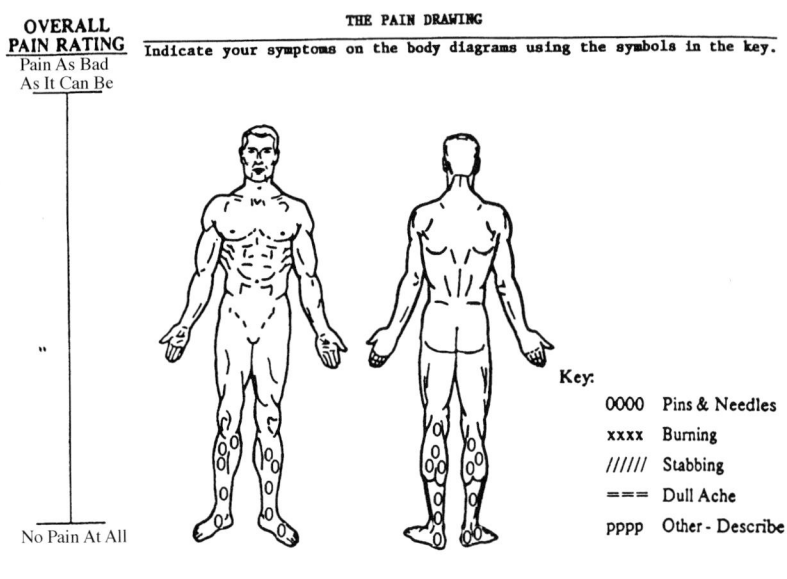

Key:

0000   Pins & Needles
xxxx   Burning
//////   Stabbing
===   Dull Ache
pppp   Other - Describe

Pain Rating

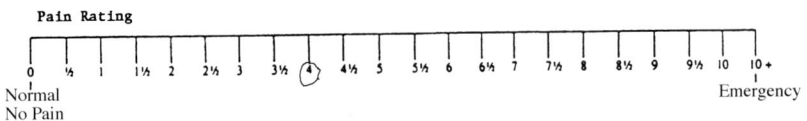

0   ½   1   1½   2   2½   3   3½   ④   4½   5   5½   6   6½   7   7½   8   8½   9   9½   10   10+

Normal No Pain   Emergency

Rate of Perceived Exertion

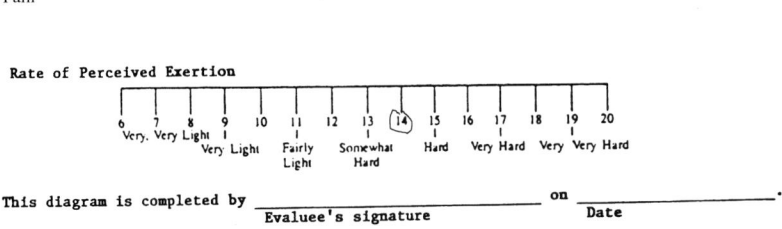

6   7   8   9   10   11   12   13   ⑭   15   16   17   18   19   20
Very, Very Light   Very Light   Fairly Light   Somewhat Hard   Hard   Very Hard   Very Very Hard

This diagram is completed by _____ on _____.
                                       Evaluee's signature   Date

INDEPENDENT MEDICAL EXAMINATION/FUNCTIONAL CAPACITY EVALUATION

PHYSICAL ASSESSMENT:

Height: 6'3"
Weight: 255 lb.

Aerobic Capacity	Heart Rate	Blood Pressure	Respiratory Rate	% of Max.HR
Pre-test	72	138/98	WNL	42
Post-test	100	131/92	WNL	58
Method of exercise:	Treadmill x 25 min. @ 2.1 m.p.h.			

THE EVALUATION DATA IS WNL <u>UNLESS</u> NOTED BELOW:

POSTURE: 83/100 on the Reedco Posture Assessment with his left shoulder depressed, rounded neck and upper back, protruding abdomen and hollow low back.

PALPATION: Unremarkable

AROM: Bilateral neck lateral flexion decreased 25%. Remaining ROM within normal limits.

MUSCLE STRENGTH: 5/5 except left ankle dorsiflexion, plantar flexion and eversion = 3+/5. Right ankle dorsiflexion, plantar flexion = 3+/5, eversion = 4-/5.

SACROILIAC JOINT: N/T

SKIN CONDITION: Appears intact and pliable.

*Hand dominance: Right

Hand grip strength:	lb.	%ile
Right	116	57
Left	103	53

Coordination: fine motor: Purdue Pegboard testing indicates the right upper extremity = 28th percentile, left upper extremity = 3rd percentile, and both hands working together on an assembly task = 37th percentile when compared with other males.

gross motor: Bilateral upper extremities within normal limits on alternate finger-to-nose testing and bilateral lower extremities as demonstrated by alternate heel-to-knee/heel-to-toe testing.

Balance: Standing balance static = G, dynamic = G. Unable to sustain any high level balance testing (Romberg, Sharpened Romberg or Stand-On-One-Leg). Balance was within functional limits throughout functional activities with no loss of balance.

Mobility: Bed mobility   Independent

Transfers   Independent

Gait: direct observation: Somewhat high steppage gait with decreased heel strike.

indirect observation: As above

Observations:

Mr.   appeared to put forth consistent effort throughout this evaluation process, attempting all tasks requested by the examiners.

FUNCTIONAL ASSESSMENT

ITEM	MAX. EFFORT	RESTRICTIONS	COMMENTS
Weight Capacity in lb. Lift: Floor-to-waist Waist-to-eye level Horizontal Push: dynamic-10' Pull: dynamic-10' Carry: Front-at-waist-50'	30 lb. 30 lb. 30 lb. 30 lb. I.F. 30 lb. I.F. 30 lb.		Maximum effort Maximum effort Maximum effort Maximum effort Maximum effort Maximum effort
Flexibility/Positional Elevated Work-10 min. Trunk Flexion Work Sitting-10 min. Standing 10-min. Unweighted Rotation Sitting Standing Crawl-30' Kneel-1 min. Crouch-deep static-1 min Repetitive Squat (10 reps.-1 min.) Repetitive Foot Movement 10 min.	WNL 10 min. 10 min. WNL WNL Avoid}Able to get in & }out of positions; }however, lack of }sensation in bi- }lateral feet & }pain in feet if }dorsiflexed }excessively }limits }activities. WFL	None None	
Static Work Sitting-30 min. Standing-15 min.	30 min. 15 min.	None None	WNL by pt. report 1-2 hr. max. by pt. report
Ambulation Walking-15 min. Stairs-100 Ladders Uneven Terrain	25 min. on treadmill WFL for several flights with handrail for balance. Avoid Avoid	None	1-2 hr. max. by pt. report

Observations during activities:

Body mechanics inappropriate secondary to inability to squat.

Reported change in symptomatic response with activities:

If ankle and feet fully dorsiflexed, increased foot pain in position such as kneeling or crouching.

INDEPENDENT MEDICAL EXAMINATION/FUNCTIONAL CAPACITY EVALUATION

NARRATIVE SUMMARY

Behavior/Observations:

Mr.   is a 49-year-old male referred to Bryn Mawr Rehab's Work Hardening Clinic for a Functional Capacity Evaluation. He arrived on time and was dressed casually and appropriately for the evaluation as requested by this facility.

Mr.   was cooperative and appeared to put forth consistent effort throughout this evaluation process, attempting all tasks requested by the examiners. Movement patterns during this evaluation process were somewhat guarded due to his difficulty with high-level balance activities.

Current symptoms include discomfort in both hands and feet of varying intensity that he reports are sometimes a "dull ache" and other times more "pins and needles." He reported a pre-evaluation pain rating of 3 with a 30-day range of 3 to 5 out of a possible 10+. He reported a post-evaluation pain rating of 3½ with slightly increased foot discomfort bilaterally.

Functional Restrictions:

None noted (Dr. Kraus) at time of evaluation.

Abilities:

Mr.   was capable of performing a 30-lb. floor-to-waist level, horizontal and waist-to-eye level lift. Two-handed carrying ability was also documented at 30 lb. for approximately 50 feet. When pushed beyond 30 lb., his balance was comprised.

Mr.   was capable of walking on the treadmill for 25 minutes at 2.1 m.p.h. working at approximately 58% of his maximum heart rate. He reports a maximum walking tolerance of approximately 1-2 hours. He also negotiated 100 stairs requiring at least one handrail for balance. However, again, cardiovascular status increased quickly. He demonstrated a sitting tolerance of at least 30 minutes and reported this to be within normal limits. He demonstrated a static standing tolerance of at least 15 minutes and reported a 1-2 hour maximum before a break is required.

Gross motor coordination was within normal limits in both upper extremities as demonstrated by alternate finger-to-nose testing and both lower extremities as demonstrated by alternate heel-to-knee/heel-to-toe testing. Purdue Pegboard testing indicates the right upper extremity = 28th percentile, left upper extremity = 3rd percentile, and both hands working together on an assembly task = 37th percentile when compared with other males. Grip strength was within the 57th percentile for the right upper extremity and within the 53rd percentile for the left upper extremity when compared with males of his age. General mobility, overall, throughout this evaluation was functional.

Limitations:

Mr. had good static and dynamic standing balance. However, this balance was compromised if asked to carry greater than 30 lb., or carrying any objects while ascending/descending stairs, or when required to move into or out of awkward positions such as kneeling, crawling or crouching.

Manual muscle testing indicates below normal strength in bilateral ankles. Gait observation indicated a high-steppage gait with decreased heel strike. However, overall gait was functional, just slightly slowed cadence.

Mr. should avoid any work which requires unprotected heights or climbing ladders and be cautious when on uneven terrain.

Work Level/Impact:

Mr. reported he worked full time in the maintenance department for for approximately 24 years up until his May 1, 1996 onset. He is presently on unemployment compensation; however, he would like to attempt a part-time return to work. He reported he can work up to 8 hours per week without compromising his unemployment compensation.

Based on the results of this Functional Capacity Evaluation, it does appear Mr. is presently capable of re-entering the workforce on a part-time basis given the above outlined limitations. Work should be limited to 4 hours per day or less and can be initiated between 3 and 5 days per week. This would be in excess of the 8 hours per week he reports unemployment will allow him to work; however, this will need to be addressed with the employer.

Recommendations:

A brief work hardening program to address endurance, bilateral lower extremity strength, balance during functional activities he would encounter when in the workplace, and body mechanics education appears indicated. This program could be done in conjunction with a part-time return to work with goal of returning to full-duty work in the future.

Mr. reported his job involves being around dangerous moving equipment and given his balance difficulties, he is thinking of returning to modified duty; for example, box making or moving pallets with a manual pallet jack. This type of work seems much more suited for his present capacities.

_____

_____   _____
                                                                                    Date

JACK W. SNYDER, MD, JD, MPH, PhD

THE ROLE OF THE CLINICAL LABORATORY IN OCCUPATIONAL MEDICINE

From the Departments of
  Emergency Medicine and
  Laboratory Medicine
Thomas Jefferson University
Philadelphia, Pennsylvania

Reprint requests to:
Jack W. Snyder, MD, JD, MPH, PhD
401 Pavilion, Thomas Jefferson
  University Hospital
125 South 11th Street
Philadelphia, PA 19107-4998

The clinical laboratory plays a limited but important role in the overall assessment and management of the patient. For some patients, laboratory analyses may contribute little or nothing to the diagnosis and treatment of their illness. For others, many tests may be needed before a diagnosis is made, and repeated analyses may be required to monitor treatment over a long period. Today, there are more than 500 different tests that may be performed in clinical chemistry, hematology, microbiology, immunology, and histopathology laboratories.[1] These tests vary from the very simple, such as the measurement of sodium, to the highly complex, such as DNA analysis, screening for drugs, speciation of microbes, or differentiation of lipoprotein variants. Many high-volume tests are done on large, expensive, automated machines, and other analyses are done manually. Infrequently performed tests may be conveniently carried out by using commercially prepared reagents packaged in kit form. Increasing workloads and budgetary constraints have heightened the need for continuous reassessment of the most cost-effective way of providing the best service.

Ideally, each laboratory test should provide the answer to a question that a physician has posed about a patient. To obtain correct answers, a clinical laboratory must address issues at three stages of testing: the pre-analytic, analytic, and post-analytic stages. Pre-analytic concerns include physiologic variation, sampling errors, and specimen transport and receipt problems. Analytic concerns include assay technology, quality control, and operator errors. Post-analytic concerns focus on collation, interpretation, and reporting of results. Physicians practicing occupational medicine may benefit from a review of some of the recurring challenges faced by laboratories seeking to provide clinicians with accurate and timely information. Experience has shown that physicians who take the time to learn about the benefits and limitations of laboratory tests use the laboratory most productively and cost-effectively. This chapter emphasizes that all physicians should (1) carefully select tests to answer questions about a specific clinical situation, (2) be certain that requests are clear and that the patient is correctly identified, (3) obtain the appropriate specimen and see that it is correctly labeled and promptly transported to the laboratory, (4) review the results of all tests in a timely manner and take appropriate action, (5) integrate laboratory findings with other clinical data from the history, physical examination, and imaging studies, and (6) investigate any puzzling or unexpected laboratory result as thoroughly as one would investigate a puzzling or unexpected physical finding or imaging abnormality.[2]

PRE-ANALYTIC ISSUES

Laboratories must receive a correct and optimal specimen for the requested test as well as information that will ensure that the right test is performed and the result returned to the requesting physician with a minimum delay. There are many causes of "abnormal" test results that do not necessarily reflect the pathophysiologic state of the patient. These causes, collectively termed "pre-analytic variation," include (1) physiologic changes in the individual, (2) changes occurring during the process of collecting the specimen, (3) changes occurring between the time of collection and the time of analysis, and (4) the presence in the specimen of substances that interfere with subsequent analyses.

Numerous *physiologic factors* influence laboratory test results. For example, a result may fall outside a "reference range" if the person tested is not from the same population as the samples used to establish that reference range. Thus, the occupational physician should consider whether an individual differs in age, sex, or race from the original samples and whether that accounts for the "abnormal" result.

Use of prescription and over-the-counter products may cause changes in body fluid concentrations of various analytes. For example, caffeine is associated with increased catecholamine release. Nicotine may alter circulating concentrations of hormones that regulate glucose metabolism. Ethanol and antiepileptic drugs reproducibly increase the release of gamma-glutamyl transferase. Thiazide diuretics, calcium salts, estrogens, and vitamins A and D may cause hypercalcemia, and anticonvulsants, barbiturates, corticosteroids, gastrin, glucagon, glucose, insulin, magnesium salts, methicillin, and tetracycline may depress total serum calcium concentrations. Lithium not only causes hypercalcemia by altering the set-point for parathyroid hormone release, but it also decreases the response to antidiuretic hormone (nephrogenic diabetes insipidus). Phenothiazines and oral contraceptives increase thyroxine-binding globulin production, causing increased total thyroxine.

Exercise may cause both short-term and long-term effects on the results of laboratory tests. Patients who regularly engage in strenuous exercise often have increased serum concentrations of muscle-derived enzymes such as creatine kinase (CK), lactate dehydrogenase (LDH), and aspartate aminotransferase (AST). Female long-distance runners often have disordered production of gonadotropins and decreased circulating sex hormone levels. Serum uric acid may increase by as much as 2 mg/dl in persons who exercise within 24 hours of venipuncture.

Upright posture increases hydrostatic pressure in the legs and decreases the return of fluid from the extravascular to the intravascular space at the venous end of the capillaries. Relative hyperproteinemia (5–10% increase) may occur since proteins do not normally cross into the extravascular space. The blood concentrations of cellular elements and highly protein-bound substances, such as calcium, drugs, iron, lipids, steroids, and thyroid hormones, also may increase by a similar amount. To prevent postural changes from influencing test results, blood should be drawn soon after rising from a recumbent position or after a patient has been allowed to sit for at least 30 minutes.

The acute stress of medical illness has been associated with increased production of adrenocorticotropic hormone (ACTH), glucocorticoids, and catecholamines, and decreased serum concentrations of thyroid-stimulating hormone (TSH), triiodothyronine (T_3), aldosterone, and gonadotropins.[3] Increased production of "acute phase reactant" proteins such as haptoglobin and fibrinogen may mask their expected decrease in hemolysis or coagulopathy. Increased uptake of low-density lipoprotein (LDL) cholesterol into tissues may cause a 30–40% reduction in serum LDL cholesterol concentrations. Therefore, in general, lipid studies should not be done on hospitalized patients.[4]

Substances absorbed from food are likely to be present in higher serum concentrations immediately after a meal. By contrast, the concentration of substances that must be used for metabolism (e.g., phosphate) or that change in response to metabolism (e.g., potassium, pH) will decrease following a meal. Although most of these changes do not persist beyond 1–2 hours, a few can last for several hours. In nondiabetics, serum glucose typically returns to basal levels within 2 hours. Triglyceride (TG) concentration increases immediately after a meal, but after a transient fall due to particle clearance, serum TG rises again several hours later as very low density lipoprotein (VLDL) is released. TG typically does not return to basal levels for at least 8–10 hours. Serum bilirubin typically rises after a patient has fasted for more than 24 hours. This increase is more frequently observed in patients with Gilbert syndrome.

Collection factors also can influence laboratory test results. For example, the use of a tourniquet may cause artifactual hemoconcentration. An apparent increase in the concentration of proteins and protein-bound substances may be noted as early as 1 minute after applying the tourniquet. Within 3 minutes, the apparent concentration may have increased 8–10%. More prolonged application causes blood stagnation and increased blood ammonia, lactate, and hydrogen ion concentrations. These effects are even more pronounced if the tourniquet is released during the draw. Clenching and unclenching of the fist with the tourniquet in place can increase the apparent serum potassium concentration by 1.0–1.5 mEq/L. Hemolysis caused by turbulent, nonlaminar blood flow or by forceful expulsion of blood from a syringe into an evacuated tube also releases potassium, as well as magnesium, phosphate, LDH, and hemoglobin.

Many substances are unstable in urine or serum, and failure to collect specimens with necessary preservatives causes inappropriately low concentrations. Additives that may be appropriate for one type of specimen cause errors when used for other tests. Gel in serum separator tubes binds many drugs, while heparin activates lipoprotein lipase and causes a progressive decrease in serum triglyceride concentration. The presence in plain, red-topped tubes of small amounts of blood from a lavender-topped tube containing potassium ethylenediamine tetraacetic acid (EDTA) may increase serum potassium and decrease serum calcium, magnesium, alkaline phosphatase, and creatine kinase. Thus, the preferred order for filling Vacutainer color-coded tubes during venipuncture is blood culture, followed by plain (nonadditive, red-top), coagulation (blue-top), heparin (green-top), EDTA (lavender-top), and oxalate-fluoride (gray-top) tubes.

Clerical errors are the most common cause of erroneous laboratory results. Mislabeling of samples is more frequent in intensive care units and hospital wards than in outpatient clinics, but in all patient care settings every specimen should be labeled before the clinician leaves the patient's room.

Post-collection changes also may contribute to pre-analytic variation in laboratory results, especially in patients with hematologic disorders. For example, potassium concentrations are slightly higher in serum than in plasma because potassium is released from platelets during clotting of the blood. When the platelet count exceeds 400,000 per mm^3, the difference between serum and plasma potassium increases by about 0.1 mmol/L for each 100,000 increase in platelet count; thus, for platelet counts above 1 million, this difference may become clinically significant. Collection of blood in heparin will prevent clotting and decrease potassium release by platelets.

The rate of glucose utilization in blood is increased when the leukocyte count is markedly elevated. In samples from patients with white blood cell counts above 500,000 per mm^3, the glucose concentration may drop below 50 mg/dl within 20 minutes of collection. In patients with lymphocyte counts above 200,000 per mm^3, heparin causes cellular degeneration, release of potassium, and artifactual hyperkalemia, which can be prevented by collecting blood without an anticoagulant.

Within 20–30 minutes at room temperature, serum concentrations of lactate, renin, and ammonia increase, and those of catecholamines decrease. Serum glucose decreases by 3–5% per hour while serum hydrogen ion concentration increases at room temperature. At 36–48 hours, when glucose is completely consumed, cells begin to release potassium, magnesium, phosphate, AST, and LDH.

Finally, a tissue or fluid sample may contain agents that *interfere* with some of the older spectrochemical analyses. For example, falsely increased serum creatinine may be measured by the alkaline picrate (Jaffé) reaction in the presence of cephalosporins, hydantoins, ascorbic acid, ketonemia, hyperbilirubinemia, lipemia, hemolysis, and meat ingestion.[5]

REFERENCE RANGES

The term *normal* may have several meanings. Normal for serum chromium concentrations might be a committee's consensus of "approved" chromium values; the "ideal" chromium value, the most representative chromium value as defined by the mean; the most commonly encountered chromium values as defined by an interval or range; or chromium values unlikely to cause harm. Occupational physicians typically are interested in the last two definitions of normality.

The term *normal* has been replaced by the term *reference* to denote a range, set of limits, or interval because these values merely provide a frame of reference for interpreting other results. Normal values are influenced by many nondisease factors, including gender, race, age, diet, physical activity, drugs, heredity, intelligence, and socioeconomic status. Thus, a "normal" interval must be defined in terms of a specific reference population.

Proper interpretation of a patient's laboratory test values requires appropriate comparison values. These values are obtained from *reference individuals* who are selected for comparison using defined criteria. Reference individuals (or subgroups) can be defined using one or more of the factors mentioned above (selection or partition criteria), or they can be a source of reference values for themselves ("subject-based" reference values). A *reference value* may then be defined as a value obtained by observation or measurement of a particular type of quantity on a reference individual.[6] An example of a set of reference values would be triglyceride concentrations in sera collected from a group of reference individuals selected for comparison according to a sufficiently exact set of criteria. By contrast, an *observed value* is defined as a value of a particular type of quantity obtained by observation or measurement and produced to make a medical decision.[6] Observed values can be compared with reference values, reference distributions, reference limits, or reference intervals. In simpler terms, an observed value is the laboratory result obtained by analysis of samples collected from an individual under clinical investigation.[8]

CHEMICAL ANALYSES

Blood Tests of Renal Function

The blood urea nitrogen (BUN) and serum creatinine concentrations, as surrogates for measurements of urea or creatinine clearance, are commonly used to assess glomerular filtration rate (GFR), a measure of kidney function. The use of serum creatinine as an index of the GFR assumes that creatinine (1) is produced at a constant rate and released only from muscle, (2) is distributed throughout body water, (3) is not metabolized in the body, and (4) is excreted unchanged exclusively by glomerular filtration in the kidneys.[9] Unfortunately, these assumptions are imperfect because creatinine is ingested in cooked meat, secreted by renal tubules, and degraded in the gut.[10] Despite these limitations, the serum creatinine is favored over BUN as an estimate of GFR because changes in nitrogen load and the rate of urine flow exert greater influence on BUN than on serum creatinine in the absence of significant changes in glomerular function. To approximate the creatinine clearance from serum creatinine, the physician can use the following formula:

$$\text{creatinine clearance} = [(140 - \text{age}) \times (\text{weight})]/(K \times S_{Cr})$$

where weight is expressed in kilograms and serum creatinine (S_{Cr}) in milligrams per deciliter, and K is 72 for males and 85 for females.[11]

In acutely ill patients, BUN and creatinine are not sensitive tests because an acute fall in GFR is not accompanied by an instant rise in BUN or serum creatinine concentrations. Instead, urea and creatinine accumulate over hours to days until production rates equal excretion rates and new steady-state concentrations are attained. BUN or creatinine values obtained before steady-state is achieved are likely to underestimate any changes in GFR. In clinically stable patients where GFR is measured by inulin clearance, the sensitivities of BUN and creatinine are poor (14% for BUN, 19% for creatinine) for mild loss of GFR (46–72 ml/min), better (34% for BUN, 84% for creatinine) for moderate loss of GFR (20–45 ml/min), and best (above 90% for both) for severe loss of GFR (< 20 ml/min).[12] However, the specificity of serum creatinine as an index of GFR is sufficient to suggest that high serum creatinine or low creatinine clearance should be regarded as strong evidence that GFR is reduced.[13]

To assess the significance of any BUN value, it must be compared to a simultaneous serum creatinine value. The expected ratio between BUN and creatinine is approximately 10 when protein intake is 1 g/kg/body weight per day, urine output is 1 ml/min, and creatinine production and fluid intake are otherwise "normal."[14] When urine flow is low, as in gastrointestinal bleeding, cirrhosis, nephrosis, congestive heart failure, or acute post-renal obstruction, or nitrogen load is high, as in extreme catabolism or steroid therapy, the BUN/creatinine ratio may exceed 10 (pre-renal azotemia); when urine flow is high, nitrogen load is low, or when creatinine production rises after severe muscle injury, the ratio may be considerably less than 10. A ratio of 10:1 or less also may be observed in patients with interstitial nephritis, tubular necrosis, chronic renal failure, or chronic liver disease. In patients with water intoxication or the syndrome of inappropriate secretion of antidiuretic hormone, slightly low serum creatinine values (0.7–0.8 mg/dl) tend to be associated with low BUN values (4–8 mg/dl).

The recommended frequency of BUN and serum creatinine measurements depends on the purpose of the tests. Guidelines from Blue Cross/Blue Shield and the American College of Physicians suggest that annual or biannual serum creatinine, with or without BUN, may be useful in screening unselected, asymptomatic, ambulatory persons because antihypertensive treatment and dietary protein or phosphorus restriction may slow progression of established chronic renal disease.[16] Any patient with diabetes mellitus, hypertension, or proteinuria should have an initial determination of BUN and creatinine, followed by creatinine clearance measurement if the blood tests are abnormal. Follow-up BUN and creatinine should be obtained every 1–2 years in patients with uncomplicated hypertension, every 4–6 months in patients with chronic renal disease, 2–3 times per week in patients receiving aminoglycosides, every 1–2 days in patients with acute renal failure, and weekly in seriously ill patients.

Urine Tests of Renal Function

Examination of the quality, quantity, and composition of the urine is vitally important in understanding renal disease. There are pitfalls, however, in urine testing that occupational physicians must keep in mind.

A clean catch specimen is always preferred. Both males and females need instruction in cleansing the urethral meatus. Midstream collections are performed by starting urination into the toilet and then bringing the collection device into the urine stream to catch the midportion of the void. First-voided early morning specimens obtained in the upright position increase the likelihood of detection of casts and protein. Urine should not be analyzed in the presence of fecal contamination, decomposition, bacterial overgrowth, or undue delay (more than 6 hours) in transport.

Qualitative screening of urine using teststrips or automated analyzers (e.g., Yellow IRIS) can suggest the presence of various urologic problems, including renal disease, urinary tract infection or neoplasm, systemic disorders, toxicologic disorders, and inflammatory or neoplastic disease adjacent to the urinary tract. Although automation has improved the consistency of microscopic examination of the urine, 95% of urine samples that are unremarkable by inspection and dipstick will have normal sediment by automated or manual microscopy.

Clinicians seeking consistency in their diagnostic approach to urine should focus on the six Cs of urinalysis: Color, Crystals, Cells, Casts, Critters, and Chemistry.[17]

The *color* of urine can vary considerably. Dark brown or smoky urine suggests a renal source of hematuria, but pink or red urine suggests an extrarenal source. Color also may be altered by the presence of drugs such as rifampin, methylene blue, and pyridium.

Crystals may be detected by instruments or interpreted by technologists or physicians. Warm, freshly-voided urine sediment from normal patients almost never contains crystals due to the presence of crystal inhibitors and the lack of an available nidus, whereas crystalluria is frequently observed in urine stored at room temperature or refrigerated. By contrast, consistently acid urine (pH < 5.0–5.6) favors the formation of xanthine, cystine, tyrosine, leucine, and uric acid crystals (and stones), whereas consistently alkaline urine (pH > 7.0) favors the formation of calcium magnesium ammonium (triple) phosphate, calcium carbonate, and calcium phosphate crystals (and stones). Calcium oxalate and calcium apatite crystals may form at any pH. Massive amounts of calcium oxalate or hippurate crystals may suggest ethylene glycol ingestion, especially in patients with anion gap acidosis and neurologic abnormalities. Acyclovir, cholesterol, bilirubin, hemosiderin, xanthine, sulfa, triamterene, iodinated contrast medium, and acetaminophen crystals also have been described in urine sediment.

Cells in urine sediment, especially leukocytes and dysmorphic erythrocytes, may indicate chemical injury, bacterial infection, glomerulonephritis, autoimmunity, appendicitis, diverticulitis, or other inflammation adjacent to or within the urinary tract.

Casts are cylindrical masses of mucoprotein in which cellular elements, protein, or fat droplets may be entrapped. Hyaline casts, seen best with reduced illumination or in phase contrast microscopy, occur in physiologic states (e.g., after exercise) and in many types of renal disease. Renal tubular (epithelial) casts typically are seen in acute tubular necrosis but also are observed in eclampsia, heavy metal poisoning, ethylene glycol intoxication, and acute allograft rejection. Finely granular casts are seen after exercise but also in glomerular and tubulointerstitial disorders. Coarsely granular casts are considered abnormal and are seen in many renal diseases. Red blood cell casts are virtually pathognomonic of glomerulonephritis, whereas bacterial or leukocyte casts strongly suggest pyelonephritis. Waxy and broad casts, which are formed in the distal nephron, suggest diffuse, widespread advanced renal disease. Fatty casts with oval fat bodies, which are formed in tubular cells that have exceeded their capacity to reabsorb protein, typically are observed in nephrotic syndrome, glomerulonephritis, and diabetic nephropathy.

Critters observed in urine include trichomonads, schistosomes, lice, mites, and worms. Various *chemicals* (see crystals above) and artifacts, including talc, starch, fibers, diatoms, plant cells, and corpora amylacea, also have been reported.

Regarding urine *chemistry*, common clinical conditions associated with acidic urine include starvation, dehydration, diarrhea, high protein diets, prolonged sleep, fat metabolism, acid-producing bacteria, and diabetic, respiratory, or metabolic acidosis. Common causes of alkaline urine include vegetarian diets, chronic renal failure, vomiting, ammonia-producing (urea-splitting) bacteria, renal tubular acidosis, and respiratory or metabolic alkalosis.

Low-molecular-weight urinary proteins, such as beta$_2$-microglobulin, metallothionein, and retinol-binding protein, have been used as indirect markers of cadmium exposure. When urine beta$_2$-microglobulin exceeds 1500 µg/g of creatinine and urine cadmium exceeds 3 µg/g of creatinine, Occupational Safety and Health Administration standards indicate that the employee must be removed from work-related exposure to cadmium. Even if exposure ceases, however, low-molecular-weight proteinuria may worsen and be accompanied by an accelerated decrease in glomerular filtration rate.[18]

TESTS OF LIVER FUNCTION

In general, clinical laboratory tests have been designed to (1) screen for abnormalities in liver function, (2) document a liver abnormality, (3) determine the type and site of hepatic injury, (4) determine prognosis, and (5) facilitate follow-up of patients with liver disease. The variety of established as well as novel tests designed to assess hepatic integrity attests to both the complexity of liver function and the need for simpler, more reliable tests.[19] Traditional liver function tests (LFTs), which measure substances synthesized or degraded by the liver, substances released from damaged tissue, or substances cleared from plasma by the liver, are rather crude indices of hepatic structure, cellular integrity, and function but often are the best available for screening populations of workers.

LFTs have been offered in combination because no single test can satisfy all of the objectives mentioned above. There are significant variations in the sensitivity, specificity, and selectivity of LFTs, but they continue to be valuable initial discriminators that complement the history and physical examination and guide the selection of more definitive or invasive tests for the patient with suspected or proven hepatic disease.

Algorithms for the interpretation of LFTs have been developed, and numerous reports show statistically significant differences in laboratory values among disease states, but statistical significance and clinical usefulness are not the same thing. Although each disease does produce a characteristic pattern of test abnormalities, the patterns overlap considerably. Thus, while LFTs are excellent for suggesting dysfunction, they are of limited value in distinguishing between types of liver disease, except within broad categories. Like all laboratory tests, LFTs are of greatest value when interpreted in light of the clinical findings and impressions.

Another important limitation of LFTs is that published sensitivity and specificity figures potentially overstate the value of the tests. Ideally, LFTs should identify disease that is otherwise inapparent, but disease prevalence actually is lower in a population *without* clinical evidence of disease than in a population *with* clinical manifestations. Also, the predictive value of a positive result decreases with a decrease in disease prevalence because specificity is almost never 100%. Thus, LFT results have the poorest predictive value in patients without clinical evidence of disease, and these are the patients in whom testing may provide the only clue to early disease! Furthermore, patients without clinical evidence of disease may carry a lower disease burden that may not be detectable by less sensitive tests.[20]

Specific Tests

Aspartate Aminotransferase

The aminotransferases catalyze the transfer of an amino group from an amino acid to a keto acid. Aspartate aminotransferase (AST), which catalyzes a transfer from aspartate to alpha-ketoglutarate, is found in highest concentration in heart, followed by liver, skeletal muscle, kidneys, and pancreas. One isoenzyme of AST is found in mitochondria and another is found in cytosol, but measurement of AST isoenzyme activity is not clinically useful. Although serum AST lacks specificity for liver disease, it is a highly sensitive indicator of acute hepatocyte necrosis and a somewhat less sensitive indicator of infiltrative or cholestatic disorders. The magnitude of the rise of AST typically does not correlate with prognosis and may not correlate with the extent of damage seen under the microscope. Specificity for liver disease may improve 90% when AST values exceed five times the upper reference limit (typically 30–40 U/L). Simultaneous measurement of alanine aminotransferase and creatine kinase (CPK) may further improve specificity, prognostication, and differential diagnosis. Unfortunately, lysis of 1% of erythrocytes will increase apparent AST by 200% because AST activity in red cells is 40 times greater than in serum.

ALANINE AMINOTRANSFERASE

Alanine aminotransferase (ALT), which catalyzes the transfer of an amino group from alanine to alpha-ketoglutarate, is widely distributed in tissues, but unlike AST, ALT is found in highest concentration in the liver. Hepatocellular ALT activity is greater than that of AST in cytosol, but ALT is not present in significant amounts in mitochondria. Overall, liver cells contain three times as much AST as ALT. Serum AST and ALT values that both exceed 10 times the reference limit are virtually diagnostic of severe liver cell damage. If both values are increased to the same extent, liver disease is likely because most other organs having AST in high concentrations have relatively little ALT.[21]

GAMMA-GLUTAMYL TRANSPEPTIDASE

Gamma-glutamyl transpeptidase (GGT) is a membrane-bound glycoprotein involved in the transport of amino acids across membranes and in the cleavage of glutathione to glutamic acid and cysteinylglycine. GGT is most abundant in the brush border of renal tubular cells, but serum GGT is not increased in renal disease. GGT is also found in liver, pancreas, duodenum, and endothelial cells, and normal serum activity is derived primarily from the liver, where the enzyme is found on the canalicular surface and in the microsomes. Therefore, increased serum GGT most often is observed with canalicular damage and with exposure to ethanol, barbiturates, phenytoin, carbamazepine, and other agents that induce microsomal enzymes. The pattern of alcohol consumption may influence the rise in serum GGT; binge drinkers and those who consume less than 2–3 drinks per day are less likely to have increased GGT than chronic, heavy drinkers. Increased GGT also is reported in biliary tract and infiltrative disease, and extrahepatic obstruction tends to produce greater increases than intrahepatic obstruction. GGT is a highly sensitive indicator of liver disease—a GGT value within the reference range not only provides strong evidence against liver disease but also suggests that the liver is not the source of a rise in serum alkaline phosphatase.

ALKALINE PHOSPHATASE

Alkaline phosphatase (ALP), which catalyzes the hydrolysis of phosphate esters at an alkaline pH, is a plasma membrane-bound enzyme required for energy-dependent transfer of substances across cell membranes. Serum ALP activity is derived primarily from liver, bone, intestine, and placenta, with each source producing a different isoenzyme. At canalicular surfaces in the liver, ALP requires zinc as a cofactor to be able to transport substances in bile.[22] When the canalicular surfaces of hepatocytes are injured by viruses, drugs, or obstruction, ALP synthesis increases and serum levels rise in 1–2 days. The extent of increased ALP activity reflects both increased synthesis and decreased biliary secretion with regurgitation into blood. In patients with infiltrative disease or localized, incomplete, or intermittent obstruction, increased ALP may not be accompanied by hyperbilirubinemia because the noninvolved liver tissue can more readily excrete the smaller (regurgitated) bilirubin molecule.

Serum ALP is a sensitive indicator of cholestatic and/or infiltrative disorders, but ALP is not specific for liver disease. Analysis of ALP isoenzymes may improve specificity if the laboratory has an accurate and reliable method for separating and measuring the liver, bone, placental, and intestinal fractions. The lack of a consensus reference range makes interpretation of serum ALP difficult. Age, gender, diet, and secretor status influence ALP activity. The best indicator of "normal" is a patient's own prior laboratory values.

BILIRUBIN

Unconjugated bilirubin (loosely bound to albumin) is the orange-yellow waste product of heme metabolism that is transported to the liver from the reticuloendothelial system. Hepatocytes attach two molecules of glucuronic acid to each bilirubin molecule to form conjugated bilirubin. The water-soluble diglucuronide is secreted into the bile and passes into the intestine. A relatively constant percentage of bilirubin is converted to colorless urobilinogen by bacteria, and the urobilinogen is reabsorbed and subsequently excreted into the bile (enterohepatic circulation). Excess urobilinogen is excreted in the urine. When excretion of bilirubin into bile is blocked, it passively diffuses into plasma, where a portion is covalently bound to albumin to form biliprotein or delta-bilirubin.

Unconjugated bilirubin should be the only form of bilirubin found in the sera of patients free of hepatobiliary disease. By contrast, all four types of bilirubin (unconjugated, monoglucuronide, diglucuronide, and biliprotein) may be detected in sera from diseased patients. Most laboratories, however, do not report the concentration of each fraction. Rather, they report total, direct, and indirect bilirubin concentrations. Total bilirubin reflects all bilirubin fractions and is measured by adding caffeine or methanol to accelerate the reaction of water-insoluble bilirubin with aqueous diazotized sulfanilic acid to form a colored product. Direct bilirubin reflects the end-product of directly mixing serum and diazo reagent (without adding an accelerator), while indirect bilirubin is indirectly calculated by subtracting direct bilirubin from total bilirubin. Direct bilirubin does not equal conjugated bilirubin because 5% of unconjugated, 70–90% of conjugated, and 100% of delta-bilirubin will react "directly."

Total bilirubin is a nonspecific and insensitive test for liver disease, whereas direct bilirubin is a highly sensitive and specific indicator of hepatic dysfunction. In patients with increased production or decreased conjugation of bilirubin, the unconjugated fraction accumulates and the total and indirect bilirubin concentrations increase. Common causes of unconjugated hyperbilirubinemia include hemolysis, hematomas, rhabdomyolysis, and Gilbert syndrome.[23] By contrast, when excretion of conjugated bilirubin is impaired, both conjugated and delta-bilirubin accumulate and cause a greater increase in direct bilirubin. With chronic defects, the proportion of delta-bilirubin increases.[24] Direct hyperbilirubinemia, which occurs when the direct fraction is more than 20% of the total, is frequent in patients with liver cell necrosis, intrahepatic cholestasis, and extrahepatic cholestasis, but the extent of the rise does not correlate well with the severity of disease.

Urine bilirubin usually parallels serum conjugated bilirubin because binding of unconjugated bilirubin by albumin prevents urinary excretion of the indirect fraction.[25] Urine urobilinogen typically rises with increased bilirubin production and falls in posthepatic jaundice, a condition in which less bilirubin reaches the intestine.[26]

OTHER TESTS OF LIVER FUNCTION

Regarding other tests of hepatic function, serum bile acid concentrations rarely add useful information if liver disease has already been detected by other tests. Increased bile acid values may, however, indicate liver disease when other LFTs are unremarkable. Prothrombin times and serum albumin values are not sensitive measures of liver disease, but they can reflect significantly impaired synthetic function.

Serum globulin concentrations are highest in chronic active (autoimmune) hepatitis, and determination of the predominant immunoglobulin class may help distinguish among primary biliary cirrhosis (IgM), chronic active hepatitis (IgG), and alcoholic liver disease (IgA).

Viral Hepatitis Testing

Chemical, serologic, and molecular tests can help the physician distinguish viral hepatitis from other causes of liver injury. In patients infected with hepatitis A virus (HAV), serum aminotransferase concentrations often exceed 1000 U/L at the time of presentation. The total serum bilirubin rises, and most of it is direct-reacting, reflecting the capacity of the liver to conjugate but not excrete bilirubin. The detection of HAV-IgM antibodies usually indicates infection within the preceding 6 months. When the IgM assay is negative, increased total anti-HAV reflects the lifelong presence of HAV-IgG, which confers protection against reinfection, confirms recent or remote HAV infection, confirms receipt of HAV vaccine, or confirms receipt of immune globulin prophylaxis within the preceding 2 months.[27]

In patients infected with hepatitis B virus (HBV), the HBV surface antigen (HBsAg) is detected in serum during active viral replication. Antibody to HBsAg (anti-HBs) reflects effective, but incomplete, clearance of the infection. HBsAg may become undetectable several weeks before the appearance of measurable anti-HBs. This "window period" probably reflects the inability of many assays to detect low concentrations of antigen and antibody during seroconversion. When HBsAg and anti-HBs are detected simultaneously, the antibody is not protective and the patient should be considered to have active HBV infection.

HBV core antigen, which is not detectable in serum, elicits anti-core IgM (anti-HBc IgM) and total anti-core antibody (anti-HBc total). Anti-HBc IgM aids the diagnosis of HBV infection because it may be detected during the previously mentioned "window period" and because it can help distinguish acute from chronic HBV infection in patients with transaminasemia and detectable HBsAg. Patients with acute HBV infection have relatively high titers of anti-HBc IgM, and patients with chronic HBV typically have low titers. Like anti-HBs, anti-HBc total indicates prior HBV exposure and typically persists indefinitely, but anti-HBc total does not enable the physician to distinguish immunity from chronic low-grade infection.

The detection of hepatitis B e antigen (HBeAg) in serum is no longer used to establish infectivity in patients with HBV. On the other hand, HBeAg and anti-HBe testing may be used to evaluate flares of disease or to identify patients with active viral replication who may be candidates for interferon therapy. Direct measurement of serum HBV-DNA has been advocated for predicting and evaluating the response to interferon treatment.

In patients infected with hepatitis C virus (HCV), a second-generation enzyme immunoassay (EIA-2) detects antibodies to the c100-3, c33c, and c22-3 viral antigens. The EIA-2 has adequate specificity in patients with transaminasemia and identifiable risk factors for HCV. However, in those with a low pretest probability of HCV infection, confirmatory tests are required because the EIA-2 produces significant numbers of false positive results, especially in patients with autoimmune hepatitis or chronic alcoholism. The two confirmatory tests are the second-generation recombinant immunoblot assay (RIBA-2) and the detection of viral RNA in blood by polymerase chain reaction (PCR). The sensitivities and specificities of both tests exceed 90%. Many physicians rely on the RIBA-2 for confirmation of HCV and use PCR to sort out the occasional indeterminate RIBA-2 result. False negative EIA-2 results may occur during the first 6 months of HCV infection or in patients who are immunosuppressed or receiving dialysis. When the index of suspicion is high and the EIA-2 is negative, PCR testing is appropriate. Serum transaminases in patients with chronic HCV infection can range from normal to four times the upper limit of the reference range, whereas serum bilirubin and alkaline phosphatase typically fall within the reference range. In general, transaminasemia associated with acute viral (HAV, HBV, HCV) injury returns to normal over several weeks, whereas transaminasemia associated with toxic or ischemic insults normalizes in hours to days.

THYROID SCREENING

Some occupational health services offer screening for thyroid conditions. The advent of sensitive TSH (sTSH) assays in the 1980s caused a shift from a thyroxine (T_4)-based testing strategy to one that is sTSH-based.[28] The American Thyroid Association has recommended that "measurement of serum TSH level, complemented by an appropriate free thyroxine index (FT_4I) estimate, represents the best and most efficient combination of blood tests for the diagnosis and follow-up of most patients with thyroid disorders."[29]

Commercially available sTSH assays vary in their level of analytic sensitivity. "First-generation" assays detect TSH only to a limit of 1.0 milli-international units (mIU) per liter. Second-generation tests can detect to 0.1 mIU/L, while third- and fourth-generation assays can detect to 0.01 mIU/L and 0.001 mIU/L, respectively. In most patients, the first- and second-generation assays are sufficient to diagnose hyperthyroidism when TSH is low and free T_4 (FT_4I) is increased. However, when the clinical presentation and laboratory values are not as clear-cut, the third- and fourth-generation tests may offer significant additional information.

For example, using the newer tests, clinically hyperthyroid patients typically have serum TSH concentrations below 0.005 mIU/L. As many as 10% of hospitalized or chronically ill persons may have depressed serum TSH but no definable thyroid disease.[30] In sick euthyroid patients, the sTSH by second-generation assay may fall below 0.1 mIU/L. Third-generation tests show that the depressed sTSH values in these patients fall only slightly below the 0.1 mIU/L detection limit.[31] Thus, some physicians may wish to use the third- or fourth-generation assays to distinguish a sick euthyroid individual (with a slightly depressed sTSH) from a hyperthyroid individual with a significantly depressed sTSH, especially if these newer tests eliminate the need for further work-up of a patient who lacks thyroid disease.[32]

Importantly, the functional sensitivity and specificity of the newer immunometric sTSH tests may not be as great as some manufacturers claim. Nevertheless, assays claiming "third-generation sensitivity" (0.01–0.02 mIU/L) may have a lower incidence of miscalculations of low TSH sera as "normal" compared to second-generation (0.1–0.2 mIU/L) assays.[33] In 1997, several large reference laboratories routinely perform second-generation tests, while third- and fourth-generation tests are limited to samples with a TSH concentration below 0.1 mIU/L.

CREATINE PHOSPHOKINASE VERSUS TROPONIN

An ideal biochemical marker of myocardial injury would (1) be found in high concentration in the myocardium, (2) not be found in other tissues, (3) be released rapidly and completely after myocardial injury, (4) be released in direct proportion to the extent of the myocardial injury, and (5) persist in plasma for several hours to provide a convenient diagnostic time window but not so long that recurrent injury would not be identified.[34] Several less-than-ideal markers have surfaced in the last 25 years. Some are commercially available and widely used (e.g., creatine kinase, heart-specific CK isoenzymes, myoglobin, lactate dehydrogenase), while others have been more recently introduced into clinical use (e.g., troponin-T, troponin-I, glycogen-phosphorylase-b). One or more of these markers may have clinical utility for the diagnosis of acute myocardial infarction (AMI), for the noninvasive detection of coronary artery recanalization after treatment with thrombolytic agents, or for the early identification of cardiovascular events in unstable angina.[35]

Measurement of cardiac troponin subunits I and T has been proposed frequently as an alternative to traditional testing for the MB isoenzyme of creatine kinase (CK-MB). In the last 5 years, dozens of hospital-based clinical laboratories have supplemented or replaced CK-MB tests with analyses of troponin-I or troponin-T. The role of these cardiac injury markers must be clearly understood by practitioners of occupational medicine.

Troponin is the contractile regulatory protein complex that interacts with tropomyosin along the thin filaments of striated myofibrils. Troponin is a complex of three proteins: troponin I (cTnI), which inhibits the coupling of actin to myosin; troponin T (cTnT), which binds the tri-protein complex to tropomyosin; and troponin C (cTnC), which binds to calcium, induces a steric shift, and reverses the inhibitory activity of cTnI. There are tissue-specific isoforms of the troponins, and cardiac myocytes contain a minor cytosolic and a major myofibrillary-bound fraction. While cTnI is highly specific for cardiac muscle, cTnT is found in skeletal muscle during human development and has recently been identified in patients with polymyositis or Duchenne muscular dystrophy.[36] Importantly, in patients who do not have cardiac disease, serum cTnI and cTnC values are low or undetectable.

The concentrations of cTnI and cTnT increase above the reference range within 4–8 hours of the onset of chest pain due to myocardial ischemia. Values peak at 12–48 hours and remain increased for 9 days. By contrast, CK-MB values increase 4–8 hours after onset of pain of cardiac origin, peak within 16–24 hours, and normalize in 48–72 hours. The troponins are bound mostly to myofibrils (97%), while CK-MB is virtually all free in the cytoplasm. Thus, the initial release kinetics of both markers may reflect cytoplasmic release of free protein, while slow continuous release of myofibril-bound protein may account for prolonged increases over several days.[37]

Many studies show that the sensitivity of cTnI for detection of AMI is equal to that of CK-MB.[38] Moreover, the cardiac specificity and duration of elevation after infarction make cTnI an ideal replacement for LDH isoenzymes to rule out AMI with a delayed presentation. Measurement of cTnI will likely replace CK-MB testing whenever the specificity of CK-MB is in doubt, as in polymyositis, muscular dystrophy, chronic renal failure with dialysis, or any cause of acute or chronic muscle injury.

For the diagnosis of AMI in the first 48 hours, cTnT has a similar sensitivity but lower specificity and diagnostic efficiency than CK-MB.[39] The value of this sensitivity is impaired, however, because the specificity of cTnT is poor when skeletal muscle is regenerating; thus, measurement of cTnI is preferred in this subset of patients. Both cTnT and cTnI are useful indicators of prognosis in unstable angina.[40] The cumulative 6-month probability of suffering cardiac death or AMI may be significantly higher in the subgroup of ischemic heart disease patients with serum cTnT concentrations exceeding 0.2 μg/l.

TOXICOLOGIC TESTING

Testing in General

Although most toxicologic diagnoses and therapeutic decisions are based on clinical assessment, laboratory analysis of body fluids can improve management in selected patients.[41] In acute toxicologic episodes, the time required for analysis often exceeds the critical time course of the illness; thus, the clinical value of laboratory testing is severely limited. By contrast, in patients with chronic exposures, selective testing may not only aid diagnosis and treatment but may be required by law. Physicians treating work-related health problems in America today must understand that the cost of maintaining procedures, instruments, and appropriately trained personnel cannot justify toxicologic testing in more than a few hundred laboratories nationwide.[42]

Monitoring, diagnostic confirmation, and screening are the three basic reasons for requesting a laboratory test in the care of patients with actual or potential exposure to toxic agents. Each reason is associated with a different clinical setting, a different "prior probability" that the test condition exists, and a different analytic attribute necessary for analysis. In monitoring a patient, the change in a highly prevalent test condition (e.g., the body fluid concentration of a therapeutic drug) is being followed. Thus, analytic precision, or ability to detect a change, is required of the test. For example, detection of altered theophylline concentrations in patients who develop abnormal liver function requires a precise test.

By contrast, tests that confirm a diagnosis are performed when multiple diagnoses, including toxicologic disorders, are being considered. Analytic specificity is required to accurately categorize the patient's condition among a few diagnostic alternatives, assuming that moderate prior probabilities of these alternative conditions are present. Such diagnostic confirmatory testing may help the clinician determine whether the patient's condition is due, at least in part, to the presence of one or more drugs or toxic agents.

In the process of screening in general, there typically is no prior suspicion of exposure or preselection of patients with a greater risk of exposure. All persons are tested for the presence of a low-prevalence condition, such as phenylketonuria or the presence of illicit substances, that is often difficult to detect clinically. Finding all cases of the test condition (i.e., maximizing sensitivity) is given highest priority so that effective intervention becomes possible. Low rates of false positives (nonspecificity) are tolerated because the results can be excluded or confirmed by secondary testing.[43]

The prevalence or prior probability of an agent's presence in body fluids strongly influences the reliability (i.e., the posterior probability or predictive value of a positive or negative test) at a given sensitivity and specificity. For example, in employee populations with low prior probability of drug presence, screening methods are adapted for increasing sensitivity (by detecting low concentrations) while maintaining adequate specificity for only 5–10 substances.[44] Without such modifications, the ratio of false positives to true positives would be unacceptably high in this low-prevalence setting (low positive predictive value but high negative predictive value). By contrast, in toxicologic emergencies where clinical suspicion suggests high prior probabilities of analyte presence, testing is designed to increase specificity by identifying more substances at higher concentrations while excluding others. Similarly, in cases involving a medical examiner, the acquisition of drug paraphernalia or other nonlaboratory evidence also increases the prior probability of drug presence as a factor in the cause of death. Although postmortem tissue changes may influence analyte detection, body fluid concentrations of drugs or toxins are often very high in death cases, and therefore sensitivity may not be given highest priority. Finally, in methadone maintenance programs, drug testing occurs in selected populations with high prior probabilities not only of a drug's presence but also of high concentrations of a small number of drugs, such as opiates or opioids.

Techniques

Drug identification or quantitation by chemical "spot" or color tests, spectrometry, immunoassay, or chromatography requires at least two steps. First, the analyte must be isolated from the biomatrix (e.g., blood, hair, sweat, tissue, or urine), which may contain agents that interfere with analysis. Second, the analyte must be characterized by matching the properties or behaviors of the unknown substance with those of valid reference compounds.

Chemical spot or color tests, which rely on the chemical reactivity of the analyte with specific reagents, are often used for direct, rapid, and easy but nonspecific detection of salicylates, metals, phenothiazines, and other agents in selected toxicologic emergencies.

Spectrophotometric assays, which may require a chemical reaction to convert the target drug to a light-absorbing species, provide acceptable accuracy for measurement of metals, carboxyhemoglobin, methemoglobin, cyanide, salicylates, borates, and acetaminophen. In particular, atomic absorption spectrophotometry and inductively coupled plasma atomic emission spectroscopy have become the mainstays of metal analysis. The use of spectrophotometry for some analytes has decreased, however, because various interferences have been described.[45]

Immunoassays, which currently measure at least 12 drugs in serum and 10 drugs or classes of drugs in urine, rely on specific antibodies that bind either to drug in a patient's sample or to "labeled" drug added to that sample. (Labeled drug is bound to an enzyme, a solid matrix, or to a fluorescent so-called "reporter" molecule.) As the concentration of drug in the patient's sample increases, the amount of antibody that binds to known concentrations of labeled drug decreases. Measurable endpoints include products of enzymatic catalysis in EIA or EMIT by Syva, aggregation-light transmission in KIMS by Roche, and fluorescence polarization in TDX by Abbott. Prepackaged, disposable immunoassays have been marketed for onsite patient testing, but the validity, reliability, and clinical utility of these devices have not been fully established.[46] Onsite devices may provide speed and convenience for health care professionals, but there is no evidence that patient outcomes are significantly improved.

Chromatographic assays are used for monitoring, screening, and diagnostic confirmation. Following isolation of drug from biomatrix, chemical derivatization may be necessary to produce molecules compatible with some chromatographic phases or detection systems.[47] Derivatized extract is then separated from other solutes as the constituents of the mobile phase differentially interact with the chromatographic stationary phase. The most common types of chromatography are thin-layer chromatography (TLC), high performance liquid chromatography (HPLC), and gas chromatography (GC).

In TLC, extracted drugs are spotted and dried onto a plate typically coated with silica gel. This plate is then placed in a closed chamber that contains a predetermined mixture of organic solvents. As solvent migrates up the plate, analytes are separated because they differentially interact with silica gel and solvent and move at different rates. Finally, the plate is sprayed or otherwise exposed to suitable reagents that allow as many as 30 drugs to be identified by color and specific positioning relative to comigrated reference compounds, or "standards." Although the combination of migration distance and staining characteristics endows TLC with specificity that may not be achieved with more elaborate procedures, the sensitivity of TLC varies with drug, detection method, and amount of starting material and seldom falls below 1.0 mg/L.

In HPLC, nonvolatile compounds are separated within tightly packed columns. High pressures (1000–6000 psi) must be applied to these columns to elute molecules for detection. Columns are typically packed with polar phases (silica gel) or nonpolar phases (alkyl groups) bonded to small particles. Polar phases are eluted with organic solvents while nonpolar phases are eluted with solvents miscible in aqueous buffers. When a mixture is injected onto the column, each component is partitioned between the stationary phase (column) and the mobile phase (liquid). Molecules with greater affinity for the column packing spend more time in that phase and therefore take longer to reach the detector. As they leave the column, drugs are detected using refractometry, conductivity, electrochemical (redox) reactions, or the absorption of ultraviolet light. The detector responds in direct proportion to the concentration of material passing through it; thus, peak heights and areas shown on the chromatogram are directly related to the concentration of each analyte. Concentrations of 0.01–1.0 mg/L are routinely measured by comparing the amplitudes of sample peaks with those of "internal" standard compounds added in constant amounts to all specimens. Drug identifications typically are based on retention times, which reflect the interval from injection to the recorded peak maximum. The high selectivity or resolving capacity of HPLC makes it especially useful for identifying or quantitating specified drugs or for screening classes of structurally similar compounds. Importantly, the range of substances identifiable by HPLC can be expanded using multiple columns or gradient systems that change the composition of eluting solvent during a single run.

In GC, injected extracts, mixtures, or their derivatives are vaporized (80°–300°C) and then forced through the column by an inert gas.[48] The components of the mobile vapor phase interact with the "liquid" stationary phase, and the analytes are separated along the length of the column. Drugs are detected using ionization, thermal conductivity, combustibility, electron donation, or capture of beta particles. Detection limits vary from 0.1–0.5 mg/L. GC is frequently combined with mass spectrometry (GC-MS), where effluent gases from the GC are ionized and fragmented following bombardment by electron beams. GC-MS provides great specificity because it produces a unique set of molecular fragments for each eluting drug. When only the unique fragments are monitored, sensitivity may extend to the nanogram per liter range.[49]

Preferred Biomatrices

Urine is the preferred specimen for drug analysis because (1) large volumes are easily and noninvasively collected and analyzed, (2) molecules typically are present in higher concentrations than in other bodily fluids, and (3) analytes usually are stable for weeks to months in frozen samples. Analysis of hair is more controversial. Hair is an attractive specimen for analysis because it is easy to collect, preserve, and store and because many drugs are stable in hair for weeks. Unfortunately, it is not always clear whether the drug originates from inside the hair shaft or from external contamination.[50] Compounds that have been detected in hair include cocaine, cocaethylene, amphetamines, phencyclidine, cannabinoids, codeine, morphine, monoacetylmorphine, heroin, fentanyl, barbiturates, antidepressants, meprobamate, ephedrine, buprenorphine, haloperidol, caffeine, and nicotine.[51]

Specific Tests

ALCOHOL

Alcohol is measured in body fluids to screen comatose and other impaired patients, to diagnose alcohol intoxication, to monitor ethanol concentrations during methanol or ethylene glycol intoxication treated with ethanol, and to detect recent ingestion by employees or job applicants. Established methods for ethanol analysis include gas chromatography, freezing-point osmometry, and oxidation by alcohol dehydrogenase, but only GC can reliably separate, identify, and quantitate all of the clinically significant alcohols, which include ethanol, methanol, isopropanol, and ethylene glycol.

Physicians should remember several key points when interpreting alcohol analyses. First, blood concentrations of ethanol may be 15–30% lower (postabsorption) or higher (preabsorption) than tissue or fluid values.[52] Second, urine results should never be used to extrapolate to corresponding blood alcohol concentrations or to determine the level of intoxication or impairment. Third, patients with blood alcohol concentrations of 50–100 mg/dl typically show mild degrees of muscular incoordination, slowed reaction time, visual impairment, emotional lability, and exhilaration.[53]

CARBOXYHEMOGLOBIN

Measurements of blood carboxyhemoglobin (COHb) may be appropriate in the evaluation of headache, irritability, nausea, vomiting, vertigo, dyspnea, collapse, coma, convulsions, or exposure to methylene chloride. COHb determinations also may influence the management of smoke inhalation or fire victims, but this test should not be used to screen workers for tobacco use. Importantly, COHb may reach 10–12% in newborns (elimination is slower than in adults), 8–9% in heavy smokers (> 2 ppd), and 4–5% in other smokers (1–2 ppd), but COHb seldom exceeds 3% in nonsmokers unless they are occupationally exposed in enclosed spaces, near incomplete combustion, or work as toll collectors, tunnel workers, or furniture strippers.

CHOLINESTERASE

Occupational physicians typically rely on cholinesterase measurements to confirm exposure to carbamate or organophosphate pesticides. Two types of cholinesterase are found in blood: (1) acetylcholinesterase (or "true" cholinesterase) in erythrocytes and (2) acylcholine acylhydrolase (or "pseudocholinesterase") in serum or plasma. The cholinesterase activity in human red cells arises during erythropoiesis and primarily hydrolyzes acetylcholine, while the cholinesterase activity in serum/plasma originates in the liver and hydrolyzes both choline and aliphatic esters. Red blood cell (RBC) or serum cholinesterase measurements may facilitate detection of atypical forms of the enzyme or confirm exposure to organophosphate or carbamate pesticides. Inherited low levels of serum cholinesterase have been associated with prolonged anesthesia and apnea following administration of low-dose succinylcholine (0.04–0.06 mg/kg). Determination of dibucaine and fluoride numbers can facilitate the phenotyping of homozygous and heterozygous patients who are sensitive to succinylcholine. Pseudocholinesterase activity also may be decreased following plasmapheresis or estrogen therapy and in patients with cirrhosis, hepatitis, malnutrition, congestive heart failure, or metastases.

Cholinesterase activity is measured by colorimetry, fluorimetry, or spectrophotometry as the rate of hydrolysis of an ester. The organophosphates typically inhibit serum cholinesterase more than RBC cholinesterase, and the serum enzyme activity returns to normal sooner than the RBC enzyme activity.

METHEMOGLOBIN AND SULFHEMOGLOBIN

Methemoglobin (MetHb) is formed when the iron in hemoglobin is oxidized to the trivalent state. MetHb cannot carry oxygen or carbon dioxide, and the presence of oxidized iron decreases oxygen release in tissue. Methemoglobinemia may be caused by the presence of strong oxidizing agents, by variants of hemoglobin M, or by deficiency of NADH-dependent MetHb reductase (diaphorase I), which reduces endogenously formed MetHb back to oxyhemoglobin. Occupational physicians may never see a patient with a hereditary form of methemoglobinemia, but they may encounter cyanosis in some patients who have been exposed to strong oxidizing agents.

MetHb is a dark brown pigment that causes venous blood to appear chocolate in color. Bubbling oxygen through the sample should not change its color, but a crystal of potassium cyanide added to a sample diluted 1:100 with deionized water should produce a pink color due to formation of cyanohemoglobin. In arterial blood, measured O_2 saturation is decreased, but laboratories that calculate O_2 saturation from pO_2 will report normal saturation in samples that contain excess MetHb. Measurement of the MetHb concentration takes advantage of its small but characteristic peak in the absorbance spectrum at 630–635 nm. Addition of cyanide eliminates this peak by converting MetHb to cyanMetHb. The decrease in absorbance is proportional to the MetHb concentration. Any MetHb value exceeding 1.5% of total Hb should be considered abnormal, and cyanosis may be observed at values of 10–15% (unless the patient is severely anemic), but symptoms are unusual in otherwise healthy persons if MetHb values do not exceed 30%.

Unlike MetHb, sulfhemoglobin (SulfHb) is not a normal constituent of blood. The appearance of SulfHb in blood is due to replacement of one nitrogen atom in the pyrrole ring of Hb by one sulfur atom. The in vivo mechanism by which this substitution occurs is not understood, but green SulfHb pigment can be formed in vitro by incubating hemoglobin with an oxidizing agent and a sulfhydryl donor,[54] and SulfHb can be found in concentrations of 1–10% following exposure to oxidant drugs. SulfHb may exist in the Fe(II) or Fe(III) state, and sulfhemoglobin may bind to oxygen or carbon monoxide reversibly. Once formed, SulfHb persists for the life of the red cell.

The normal absorbance spectrum of oxyhemoglobin shows little absorbance above 600 nm. However, if SulfHb is present in a hemolysate, a broad increase in the absorption curve occurs in the range of 600–620 nm. This plateau is not abolished by treatment with cyanide. Any SulfHb value exceeding 0.37–0.50% should be considered abnormal, and SulfHb produces a more intense cyanosis than MetHb, but SulfHb seldom occurs in concentrations that will produce serious hypoxia.[55]

METALS AND TRACE ELEMENTS

Practitioners of occupational medicine occasionally request the detection or quantitation of metals and other trace elements in biologic specimens. Accurate determination of these elements presents special analytic challenges and requires special precautions. The major pre-analytic problem is external contamination. The presence in the laboratory environment of trace metals in nanogram to microgram amounts probably contributes to the wide variation in reported reference values. Common sources of contamination include dandruff, hair, skin, metal surfaces, dust, paper products, rubber, and wood. For valid and reliable trace elemental analysis, current standards of laboratory practice include use of fluorocarbon, polyethylene, or polypropylene plastics; regimented cleaning and rinsing of glassware using metal-scavenging solutions and water that meets the standards of the American Chemical Society; measurement of trace elements in all reagents and anticoagulants; and selective use of stainless steel equipment.

Any method used to measure trace elements in biologic specimens should be sensitive, specific, precise, accurate, and relatively fast. The most popular techniques for analysis of metals include flame photometry, atomic absorption spectrophotometry (AAS), and inductively coupled plasma atomic emission spectroscopy (ICPAES). The method of choice frequently depends on the type of sample as well as the element to be determined.

In *flame photometry*, sodium, potassium, lithium, rubidium, and magnesium atoms supplied with energy from a hot flame will emit this energy at wavelengths or line spectra characteristic for each element. The specific wavelength used to measure each element is one that provides a line both free from interference and of sufficient intensity for reliable detection. Under constant and controlled conditions, the light intensity of the characteristic wavelength produced by each of the atoms is directly proportional to the number of atoms that are emitting energy.[56]

In *atomic absorption spectrophotometry*, diluted serum or plasma is nebulized or aspirated directly into a flame, where the element of interest is dissociated from its chemical bonds and placed in the unexcited, ground, or neutral state, i.e., a low energy level where the atom can absorb narrow bandwidth radiation corresponding to that element's line spectrum.[56] When light of appropriate wavelength (produced by a hollow cathode lamp) enters the flame, some of it is absorbed by the ground state atoms in the flame—hence the term "atomic absorption." As the number of atoms absorbing light increases, the intensity of light reaching a detector decreases. On most instruments, the power to the lamp can be "pulsed" so that light is emitted at a specified number of pulses per second. By contrast, light emerging from the flame is continuous and composed of pulsed unabsorbed light from the lamp, sample emission, and unpulsed flame spectrum. The detector senses all light, but an amplifier that is electrically tuned to accept only pulsed unabsorbed light from the lamp largely excludes the other sources. AAS is considered a sensitive, accurate, precise, and highly specific laboratory test. Chemical, ionization, and matrix interferences have been reduced through improved extraction techniques and the addition of competing ions that facilitate release of the analyte from complexing or chelating anions. Electrothermal, or "flameless," AAS may be used to detect nanogram per gram concentrations in small volume samples (as little as 10 µl).

Unlike AAS, which detects only one element at a time, *inductively coupled plasma atomic emission spectrometry* simultaneously detects up to 20 elements over a 1000-fold linear dynamic range. ICPAES may replace flame AAS as the method of choice for some trace element analyses because ICPAES is more sensitive, accurate, and precise and has fewer interferences. On the other hand, ICPAES requires more rigorous quality assurance, contamination control, and computerized data management.[58]

TESTS OF IMMUNE FUNCTION

Clinical laboratory assessment of the immune response may be appropriate in allergic, autoimmune, infectious, neoplastic, or immunodeficiency disorders. The role of immune function testing in toxicologic and occupational disorders has not been well defined, but the fact that immune cells removed from humans can function in vitro allows the analyst to evaluate the possibility that cellular, biochemical, and molecular changes may be causally related to exposure to environmental agents.

Modern assessment of immunocompetence includes methods designed to (1) characterize and quantitate immunoglobulins, (2) detect and quantitate specific antibodies, (3) evaluate lymphocyte, monocyte, and neutrophil function, (4) assess complement, and (5) examine immediate hypersensitivity. This chapter reviews analytic principles that can help occupational physicians improve their selection and interpretation of these increasingly sophisticated tests.

Immunoglobulins

Commonly employed techniques for assay of immunoglobulins include electrophoresis, immunoprecipitation, and nephelometry. In *zone electrophoresis*, serum proteins migrate at different rates in an electrical field. These molecules separate into five zones or bands, identified as albumin and as alpha-1, alpha-2, beta, and gamma globulin fractions. The concentration of each band is measured by scanning the electrophoretic strip in a densitometer, which is a modified spectrophotometer. This semiquantitative method is used primarily to screen for monoclonality. To identify myeloma, Bence-Jones, or other monoclonal immunoglobulins, analysts use *immunoelectrophoresis*, a two-step technique wherein electrophoretic separation of proteins in a gel is followed by the addition of specific antisera to troughs cut parallel to the separation migration. The antisera diffuse throughout the support medium at right angles to the separated proteins. Interaction between antibody and separated, specific antigens leads to precipitation of antigen-antibody complexes in regions where antigen and antibody concentrations are fairly equal. To enhance the detection of monoclonal proteins in low concentrations in body fluids, *immunofixation electrophoresis* combines electrophoresis with an overlay of monospecific antibodies on the surface of the gel. Precipitated immune complexes can be stained to distinguish the wide (diffuse) bands of polyclonal proteins from the narrow bands of monoclonal or oligoclonal proteins. Immunofixation offers greater sensitivity, more rapid diffusion, and easier interpretation than immunoelectrophoresis, but detection by fixation is poor when excess antigen is present, and proteins with similar electrophoretic mobility are more difficult to distinguish.

To measure the concentration of specific immunoglobulins in body fluids, three techniques have been described: radial immunodiffusion, electroimmunodiffusion, and nephelometry. In *radial immunodiffusion*, a biologic fluid sample is placed in a well cut into agarose that contains specific antiserum. The protein antigen diffuses into the agarose, and an immunoprecipitate forms in the region of antigen-antibody equivalence. Since the antibody level is fixed, the diameter of the precipitin ring varies with antigen concentration. The ring can be evaluated when it has reached its endpoint or at a fixed time prior to reaching endpoint equivalence. In the former, the antigen concentration varies with the square of the ring diameter, and in the latter, the log of the antigen concentration varies with the ring diameter. Commercially available kits have lowered the detection limits to 0.03 milligrams of protein per liter, but radial immunodiffusion is slow (1–3 day turnaround), labor-intensive, and subject to false positive or false negative results in some patients with Waldenstrom's macroglobulinemia, ataxia telangiectasia, IgA deficiency, or high concentrations of IgG rheumatoid factor. *Electroimmunodiffusion*, or "rocket electrophoresis," is a faster variant of radial immunodiffusion in which multiple dilutions of a sample are placed in a series of wells cut in agarose gel containing specific antibody. The samples migrate in an electrical field, and the immunoprecipitates form spurs in the shape of a rocket. The concentration of antigen is directly proportional to the length of the "rocket."

In modern clinical laboratories, immunodiffusion systems have been replaced by automated nephelometers. In *nephelometry,* after a specific antibody is mixed with the biologic fluid containing the antigen of interest, the amount of incident light scattered by immune complexes is measured in the presence of antibody excess, a condition that maintains the complexes in solution. The concentration of antibody added to each sample is constant, and changes in light scatter therefore correlate with changes in antigen concentration. Rate nephelometry measures light scatter associated with the peak rate of immune complex formation, while fixed-time nephelometry measures light scatter at the same time point in all reaction mixtures.

Specific Antibodies

The detection and quantitation of autoantibodies, microorganism-specific antibodies, drug-specific antibodies, and toxin-specific antibodies has become a national obsession. Semiquantitative methods include immunodiffusion, immunodiffusion with electrophoresis, agglutination, indirect immunofluorescence, and Western blotting. The preferred method of quantitation is the enzyme immunoassay (EIA).

In Ouchterlony *immunodiffusion*, sample or control antibodies are placed in wells surrounding a central well cut in agarose. As antibodies diffuse into the support medium, they immunoprecipitate with antigen diffusing from the center well. The pattern formed at the intersection of the reference antibody-antigen precipitin band and the sample antibody-antigen precipitin band is then evaluated. Fusion of the bands at the point of intersection means a "reaction of identity," crossing of both bands means "nonidentity," and crossing of only one band means "partial identity." Two-dimensional double gel immunodiffusion is a fast, easy, and highly specific screening test that does not require purified antigen preparations.

"Counter" immunoelectrophoresis (CIE) is a combination of *immunodiffusion with electrophoresis*. Antigen is placed in a cathodal well and antibody into an anodal well within a gel. In an electric field, negatively charged antigen moves toward the anode, while relatively neutral antibody migrates toward the cathode due to endosmotic flow. Compared to the passive immunodiffusion of Ouchterlony, the active immunodiffusion of CIE provides faster turnaround. CIE has been used primarily for diagnosis of infectious diseases, and Ouchterlony has been used to detect Sm, SS-A, SS-B, ribonucleoprotein, and other autoantibodies.

One antibody molecule may combine simultaneously with more than one antigen molecule to cause visible clumping or *agglutination*. Direct agglutination assays typically use red cells that express the antigen of interest, whereas indirect assays rely on latex spheres or other inert particles coated with antigen. Various dilutions of sample are incubated with a source of antigen and observed for the presence of visible clumping. Agglutination assays are used routinely for RBC crossmatching and the detection of rheumatoid factor and CMV antibody.

Antibodies to antigens expressed on a solid phase also can be detected using *indirect immunofluorescence*. Cultured cells or tissue fixed on a glass slide are overlaid with sample to allow specific antibodies to bind to tissue antigens. The slide is washed and treated with a fluorochrome-labeled antibody to human immunoglobulin. Anti-nuclear, anti-centromere, and antiviral antibodies can then be detected with reasonable sensitivity using a fluorescence microscope.

The *Western blot* is a semiquantitative but extremely sensitive technique that can identify 10–100 pg (10^{-12} g) of protein and simultaneously characterize the pattern of antibody reactivity to multiple distinct antigens.[59] Following electrophoretic separation in sodium dodecyl sulfate-polyacrylamide gel, proteins are transferred (blotted) from the gel to nitrocellulose paper, cyanogen-bromide activated paper, or a cationized nylon-based membrane. These synthetic membranes adsorb or covalently bind proteins over a wide range of concentrations. The patient's sample is overlaid on the membrane containing the separated antigens. Specific antibody bound to appropriate antigen is then detected using radioactive or enzyme-labeled antibody directed against human immunoglobulin. The general location and molecular weight of the separated protein antigens are known, and a control membrane is stained with colloidal gold or amido black to identify the specific location of these antigens.

Enzyme immunoassay uses the catalytic properties of enzymes to detect and quantitate immunologic reactions. Two types of EIA are commercially available: the indirect assay and the "sandwich" assay. The indirect method most often is used to detect antibodies by allowing a biologic fluid to bind to antigen that coats polystyrene beads, tubes, or microtiter plates (solid phase). The bound immunoglobulin is detected by adding an enzyme-labeled anti-human immunoglobulin followed by a chromogenic substrate to produce a color. Washing is required between each individual step to remove unbound reactants. The optical density of the colored end-product is proportional to the antibody concentration. In the alternative "sandwich" technique, the patient's antibodies are detected by adding an enzyme-labeled antigen rather than anti-human immunoglobulin. The sandwich assay also can be used to detect antigen by initially binding antigen-specific antibody onto the solid phase prior to adding patient sample, enzyme-labeled specific antibody, and chromogenic substrate. EIAs are highly sensitive tests, but all solid phase assays are plagued by nonspecific binding to the solid phase, which can be reduced using specific blocking steps.

HIV Testing

The most widely used test for confirmation of the diagnosis of HIV infection involves detection of antibodies to proteins unique to the human immunodeficiency virus. The most widely used screening test is the enzyme immunoassay. Several variations of EIA for HIV are commercially available. A positive result requires that the serum be retested to confirm the reaction. Sensitivities and specificities in excess of 99% are reported for EIA.

All positive EIA results are confirmed by Western blot analysis. Not all Western blots produce unequivocal results. The test is not interpreted as positive unless there are multiple protein bands that can be considered truly independent.[60] Various criteria have been suggested for determination of positive Western blots;[61] unfortunately, the lack of uniformity among laboratories in applying these criteria has made comparison among test results difficult. Indeterminate Western blots with only 1 or 2 bands occur in 10–20% of sera that are reactive by EIA.[62] The risk of developing AIDS for persons with a repeatedly reactive EIA and an indeterminate Western blot depends on the risk factors for that individual. If there are no risk factors for HIV infection, the patient does not require further follow-up. False positive and false negative Western blots do occur, but they are rare.

Both EIA and Western blot detect antibodies in the patient's serum. Since these antibodies may not appear in serum for at least 6 weeks after initial exposure to HIV, other techniques must be used to diagnose acute HIV infection. Viral cultures provide a sensitive method for detecting HIV, but culture is cumbersome, costly, and currently confined to research laboratories. Perhaps the most widely used test for diagnosing acute HIV infection is the p24 antigen test. This viral protein is the first marker to be detected in serum, often within a few days of infection. Unfortunately, despite its high specificity, the p24 test is not considered particularly sensitive.

Autoantibodies

The clinical relevance of the detection and quantitation of autoantibodies is not well understood. The development of immunologic responsiveness to self is called autoimmunity and reflects the impairment of self-tolerance. Central to the concept of autoimmunity is a breakdown in the ability of the immune system to distinguish between self and nonself antigens. Autoimmunity was classically interpreted as an abnormal immune response that invariably caused disease. However, it is now clear that autoimmune responses are common and are necessary for the regulation of the immune system.[63] For example, the normal development of anti-idiotype antibodies (antibodies against immunoglobulins), which serve as regulatory proteins for the immune response, is by definition an autoimmune response. Thus, the regulated production of autoantibodies is a normal event.[63] By contrast, when these regulatory mechanisms are altered, the *uncontrolled* production of autoantibodies, or the appearance of abnormal cell-cell interactions, may produce disease. The mere presence of autoantibodies, however, is not sufficient to make a diagnosis of autoimmune disease—there must be evidence that the autoimmune reaction is a cause (and not an epiphenomenon[66] or effect) of an objectively verifiable disease process.

As noted above, autoantibodies can be found in the serum or tissues of many normal individuals. Apparently, innocuous autoantibodies also are formed following damage to tissue and may serve a physiologic role in the removal of tissue breakdown products. Thus, it is difficult to distinguish normal, physiologic autoimmunity from pathologic autoimmunity. Ideally, at least three requirements should be met before a disorder can be categorized as truly due to autoimmunity. These include (1) the presence of an autoimmune reaction, (2) clinical or experimental evidence that such a reaction is not secondary to tissue damage but is of primary pathogenetic significance, and (3) the absence of another well-defined cause of the disease.[65]

An abnormal immune response to self-antigens implies that there is a loss of immune tolerance, which is best viewed as an active process in which the immune response is blocked by inhibitory molecules. There are various ways by which tolerance can be lost or bypassed, thus terminating a previously unresponsive state to autoantigens. Among the most popular theories explaining the loss of tolerance are (1) polyclonal B-cell activation, in which B lymphocytes are directly activated by complex substances that contain many antigenic sites, such as bacteria and viruses; (2) abnormal T-cell function, including alterations in the number or functional activities of helper or suppressor T cells; (3) biologic mimicry, where antibodies formed against foreign antigens are found to cross-react with self-antigens; and (4) reactions to sequestered antigens, where antibodies are produced when self-antigens typically not present in the circulation are released into the bloodstream following tissue injury. Although some evidence suggests that a numerical decrease in suppressor T-cells may be a contributing factor in autoimmune diseases, the precise role (if any) of the other hypotheses in the causation of autoimmune disorders remains to be determined. Most importantly, occupational physicians who request laboratory tests of immune function should not base a diagnosis of an occupational or environmental autoimmune disorder merely on reported symptoms and the presence of antibodies to either foreign- or self-antigens. It also deserves emphasis that current scientific information does not enable the occupational physician to determine if the result of any laboratory test of immune function represents a cause, effect, or epiphenomenon in the context of potentially work-related health problems.[66]

AUTOMATED COMPLETE BLOOD COUNTS

The automated complete blood count (CBC) currently has 10 parameters: the white blood cell count (WBC), red blood cell count (RBC), hemoglobin (HGB), hematocrit (HCT), mean cell volume of red cells (MCV), mean cell hemoglobin content (MCH), mean cell hemoglobin concentration (MCHC), red cell distribution width (RDW), platelet count (PLT), and mean platelet volume (MPV). Analysis begins with the automatic aspiration of a specific amount (up to 300 µl) of a well-mixed blood specimen. Following automated assessment of specimen integrity (absence of clots) and adequacy, the aspirated specimen is aliquoted, diluted with appropriate diluent(s) with or without the added red cell lysing agent, and channeled to specific counting chambers (or baths or flow cells) for actual cell counting and sizing, and to a cuvette for hemoglobin quantitation by the spectrophotometric cyan-methemoglobin method.[67]

Modern analyzers count and size cells using electrical impedance or light scattering technology. *Impedance* instruments allow diluted blood sample to flow through a small aperture located between two sensing electrodes. As each cell passes through the aperture, a momentary increase in impedance is recorded in the form of an electrical pulse. The amplitude of each pulse is proportional to the cell volume, and the number of pulses generated is proportional to the number of cells passing through the aperture. Different cell populations are categorized on the basis of cell volume. The RBC count is based on the number of pulses of cell size exceeding 36 fl, while PLT counts are based on a size range of 2–20 fl. In the hemolyzed aliquot, the WBC count is determined by the number of pulses of cell size exceeding 35 fl. The mean size of all pulses included in the RBC histogram is reported as the MCV, and the coefficient of variation (CV) or standard deviation (SD) of the distribution of RBC pulses is reported as the RDW. Similarly, the MPV reflects the mean size of all pulses included in the PLT histogram, and platelet distribution width (PDW) (not reported) can be computed as the CV or SD of the distribution of pulses composing the PLT histogram.[68] The HCT, MCH, and MCHC are calculated (not measured) values.[69]

Light-scattering instruments hydrodynamically focus a specific amount of diluted blood sample in a flow cell that is illuminated by a narrow beam of light. As a cell passes through the sensing zone (lighted area) of the flow cell, it scatters light that is photodetected and converted to an electrical pulse whose amplitude is proportional to the cell volume. The number of pulses generated is proportional to the number of cells passing through the sensing zone. In the Technicon light-scatter analyzer, red cells are isovolumetrically sphered and fixed prior to their passage through the sensing zone. The data are displayed as histograms of RBC volume, HGB concentration, and PLT volume, respectively. As with impedance technology, the MCV and MPV are means, the RDW and PDW are CVs derived from histograms, and the

HCT, MCH, and MCHC are calculated values. In the hemolyzed aliquot, leukocytes are fixed and stained for myeloperoxidase activity and hydrodynamically focused in a second flow cell. For leukocytes, light scatter and light absorption are measured with a pair of photodetectors, and data are displayed as a two-dimensional cytogram, a WBC count, and a differential in relative and absolute numbers.

CBC results obtained by processing appropriately collected and anticoagulated blood specimens through properly calibrated, maintained, and quality-controlled automated analyzers are considered accurate and precise over a relatively wide range of values.[70] The occupational physician should be aware, however, that HGB, MCH, and MCHC may be falsely elevated if the plasma is lipemic or if WBC count exceeds 50,000 cells/mm^3. "Spun" (manually centrifuged) HCT may be 3–12% higher than automated HCT due to plasma trapping, especially in polycythemic patients with hypochromic, microcytic red cells (MCV < 70 fl). High titers of cold agglutinins may cause spurious macrocytosis (MCV > 95–100 fl), low RBC count due to RBC autoagglutination, and low WBC count due to leukoagglutination.[71] Cryoproteinemia may cause pseudoleukocytosis or pseudothrombocytosis or both, while red cell fragments, extremely microcytic red cells, or both, may increase falsely the PLT count.

Further evaluation may be required when HGB is < 10 g/dl or > 18 g/dl, MCV is < 80 fl or > 100 fl, MCHC is > 37%, or the WBC is < 2000/mm^3 or > 20,000/mm^3. The presence of eosinophilia (> 10%), monocytosis (> 15%), sickle cells, spherocytes, stomatocytes, oval macrocytes, schistocytes, "tear drop" cells, or basophilic stippling should prompt concern. Observation of agranular or hypersegmented (five or more nuclear segments) neutrophils, Auer rods, Döhle bodies, marked toxic granulations, monocytes with prominent nucleoli (blasts), immature granulocytes, plasma cells, or a large number of atypical lymphocytes also should raise clinical suspicion. If the RBC count multiplied by three does not approximate the HGB, or if the HGB times three does not approximate the HCT, the clinician should check for abnormalities in the peripheral smear and RBC indices.

The clinical utility of the RDW and MPV has been debated for many years.[72] Some physicians believe that analysis of MCV plus RDW can facilitate the classification of anemias,[73] while others emphasize the limitations of using both parameters.[74] Despite significant controversy, MCV plus RDW has been used to separate patients with iron deficiency (MCV low, RDW increased) from those with thalassemia minor (MCV low, RDW normal) or anemia of chronic disease (MCV low, RDW normal). On the other hand, RDW should not be used to distinguish alcohol-related macrocytosis from B_{12} or folate deficiency. The clinical utility of the MPV has not been demonstrated. A single reference range has not been established,[75] and significant changes in MPV occur with time if the sample has been anticoagulated in the tripotassium salt of EDTA.[76] Alterations of MPV in various clinical conditions have been documented, but the value of these changes in clinical decision making has not been determined.[77]

AUTOMATED MULTICHANNEL CHEMISTRY PANELS

Significant changes are occurring in the performance, billing, and reimbursement of automated multichannel chemistry tests. Occupational physicians who frequently request electrolyte, metabolic, liver function, or general chemistry screening panels increasingly will find that the particular group of analytes whose values they have come to rely upon is no longer provided by many clinical laboratories. On Jan. 1, 1998, laboratories no longer will be able to use current procedural terminology (CPT) codes 80002–80019 to bill Medicare for the automated multichannel tests they now perform as customized panels or profiles because the American Medical Association has officially eliminated these codes from the 1998 version of the CPT manual. In place of the traditional 20- and 22-test profiles, laboratories may choose to adopt up to four new specific panels.[78] Requests for these new panels will carry a presumption of medical necessity, which means that clinicians and laboratories may not have to provide medical necessity documentation unless otherwise required by local medical review policy. Other advantages of the new panels include the requirement of only one billing code and potentially improved accuracy in tracking individual physician utilization of individual analytes.[79]

Among the many challenges presented by the new reimbursement scheme for AMC tests is the need to change physician behavior. With appropriate education, most physicians likely will conclude that the new panels should replace the 20- or 22-test profiles for use in screening. Some laboratories, however, may choose the route taken by the Mayo Clinic, which has decided to eliminate all panels except electrolytes. Still other laboratories may ask physicians to order tests individually. Regardless of the number of panels offered by a particular laboratory, physicians must clearly understand that their requests for testing may not be honored if they do not provide the required documentation of medical necessity.[80]

REFERENCES

1. Tietz NW (ed): Clinical Guide to Laboratory Tests. 3rd ed. Philadelphia, WB Saunders, 1995.
2. Borer WZ: Selection and use of laboratory tests. In Tietz NW, Conn RB, Pruden EL (eds): Applied Laboratory Medicine. Philadelphia, WB Saunders, 1992, pp 1–5.
3. Friedman RB, Young DS: Effect of Disease on Clinical Laboratory Tests. 2nd ed. Washington, DC, American Association of Clinical Chemistry Press, 1989.
4. Total serum cholesterol may decrease by as much as 20% in the luteal phase of the menstrual cycle. Ideally, serum cholesterol should always be measured at the same point in the menstrual cycle.
5. Young DS: Effect of Drugs on Clinical Laboratory Tests. 3rd ed. Washington, DC, American Association of Clinical Chemistry Press, 1990.
6. International Federation of Clinical Chemistry, Expert Panel on Theory of Reference Values: Approved recommendations on the theory of reference values: Part 1. The concept of reference values. J Clin Chem Clin Biochem 25:337–342, 1987; Part 2. Selection of individuals for the production of reference values. J Clin Chem Clin Biochem 25:639–644, 1987; Part 3. Preparation of individuals and collection of specimens for the production of reference values. J Clin Chem Clin Biochem 26:593–598, 1988; Part 4. Control of analytical variation in the production, transfer, and application of reference values. Eur J Clin Chem Clin Biochem 29:531–535, 1991; Part 5. Statistical treatment of collected reference values: Determination of reference limits. J Clin Chem Clin Biochem 25:645–656, 1987; Part 6. Presentation of observed values related to reference values. J Clin Chem Clin Biochem 25:657–662, 1987.
7. [Reference deleted.]
8. Solberg HE: Establishment and use of reference values. In Burtis CA, Ashwood ER (eds): Tietz Textbook of Clinical Chemistry. 2nd ed. Philadelphia, WB Saunders, 1994.
9. Kassirer JP: Clinical evaluation of kidney function—glomerular function. N Engl J Med 285:385–389, 1971.
10. Levey AS, Perrone RD, Madias NE: Serum creatinine and renal function. Annu Rev Med 39:465–490, 1988.
11. Cockcroft DW, Gault MH: Prediction of creatinine clearance from serum creatinine. Nephron 16:31–41, 1976.
12. Price M, Kottke FJ: Comparison of glomerular filtration rate, blood urea nitrogen, and serum creatinine in patients with chronic urinary tract disease. Minn Med 63:781–782, 1980.
13. Shemesh O, Golbetz H, Kriss JP, Myers BD: Limitations of creatinine as a filtration marker in glomerulopathic patients. Kidney Int 28:830–838, 1985.
14. Dossetor JB: Creatininemia versus uremia: The relative significance of blood urea nitrogen and serum creatinine concentrations in azotemia. Ann Intern Med 65:1287–1299, 1966.
15. Sox HC (ed): Common Diagnostic Tests. Use and Interpretation. 2nd ed. Philadelphia, American College of Physicians, 1990.

16. Mogensen CE: Diabetes mellitus and the kidney. Kidney Int 21:673–675, 1982; Rosman JB, Ter Wee PM, Meijer S, et al: Prospective randomised trial of early dietary protein restriction in chronic renal failure. Lancet 2:1291–1296, 1984; Maschio G, Oldrizzi L, Rugiu C: Clinical effects of long-term dietary protein and phosphorus restriction in patients with early chronic renal failure. Contr Nephrol 55:20–27, 1987.
17. Haber MH: Urinary Sediment: A Textbook Atlas. Chicago, American Society of Clinical Pathologists, 1981.
18. Roels HA, Lauwerys RR, Buchet JP, et al: Health significance of cadmium-induced renal dysfunction: A five year follow up. Br J Ind Med 46:755–764, 1989.
19. Balistreri WF, A-Kader HH, Setchell KDR, et al: New methods of assessing liver function in infants and children. Ann Clin Lab Sci 22:162–174, 1992.
20. Witkin GB, Chapman JF, Lasesne HR: Choosing liver function tests. Emerg Med 19:23–46, 1987.
21. The differing half-lives of the ALT and the isoenzymes of AST explain many of the observed patterns in patients with liver disease. ALT has a half-life of 48 hours, cytoplasmic AST has a half-life of 8 to 10 hours, and mitochondrial AST has a half-life of 8–10 days.
22. Clinical zinc deficiency or the presence of zinc chelators, such as EDTA, oxalate, and citrate, may decrease serum alkaline phosphatase activity.
23. Gilbert syndrome, a common source of patient referral to gastroenterologists and hepatologists, is seen in as many as 7% of Caucasians in the United States and Western Europe. Among these patients, serum indirect bilirubin concentrations typically do not exceed 3 mg/dl, males predominate by at least 1.5:1, and some individuals complain of fatigue, weakness, abdominal pain, and other nonspecific symptoms. Bilirubin concentrations tend to fluctuate substantially in a given individual, with higher concentrations associated with stress, fatigue, alcohol ingestion, intercurrent illness, and reduced caloric intake. In women, Gilbert syndrome may be characterized by marked premenstrual accentuation of the hyperbilirubinemia. Other conventional LFTs and liver biopsies are unremarkable in Gilbert patients. For patients and families who want further proof of the absence of liver disease, a 36- to 72-hour dietary restriction to 1680 calories per day may produce a twofold to threefold increase in total (mostly indirect) bilirubin. In normal subjects, the serum bilirubin should increase by 0.4 mg/dl. The major reason to establish the diagnosis of Gilbert syndrome is to reassure the patient and to avoid unnecessary surgical procedures. See Levinson MJ: Jaundice. In Conn RB, Borer WZ, Snyder JW (eds): Current Diagnosis 9. Philadelphia, WB Saunders, 1997, pp 41–45.
24. The clinical value of quantitating delta-bilirubin is under investigation. Bilirubin covalently bound to albumin predominates in the recovery phase of hepatitis, where direct hyperbilirubinemia will occur without bilirubin in the urine. Some laboratory methods measure delta-bilirubin as part of direct bilirubin, while others measure conjugated bilirubin exclusive of delta-bilirubin, which can then be quantitated.
25. Other than visual examination, the most common method for detecting bilirubin in urine involves use of a "dipstick" impregnated with diazo reagent. Dipstick methods can detect concentrations ≥ 0.5 mg/dl. A fresh urine specimen is required because bilirubin is unstable when exposed to light and room temperature. If the test must be delayed, the sample should be protected from light and stored in a refrigerator at 2–8°C (35.6°–46.4°F) for no longer than 24 hours.
26. Measurement of urobilinogen is currently discouraged because the results do not meaningfully add to the diagnostic information obtained from more traditional LFTs.
27. Neuschwander-Tetri BA, Bacon BR: Viral hepatitis. In Conn RB, Borer WZ, Snyder JW (eds): Current Diagnosis 9. Philadelphia, WB Saunders, 1997, pp 644–650.
28. Klee GG, Hay ID: Biochemical thyroid function testing. Mayo Clin Proc 69:469–470, 1994. A sensitive TSH assay is defined by a minimum requirement that the serum from clinically hyperthyroid patients gives results that are more than three log standard deviations below the mean value found in sera from normal subjects.
29. Surks MI, Chopra IJ, Mariash CN, et al; American Thyroid Association guidelines for use of laboratory tests in thyroid disorders. JAMA 263:1529–1530, 1990.
30. Spencer CA, Eigen A, Shen D, et al: Specificity of sensitive assays of thyrotropin (TSH) used to screen for thyroid disease in hospitalized patients. Clin Chem 33:1391–1396, 1987.
31. Nicolloff JT, Spencer GA: The clinical use and misuse of the sensitive thyrotropin assays. J Clin Endocrinol Metab 71:553–558, 1990.
32. Physicians can also use the third- and fourth-generation TSH tests to determine the dose of suppressive therapy given to patients with differentiated thyroid carcinoma. Thyroxine is given to the limit of clinical tolerance in an effort to inhibit the growth of metastatic tumor. Over-replacement may lead to reduced bone density, transaminasemia, tachycardia, dysrhythmias, and left ventricular hypertrophy. Results from newer sTSH tests may permit a more accurate titration in an attempt to balance the adverse effects of thyroid hormone excess with the inhibition of tumor growth.

33. Spencer CA, Yaksuchi M, Kazarosyan M, et al; Interlaboratory/intermethod differences in functional sensitivity of immunometric assays of thyrotropin and impact on reliability of measurement of subnormal concentrations of TSH. Clin Chem 41:367–374, 1995.
34. Adams JE, Adendschein D, Jaffe A: Biochemical markers of myocardial injury. Is MB creatine kinase the choice of the 1990s? Circulation 88:750–763, 1993.
35. Hornykewycz S, Gabriel H, Huber K: Biochemical markers of myocardial necrosis in acute myocardial infarction and thrombolysis. Ann Hematol 69(suppl 2):S59–S63, 1994.
36. Bodor GS, Porterfield D, Voss E, et al: Cardiac troponin T composition in normal and regenerating human skeletal muscle [abstract]. Clin Chem 41:S148, 1995.
37. Bodor GS, Porter S, Landt Y, et al: Development of monoclonal antibodies for an assay of cardiac troponin-I and preliminary results in suspected cases of myocardial infarction. Clin Chem 38:2203–2214, 1992; Collinson PO, Mosely D, Stubbs PJ, et al: Troponin T for the differential diagnosis of ischemic myocardial injury. Ann Clin Biochem 30:11–16, 1993.
38. Adams JE, Schechtman KB, Landt Y, et al; Comparable detection of AMI by CK-MB isoenzyme and cardiac troponin I. Clin Chem 40:1291–1295, 1994; Lance C, Calzolari C, Bertinchant JP, et al: Cardiac-specific immunoenzymometric assay to troponin I in the early phase of acute myocardial infarction. Clin Chem 39:972–979, 1993.
39. Wu AHB, Valdes R Jr, Apple FS, et al: Cardiac troponin-T immunoassay for diagnosis of acute myocardial infarction and detection of minor myocardial injury. Clin Chem 40:900–907, 1994.
40. Ravkilde J, Horder M, Gerhardt W, et al: Diagnostic performance and prognostic value of serum troponin-T in suspected myocardial infarction. Scand J Clin Lab Invest 53:677–685, 1993; Wu AHB, Feng YJ, Contois JH: Prognostic value of cardiac troponin I in chest pain patients. Clin Chem 42:651–652, 1996.
41. Osterloh JD: Utility and reliability of emergency toxicologic testing. Emerg Med Clin North Am 8:693–723, 1990.
42. Travers EM: Cost analysis in the toxicology laboratory. Clin Lab Med 10:591–623, 1990.
43. Bayes RT: An essay toward solving a problem in the doctrine of chance. Philos Trans R Soc London 53:370–418, 1763. Bayes theorem has been used for centuries to calculate the probability of a future event based on prior experience with the success of a measurement or test in predicting outcome. Bayesian analysis defines sensitivity as the percentage of positive specimens that correctly test positive and specificity as the percentage of negative specimens that correctly test negative. The positive specimens that give a positive result are true positives (TP). Positive specimens that erroneously give negative results are false negatives (FN). Thus, diagnostic sensitivity is calculated as TP/(TP + FN). Negative specimens that give a negative test result are true negatives (TN). Negative specimens that erroneously give a positive test result are false positives (FP). In turn, diagnostic specificity is calculated as TN/(TN + FP). Predictive value is defined as the probability that the test result is true or correct. The predictive value of a positive result (PPV) is calculated as (prevalence)(sensitivity)/(prevalence)(sensitivity) + (1-prevalence)(1-specificity).
44. Spiehler VR, O'Donnell CM, Gokhale DV: Confirmation and certainty in toxicologic screening. Clin Chem 34:1535–1539, 1988.
45. For example, sulfhemoglobin and methylene blue falsely increase methemoglobin concentrations measured by co-oximetry, while ketoacidosis, renal failure, phenylketonuria, phenothiazines, diflunisal, and salicylamide false increase salicylate concentrations measured by colorimetry. See Dalrymple RW, Sterns FW: Diflunisal interferes with determination of salicylate by Trinder, Abbott Tdx, and DuPont aca methods. Clin Chem 32:230, 1986.
46. Although broad immunoreactivity allows detection of multiple drugs from the same class, it also creates the potential for crossreactivity with drugs that may not be of clinical interest. Even "highly specific" antibodies have been associated with unforeseen crossreactivities or interferences that cause both false positive and false negative assay responses. See Olsen KM, Gulliksen M, Christopherson AS: Metabolites of chlorpromazine and brompheniramine may cause false-positive urine amphetamine results with monoclonal EMIT®d.a.u. assay of amphetamine. Clin Chem 38(4):611–612, 1992; Poklis A: Unavailability of drug metabolite reference material to evaluate false-positive results for monoclonal EMIT®d.a.u. assay of amphetamine. Clin Chem 38(12):2560, 1992; Wagener RE, Linder MW, VAldes R: Decreased signal in EMIT assays of drugs of abuse in urine after ingestion of aspirin: Potential for false-negative results. Clin Chem 40:608–612, 1994; Mikkelsen, Ash KO: Adulterants causing false negatives in illicit drug testing. Clin Chem 34:2333–2336, 1988.
47. For example, optimum detection of morphine by gas chromatography requires that the extracted morphine be N-acetylated to decrease polarity and increase volatility.
48. GC is commonly employed for the identification and quantitation of ethanol, methanol, isopropanol, and acetone. By contrast, analysis of ethylene glycol requires a dedicated GC procedure with a

different preparative approach. Opioids, amphetamines, antihistamines, and antidepressants also can be analyzed by GC.
49. Quality control programs are an integral part of clinical laboratory testing. Quality control provides a system for monitoring and validating the accuracy and performance of the entire analytical process. In GC or GC-MS, several distinct procedural and instrumental parameters must be verified, including column efficiency, oven temperature control, detector function, and specimen extraction protocol. The first three can be monitored daily by injecting a mixture of known drug standards onto the instrument and evaluating detector response, peak resolution, and relative retention times for individual analytes. The extraction process can be validated by extracting a control sample containing a known mixture of drugs, or by including an internal standard in the extraction protocol for each specimen. The internal standard added prior to extraction should not be a molecule that can be seen in actual patient samples. Furthermore, the chromatographic behavior of the internal standard must not interfere with identification of commonly observed drugs.
50. Baumgartner WA, Hill VA, Blahd WD: Hair analysis for drugs of abuse. J Forensic Sci 34:1433–1453, 1989; Arnold W: Radioimmunological hair analysis for narcotics and substitutes. J Clin Chem Clin Biochem 25:753–757, 1987. Cone EJ, Yousefnejad D, Darwin WD, et al: Testing human hair for drugs of abuse. II. Identification of unique cocaine metabolites in hair of drug abusers and evaluation of decontamination procedures. J Anal Toxicol 15:250–255, 1991.
51. Cone EJ: Testing human hair for drugs of abuse. Individual dose and time profiles of morphine and codeine in plasma, saliva, urine, and beard compared to drug-induced effects on pupils and behavior. J Anal Toxicol 14:1–7, 1990; Moore CM: Drug testing in the 90s. In Leikin JB, Paloucek FP (eds): Poisoning and Toxicology Handbook. Cleveland, Lexi-Comp, Inc., 1995, pp 1168–1169.
52. Garriott JC: Forensic aspects of ethyl alcohol. Clin Lab Med 3:385–396, 1983.
53. Gerson B: Alcohol. Clin Lab Med 10:355–374, 1990.
54. Carrico RJ, Peisach J, Alben JO: The preparation and some physical properties of sulfhemoglobin. J Biol Chem 253:2386, 1978.
55. Ellenhorn MJ, Barceloux DG: Medical Toxicology. Diagnosis and Treatment of Human Poisoning. New York, Elsevier, 1988.
56. Evenson MA: Photometry. In Burtis CA, Ashwood ER (eds): Tietz Textbook of Clinical Chemistry. 2nd ed. Philadelphia, WB Saunders, 1994.
57. [Reference deleted.]
58. Milne DB: Trace elements. In Burtis CA, Ashwood ER (eds): Tietz Textbook of Clinical Chemistry. 2nd ed. Philadelphia, WB Saunders, 1994.
59. Burnette WN: "Western blotting:" Electrophoretic transfer of proteins from sodium dodecyl sulfate-polyacrylamide gels to unmodified nitrocellulose and radiographic detection with antibody and radioiodinated protein. Anal Biochem 112:195, 1981.
60. Centers for Disease Control: Interpretation and use of the Western blot assay for serodiagnosis of human immunodeficiency virus type 1 infections. MMWR 38(S-7):1–7, 1989.
61. For example, the Association of State and Territorial Public Health Laboratory Directors and the CDC suggest that a positive Western blot requires detection of antibody to any two of the three major antigens (p24, gp41, or gp120/gp160). The FDA Licensed DuPont Test requires detection of p24, p31, and gp41 or gp120/gp160. The American Red Cross requires detection of three or more bands—one from each gene product group (GAG, POL, and ENV). Finally, the Consortium for Retrovirus Serology Standardization suggests detection of 2 or more bands—either p24 or p31 plus gp41 or gp120/gp160.
62. Celun CL, Coombs RW, Lafferty W, et al: Indeterminate human immunodeficiency virus type 1 Western blots: Seroconversion risk, specificity of supplemental tests, and an algorithm for evaluation. J Infect Dis 164:656–664, 1991.
63. Johnson KJ, Chensue SW, Kunkel SL, Ward PA: Immunopathology. In Rubin E, Farber JL (eds): Rubin & Farber Pathology. 2nd ed. Philadelphia, JB Lippincott, 1994, pp 97–141.
64. [Reference deleted.]
65. Cotran RS, Kumar V, Robbins SL: Diseases of immunity. In Robbins SL (ed):Robbins Pathologic Basis of Disease. 4th ed. Philadelphia, WB Saunders, 1989, pp 163–237.
66. An epiphenomenon is defined as an event that bears no known causal relationship to another event.
67. Gulati GL, Hyun BH: The automated CBC: A current perspective. Hematol Oncol Clin North Am: Diagnostic Hematology 8:593–603, 1994.
68. Some physicians find it useful to think of RDW and PDW as measures of RBC heterogeneity and platelet heterogeneity, respectively.
69. HCT, MCH, and MCHC are calculated by the following formulas: HCT (%) = RBC ($\times 10^{12}$/L) $\times$ MCV $\times$ 0.1; MCH (pg/RBC) = HGB (g/dL) $\times$ 10/RBC (x 10^{12}/L); MCHC (g/dL) = HGB (g/dL) $\times$ 100/HCT (%).

70. Bull BS, Korpman RA: Autocalibration of hematology analyzers. J Clin Lab Autom 3:111, 1983; Crawford JM, Lau YR, Bull BS: Calibration of hematology analyzers. Arch Pathol Lab Med 111:324, 1987; Gulati GL, Hyun BH: Quality control in hematology. Clin Lab Med 6:675, 1986; Gulati GL, Hyun BH, Ashton JK: Advances of the past decade in automated hematology. Am J Clin Pathol 98(suppl):S11–S16, 1992; Koepke JA, Protextor TJ: Quality assurance for multichannel hematology instruments: Four years experience with patient mean erythrocyte indices. Am J Clin Pathol 75:28, 1981; Savage RA: Calibration bias and imprecision for automated analyzers: An evaluation of significance of short-term bias resulting from calibration of an analyzer with S-Cal. Am J Clin Pathol 84:186, 1985.
71. RBC autoagglutination can be prevented by keeping blood warm and by warming the diluent before and during cell counting.
72. Bessman JD, Williams LJ, Gardner FH Jr: Improved classification of anemias by MCV and RDW. Am J Clin Pathol 80:322, 1983; Brittenham GM, Koepke JA: Red cell volume distributions and the diagnosis of anemia: Help or hindrance? Arch Pathol Lab Med 111:1146, 1987; Flynn MM, Reppun TS, Bhagavan NV: Limitations of red blood cell distribution width (RDW) in evaluation of microcytosis. Am J Clin Pathol 85:445, 1986; Karnad A, Poskitt TR: The automated complete blood cell count: Use of the red blood cell volume distribution width and mean platelet volume in evaluating anemia and thrombocytopenia. Arch Int Med 145:1270, 1985; Morgan DL, Peck SD: The use of red cell distribution width in the detection of iron deficiency in chronic hemodialysis patients. Am J Clin Pathol 89:513, 1988.
73. Bessman JD, Williams LJ, Gardner FH Jr: Improved classification of anemias by MCV and RDW. Am J Clin Pathol 80:322, 1983; Karnad A, Poskitt TR: The automated complete blood cell count: Use of the red blood cell volume distribution width and mean platelet volume in evaluating anemia and thrombocytopenia. Arch Int Med 145:1270, 1985; Robert GT, El Badawi SB: Red cell distribution width index in some hematologic diseases. Am J Clin Pathol 83:222, 1985.
74. Morgan DL, Peck SD: The use of red cell distribution width in the detection of iron deficiency in chronic hemodialysis patients. Am J Clin Pathol 89:513, 1988; Brittenham GM, Koepke JA: Red cell volume distributions and the diagnosis of anemia: Help or hindrance? Arch Pathol Lab Med 111:1146, 1987, Flynn MM, Reppun TS, Bhagavan NV: Limitations of red blood cell distribution width (RDW) in evaluation of microcytosis. Am J Clin Pathol 85:445, 1986.
75. Graham SS, Traub B, Mink IB: Automated platelet-sizing parameters on a normal population. Am J Clin Pathol 87:365, 1987.
76. Lippi U, Schinella M, Modena N, et al: Unpredictable effects of K_3 EDTA on mean platelet volume. Am J Clin Pathol 87:391, 1987.
77. Bessman JD, Williams LJ, Gilmer PR: Platelet size in health and hematologic disease. Am J Clin Pathol 78:150, 1982.
78. The four new panels are as follows: (1) a liver function panel that includes serum albumin, total and direct bilirubin, alkaline phosphatase, aspartate aminotransferase, and alanine aminotransferase; (2) an electrolyte panel consisting of serum sodium, potassium, chloride, and carbon dioxide; (3) a basic metabolic panel that includes sodium, potassium, chloride, carbon dioxide, glucose, and creatinine; and (4) a comprehensive metabolic panel consisting of serum albumin, total bilirubin, total calcium, blood chloride, creatinine, glucose, alkaline phosphatase, serum potassium, total protein, serum sodium, aspartate aminotransferase, and blood urea nitrogen.
79. Theoretically, every test billed to Medicare or a private payer will be traceable to a corresponding CPT code.
80. Many laboratories may be increasingly unwilling to provide tests results when the lack of medical necessity documentation substantially reduces the likelihood of reimbursement.

MICHAEL H. LEWITT, MD, MPH

EPIDEMIOLOGY AND BIOSTATISTICS

From Great Valley Health
Occupational Medicine
Paoli Memorial Hospital
Paoli, Pennsylvania

Reprint requests to:
Michael H. LeWitt, MD, MPH
Great Valley Health
Occupational Medicine
Paoli Memorial Hospital
255 West Lancaster Ave.
Paoli, PA 19301

The study of epidemiology and biostatistics provides the knowledge behind the scientific underpinnings for the practice of preventive medicine and its clinical specialty of occupational medicine. This chapter presents an overview of the material that the clinician must know to practice occupational medicine, whether in the clinic, workplace, military, academia, or management.

EPIDEMIOLOGY

Epidemiology is the study of the distribution of factors that affect the well being of, and illness or injury to, a population. It can be as topical as a newspaper article[38] or as detailed as a mortality study showing differential death rates for populations.[19] It is the medical science that allows the intensive follow-up study of the causative factors and conditions causing deviations from health that have been identified as such by epidemiologic means.[33] It has relevance to the practice of occupational and environmental medicine[1,35] in that it provides a framework to view targeted exposures against a background of disease occurring without additional known risks.

To study epidemiology, one needs some basic tools and concepts. This chapter provides those tools and concepts and includes a working vocabulary so that an individual may understand some of the essentials of epidemiology.

Incidence refers to the number of new cases of illness, injury, or other items of interest that may be measured and that occurs to a defined population over a specified time. An example is the number of cases of influenza occurring in Philadelphia during October, November, and December 1996. *Prevalence* refers to the current number of cases of illness or injury found in a defined population at a specified time. It may also be defined as incidence times duration, when the prevalence is uncommon (e.g., ≤ 10%). For example, one may ask how many cases of AIDS are under treatment in Philadelphia on December 31, 1996 (point prevalence), in December 1996, or during 1996. Each of these can be calculated in terms of rates or ratios, described below.

Rates express a measure of how frequently events occur. There are many rates commonly used in epidemiology. The rates are descriptive of a particular type of relationship, such as *proportional mortality rate* (*PMR*), which may also be expressed as a *ratio* (one value divided by another), an age-specific, cause-specific, gender-specific, location-specific, morbidity or mortality rate (or ratio), prevalence or incidence rates, which can be used to determine the frequency of occurrence of events under study.[19]

Endemic refers to a prevalence rate of a disease or clinical finding that is fairly constant in a population, often due to factors that are normally found in the population. *Epidemic* refers to an increased prevalence rate of an illness or clinical finding in a population, generally due to changes in the normal defense mechanisms (host), in the virulence of the organism (agent), or in the environment. *Pandemic* refers to a much larger prevalence rate of a disease or clinical finding in a population; it involves a larger percentage of the population, a wider area of spread, or both.

A number of types of epidemiologic studies look at populations, including **cross-sectional**, **cohort**, and **case-control** studies. Cross-sectional, or prevalence, studies examine relationships between an illness or injury and other variables of interest as they exist in a defined population at a particular time. Cohort, or follow-up, studies look at factors associated with the development of disease or injury, usually from an exposure perspective. A study population, initially free of the entity under investigation, is followed prospectively. Case-control studies compare cases (persons with illnesses or injuries of interest) with a control group of persons without the illness or injury. They are especially useful when the entity under study is uncommon.

Also of importance is the difference between **prospective** and **retrospective** studies (Table 1). Retrospective studies look back on a population, and prospective studies look ahead to the future of a population. A study may be *descriptive* if it reports

TABLE 1. Advantages and Disadvantages of Prospective and Retrospective Studies

Prospective (cohort, incidence, longitudinal) Studies	Retrospective Studies
Advantages	
Accurate relative risk	Short study time
Determines incidence and calculates rates	Relatively inexpensive
No problems with subject recall	Small number of subjects
Less bias in selecting controls or ascertaining exposures	Studies rare diseases
	Few ethical concerns
	No need for volunteers
	No attrition problems
Disadvantages	
Ethical problems	No incidence figures
Need volunteers, large numbers of subjects	Biased recall possible
Attrition problems	Approximates relative risk
Long study time	Possible bias in control group
Studies common rather than rare entities	
Expensive	

the findings—for example, the percentage of left-handed writers in a population[12]—or *analytic* if it assesses why findings are reported—for example, why left-handed individuals might have a higher rate of accidents or injuries.[9] Studies may be *observational* if a population is being assessed or be *experimental* if the population is undergoing some exposure or experience that is different from a control or nonexposed population.

Additional concepts that are helpful in understanding epidemiologic findings include *relative risk* (the increase or decrease that one population experiences compared to another), which is derived by dividing the incidence rate in an exposed population by the incidence rate in a nonexposed population (Fig. 1). In the case-control model, one also can calculate an *odds ratio* (see Fig. 1), which is the increased likelihood of a disease or injury in an exposed population contrasted with a nonexposed population.

An understanding of biostatistics is an integral part of epidemiologic research. As a general rule, a finding is considered *valid* if the results differ from a chance finding by some predetermined criteria (e.g., a probability of less than 0.05 or 0.01, meaning that the same results could be found by chance alone in 1 case in 20 or in 1 case in 100, respectively). The purpose of using statistics is to ascertain whether the *null hypothesis* (the statement that there is no statistical difference between the study group and control group, or different populations) has been disproved. If so, the findings may have statistical significance. More extensive discussion is found in a number of sources.[8,10,15,17,22,29,32,36,43] Several publications provide helpful information regarding the writing and publication of scientific research and review.[11,25,31] Finally, there is an excellent text on "tunnel vision" as it applies to our understanding of day-to-day interpretation of numbers and preconceived numeric and logical conclusions.[41]

Validity or accuracy describes how closely a series of observations match an actual event or finding, while *reliability* or reproducibility describes how closely a

Exposed, with disease A	Exposed, without disease C
Unexposed, with disease B	Unexposed, without disease D

FIGURE 1. Relative risk calculations in a cohort study: $RR = (A/A + C)/(B/B + D)$. Odds ratio calculations in a case-control study: $OR = (A/B)/(C/D) = AD/BC$.

series of observations, made at different times, match each other. A laboratory test that gives a cholesterol result, on repeated samplings, of 200 mg%, in a sample that is actually 200 mg%, is valid. It may also be reliable if the repeated samplings are close (within statistical measurement) to each other in value. A test may be reliable without being valid (if the repeated measurements are close to each other but not to the actual value of what is being tested) or valid without being reliable (approaching the actual value of the observation but without reproducibility to some statistical criterion), depending on the results of repeated testing.

Attributable risk is a determination of the amount of disease or injury in the population under study that can be attributed to a particular causal factor or group of factors. A breakdown of the results can be assigned various names, including *attributable fraction*, *etiologic fraction*, and *population attributable risk*. Attributable risk also can be defined as the incidence among an exposed population minus the incidence among the nonexposed population (background risk). An example is the risk of lung cancer in smokers compared to the risk in nonsmokers. The total risk in smokers compared to the risk in nonsmokers is the risk attributable to smoking, assuming that all other risks are equally distributed in the study and control populations.

Bias is a systematic error in the analysis, plan, or process of a particular study. There are a number of different types,[32] including the following:

- *Systematic bias*, where the results deviate from true values in a consistent way (e.g., rounding up, or using only even values, such as with blood pressure measurements)
- *Sampling or chance variability*, a finding that is inherent in all studies, and the reason that statistical support is so critical
- *Diagnostic bias*, where the exposed (at risk) population is studied more closely than the nonexposed population
- *Validity of diagnosis bias*, where the knowledge of the exposure could influence the diagnosis (a good reason for using an objective or blinded evaluator)
- *Interviewer bias, nonresponse bias, lost to follow-up bias, recall bias* and other characteristics of the data gathering process that may have a differential impact if one part of the study population (control or experimental/exposed) has a greater chance of being selected or not selected (violating random assignment, for example)
- *Prevalence bias*, where there is early dropout due to death or disease, or in cases in which the disease may be present but is not recorded or recognized.
- *Confounding bias*, where a variable that influences selection or analysis is associated with the endpoint under study and the factor that is being posited as causative, and other biases that may arise in study design, realization, or analysis
- *Ecologic fallacy*, a bias or error in inference that occurs when an association observed between variables in a group is assumed to be representative of an individual.

Meta-analysis is a method whereby groups of studies performed at different times, often with different populations, and by different researchers can be combined and analyzed with the goal of studying new or revisiting old problems. Meta-analysis allows a larger population than could be practically or ethically combined. A variety of studies have provided thoughtful questions about the process, the assumptions, and the conclusions.[20,28,30,34,45,46] While a number of shortcomings and deficits are associated with meta-analysis, it is often the best or only way to study important issues.

Statistical association and presumed cause-and-effect relationships should have a relationship in time (exposure precedes disease), a reasonable biologic relationship (association coherence), a strong association (statistical significance, dose relationship), medical plausibility and consistency (often a result of additional studies supporting the conclusions), and specificity of the association (exposure and disease seem to be interlinked without other exposures causing the same findings). Finally, to paraphrase Sherlock Holmes, when the impossible has been ruled out, whatever remains, however implausible, is the truth. Thus, an inability to find alternative explanations is helpful but not always conclusive in finding answers.[24]

BIOSTATISTICS

One can best use statistics if they are understood.[5,6,10,29,37] However, this understanding need not and should not be from the prospective of rote memorization or poorly understood applications of arcane formulas. In fact, computer programs have greatly facilitated the drudgery of number crunching.[4] If one, with the perspective of learning, returns to numbers,[39,40] there is found a beauty, joy, and pleasure often unequaled in other disciplines, even those less quantitative.

Measures of Central Tendency and Dispersion

Measures of central tendency and dispersion are ways of examining data and their dispersion around a common point. Data do not have meaning without a context, and measures of central tendency and dispersion provide a way of determining the relationship a particular measurement has with regard to other data obtained under similar circumstances and, also, how this might relate to information obtained under different circumstances, by applying statistical testing.

The *mean* or average (when referring to the mean of the total population, μ, and when chosen from a sample within the population, $\bar{x}$) refers to a number that is a midpoint of a group of numbers. The *arithmetic mean* is the sum of all the data, divided by the number of items included. If the sum of 10 items is 104, the arithmetic mean is 10.4. A *geometric mean*, which is used less frequently, and most commonly with data measured on a logarithmic scale, is the Nth root of the product of all the data. If the product of 10 terms is 1,048,576, for example, the 10th root is 4.0.

The *median* is the most middle value of all the data, listed in order from lowest to highest. If the number of terms (N) is odd, than the median is the middle one $[(N + 1)/2]$; if the number of terms is even, the median is the number halfway (the mean for these two values) between the two most middle terms. With the median, half the results are below and half are above the median value. With an even number of items, there may not even be a value that is the same as the median, but with an odd number, one value is the median. There is no specific symbol for the median. The median is unaffected by values that are much larger or smaller than the rest of the values; in contrast, the mean is dependent on a contribution toward its value from each item. The median represents a simple ordering of values.

The *mode* is the value or values that occur most often. When the data have sets of values that are equal in occurrence, there may be more than one mode. The mode is less helpful in making an assessment of the dispersion, but may have some value in certain settings.

The *range* is the arithmetic (subtractive) difference between the two extreme measurements, the largest and smallest.

The *standard deviation* is the most important measurement of spread about a central point. By using statistical concepts, it measures how much spread or dispersion each value has compared to the mean. A standard deviation can be measured on a population (a parameter, σ) or a sample chosen from a population (measured within the larger sample, s). The formula is found in many textbooks and is easily calculated by a variety of statistical programs and many spreadsheets. The *variance* is the square of the standard deviation. The *standard error of the mean* is the standard deviation of a sample, divided by the square root of the number in the sample. It is a measure of how much the sample standard deviation differs from the true population standard deviation.

The *bell-shaped, standard, normal,* or *Gaussian curves* (Fig. 2) are ways of describing a curve consisting of data that follow several principles. The data are continuous, distributed equally around a mean (here described as μ), and the curve that describes the distribution of data has certain characteristics. The standard deviation of the distribution (σ) is such that $\pm 1\,\sigma$ represents 68.2% of the population, $\pm 2\,\sigma$ represents 95.4% of the population, and $\pm 3\,\sigma$ represents 99.7% of the population. In addition, this curve is called a standard or normal distribution when the mean is converted to 0 and the σ is converted to 1 by means of a *Z transformation*. This transformation is described in many statistical texts and may be performed by statistical programs.[6,10,37,43]

Unlike a normal or Gaussian distribution, a *binomial distribution* does not have continuous data. Instead, each circumstance represents a choice of one or another outcome (e.g., yes–no, pass–fail, heads–tails), and the probable result can be determined by means of statistical (probabilistic) predictions. The formula allows one to make predictions about specific outcomes, such as the probability that 25% of patients receiving an antibiotic agent will have a particular side effect.[6,10,37] It answers questions about the chances of certain occurrences, given certain probabilities.

The *Poisson distribution* is used to calculate the probability of events that are uncommon, such as winning a lottery, or the chances of someone in a work population having a stroke, or the use of resources for events that occur infrequently. The

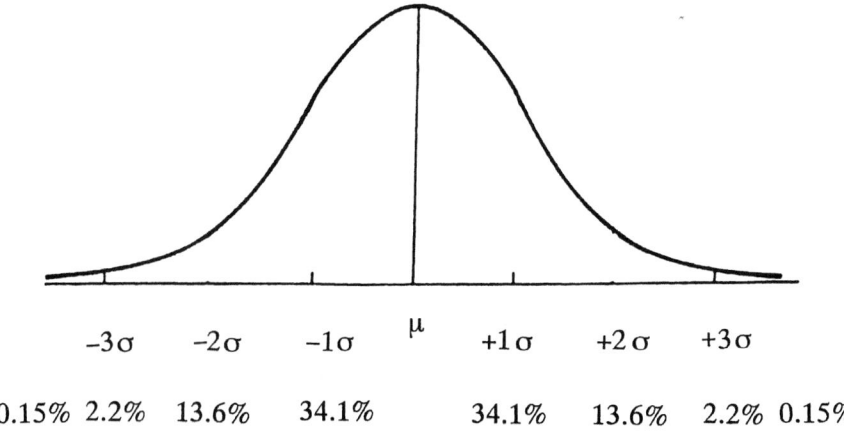

FIGURE 2. A Gaussian, normal curve.

formula has considerable value when planning for the unlikely, as may occur in many medical settings.[6,10,37]

Measures of Spread

Confidence intervals are measures of the upper and lower limits of a statistical finding (generally the arithmetic mean), expressed to a certain degree of statistical probability (often 95%), with a numeric indication of these values. An example is the expression of a mean value, 6.25, with 95% confidence limits of 5.125 and 7.375. These values are found by means of statistical manipulation of the data, and the formula is discussed in standard textbooks and in statistical programs.

The *central limit theorem* is a mathematical concept that allows us to make assumptions about sampling from a population. These include the belief, tested statistically, that repeated samplings will give a mean not significantly different from the mean of the population from which the samples are derived, that the sampling has a normal distribution if the population has a normal distribution, and that the standard error of the mean of the sample gets successively closer to the standard error of the mean of the population as the size of the sample gets larger.

Correlation

Coefficient of variation (*correlation coefficient* or *Pearson product-moment correlation*) is a measurement of closeness, or correlation, between two values and, in a general sense, a measure of to what extent a particular value fits a particular curve or equation (possibly a line). It ranges from +1, indicating perfect, positive correlation to –1, indicating perfect, but negative correlation. A value of 0 indicates no relationship. The *coefficient of determination* is the square of the correlation coefficient.

Sensitivity, Specificity, Positive and Negative Predictive Values

When a test is described, it is usually measured against a "gold standard," a finding that is considered accurate. It may consist of a histologic specimen of tissue, an angiographic or other radiographic lesion, or some other clinical demonstration that is considered highly accurate. A test is then studied to determine when it is positive in the presence of disease (*true positive*), when it is negative in the presence of disease (false negative), when it is negative in the absence of disease (*true negative*), and when it is positive in the absence of disease (*false positive*) (Fig. 3). *Sensitivity* of a test is defined as the true positives divided by the sum of true positives plus false negatives. *Specificity* of a test is defined as the true negatives divided by the sum of true negatives plus false positives. These terms sometimes have less clinical application than academic value.[44]

The positive predictive value (*PPV*) of a test describes the probability that a positive test will represent a true positive.[3,16] It is defined as the true positives divided by the sum of the true and false positives. *Negative predictive value* (*NPV*) of a test describes the probability that a negative test will represent a true negative result. It is defined as the true negatives divided by the sum of the true and false negatives. PPV and NPV are influenced by the *prevalence* of disease (Fig. 4 and Table 2). In this context, it refers to the percentage of the population that has the disease, trait, or characteristic in question. Depending on how the population is chosen, it may refer to a specific population, such as people with chest pain presenting to an emergency department; a study population; or a larger, more randomly selected population. The values change dramatically as the prevalence changes. Because of the way the statistics are derived, as

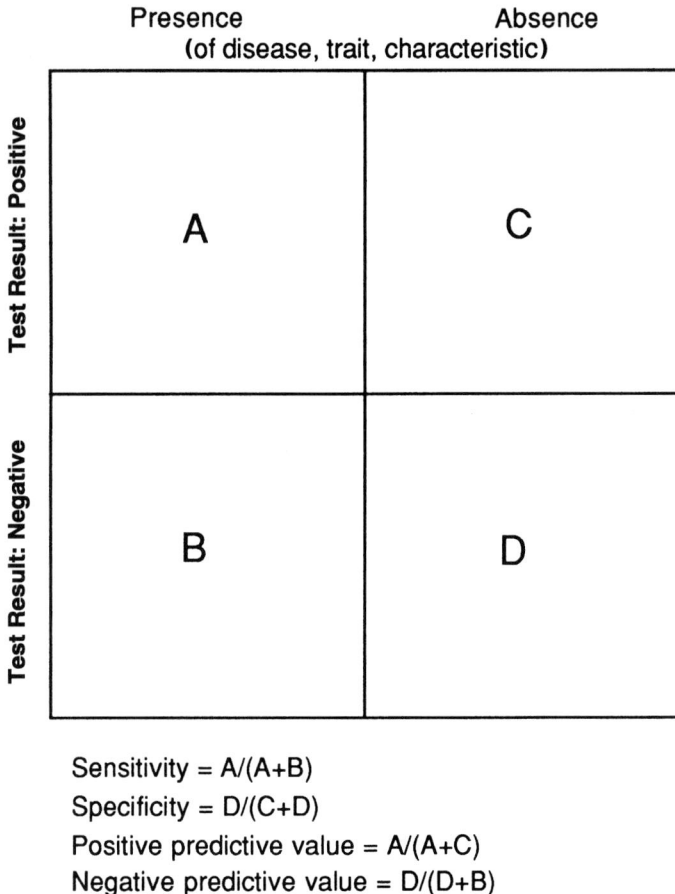

FIGURE 3. Characterization of test results. A = true positive. B = false negative. C = false positive. D = true negative.

sensitivity increases, specificity decreases, depending on what criteria are used for the definition for disease, characteristic, or trait. An example is using intraocular pressure of certain levels as the dividing line between disease and disease-free[7] (Fig. 5).

Various clinical trials use statistical principles, often applying them incorrectly or inappropriately.[26,27] A number of publications are available for assistance in developing studies[18,31,36] and even as basic a concept (too often overlooked) of determining an adequate sample size so that statistical meaning can be derived.[6,10,13] Several examples delineate applications for and uses of various statistical methods.[14,23]

Another way of showing a relationship between true/false positives is by means of *receiver operating curves (or characteristics)*, sometimes abbreviated as ROCs. The ROC is a plot of the rate of true positives against the rate of false positives (Fig. 6), and two or more curves can be compared by statistical means. It allows one to make inferences about a test and its predictive value.

Bayesian analysis is a means of estimating probabilities of one event from the probability of another, related event.[41] It is derived from statistical analyses first

	Disease Present	Disease Absent
Test Result: Positive	950	1,980
Test Result: Negative	50	97,020

Sensitivity = 950/(950 + 50) = 95%
Specificity = 97,020/(97,020 + 1,980) = 98%

Positive Predictive Value = 950/(950 + 1980) = 32%
Negative Predictive Value = 97,020/(97,020 + 50) = 99%

Prevalence = 1,000 [950 + 50]/100,000 [97,020 + 1,980 + 1,000] = 1%

FIGURE 4. Calculations of sensitivity, specificity, positive predictive value, negative predictive value, and prevalence.

TABLE 2. Increasing Prevalence of Disease with Constant Sensitivity and Specificity and with Changes in Positive and Negative Predictive Values

Prevalence	Positive Predictive Value	Negative Predictive Value
0.1%	4.5%	99.9%
1.0%	32%	99.9%
10%	84%	99.4%
25%	94%	98.3%
50%	98%	95.1%

Sensitivity = 95%
Specificity = 98%

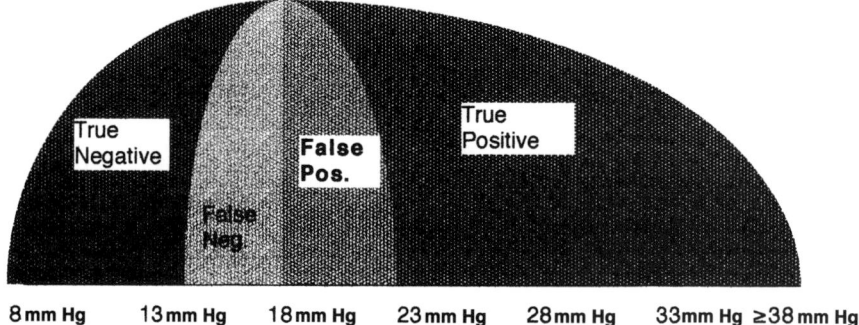

FIGURE 5. Intraocular pressures. Depending on where the criterion is set, some people without the disease may be included in the "diseased" population (false positives), while some people with the disease may be included in the "disease-free" population (false negatives). In this example, because an intraocular pressure higher than 18 mm Hg is set as the criterion, more people without the disease are excluded, specificity increases, and sensitivity decreases (more with the disease, but lower pressures, are missed). Conversely, as the criterion is lowered, more with the disease are included (sensitivity increases) but at the cost of including more who do not have the disease (specificity decreases).

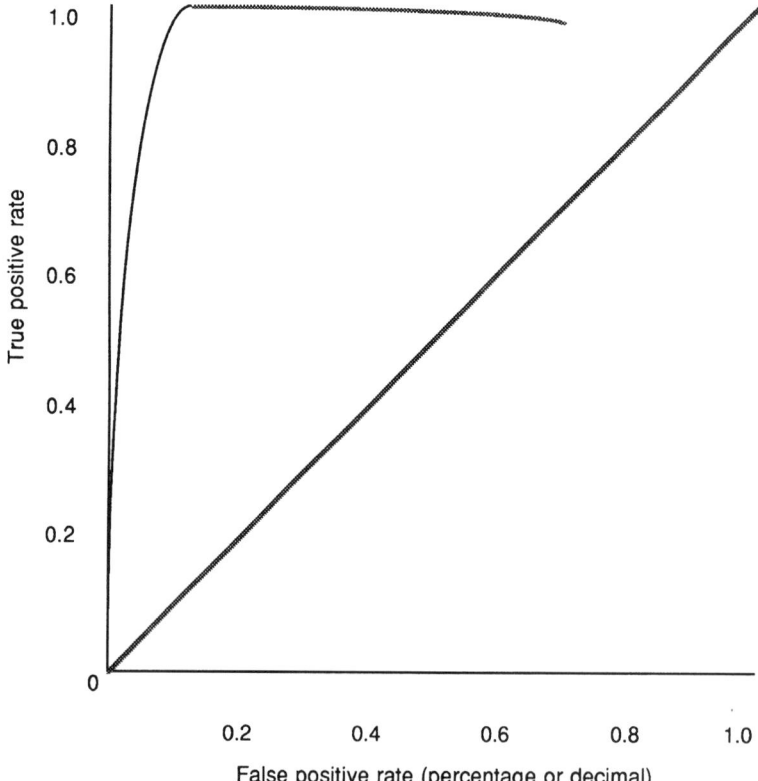

FIGURE 6. The receiver operating curve, with true and false positives.

published in the 18th century. It uses *prior probability*, the probability of an event whose value is known before the current statistical estimation, to calculate a *posterior probability*, a determination that can be made after the calculation. Bayesian analysis is a way of determining the probability of a clinical entity such as illness after knowing that the patient has had a positive test. It considers the sensitivity, false positives, and prior probability.

Cohen's *kappa* is a measurement of agreement between observers. One example is a pair of radiologists looking at films of individuals with exposure to coal or other types of industrial dust. The formula uses the observed agreement minus the chance agreement divided by the quantity of 1 minus chance agreement.[2,10]

Since much medical decision making is being influenced by cost analyses,[21] it behooves the clinician and administrative physician to understand where the information comes from, how it is obtained, and where shortcomings may occur, intentionally or inadvertently. Piatelli-Palmarini discusses preconceived errors in thinking, which may direct results into inappropriate and sometimes unfortunate directions.[41]

Types of Errors

The *type I, alpha* (α) *error* is similar conceptually to a false positive; a difference is stated to be significant where no difference of significance actually exists. It represents an error in stating that the null hypothesis is false, when it is actually true, much like the specificity in a testing situation. One should set this number as small as possible when designing a study so that the likelihood of incorrectly assessing the null hypothesis is small.

The *type II, beta* (β) *error* is similar conceptually to a false negative; no difference is stated to be significant where a significant difference actually exists. It represents an error in stating that the null hypothesis is true, when it is actually false, much like the sensitivity in a testing situation.

Power, $(1 - \beta)$, is the likelihood that the null hypothesis will be rejected appropriately, like the true positive in a testing matrix. It is an assessment of the chance of showing statistically significant differences when they exist. *Power analysis* is a means of assessing the size of a population for a study so that changes of particular statistical significance can be made without including chance as the cause. Even studies with low power[47] may have results that are important for the practice of medicine,[48] despite some statistical weaknesses. Unfortunately, much of what has been practiced in medicine has not been subjected to the same rigorous analysis as newer therapies, which often must prove themselves against a gold standard[5,42] or perhaps fall by the wayside of clinical practice.

Statistical Testing (Table 3)

The *Chi-square test* is a way to measure proportions between two or more groups and then determine whether the difference, if any, is statistically significant. It is a measure of independence and therefore should not be used for the comparison of samples that have an interrelationship. The result is compared to values in a Chi-square table to determine whether the result approaches or exceeds statistical probability. Chi-square, one of the most commonly used statistics in medical research, is used to compare populations to determine differences in some measured variable. When there is confounding, the *Mantel-Haenszel* test may be used.

T testing is a method whereby means of samples or populations, correlation coefficients, or linear regressions can be tested to demonstrate whether the null

TABLE 3. Some Situations Where Certain Tests Might Be Performed

Test	Independent Variable(s)	Dependent Variable
Chi-Square	Nominal data	Nominal data
T test	Nominal or binary data	Numerical data
Regression	Numerical data	Numerical data

Nominal scales are used when the information fits into categories or dichotomous/binary types of observations. It may be described in proportions or as percentage information. Numerical data are the actual quantified data.

hypothesis is supported or if the differences are due to more than chance alone. T testing, because of its ease of use and practicality, has widespread utilization in published research.

Analysis of variance is a statistical analysis that looks at variances within and between various groups under study to enable the researcher to assess whether the differences are related to the groups themselves or to some experimental or other variable.

CONCLUSION

There is a wide field of information concerning epidemiology and biostatistics. This chapter provides an introduction and review of many commonly used concepts.

REFERENCES

1. Bang KM: Applications of occupational epidemiology. Occup Med State Art Rev 11(3):381, 1996.
2. Beam CA, Layde PM, Sullivan DC: Variability in the interpretation of screening mammograms by U.S. radiologists. Findings from a national sample. Arch Int Med 156:209, 1996.
3. Brenner H, Gefeller O: Use of the positive predictive value to correct for disease misclassification in epidemiologic studies. Am J Epidemiol 138:1007, 1993.
4. Brown RA, Beck JS: Medical Statistics on Personal Computers. 2nd ed. Philadelphia, American College of Physicians, 1994.
5. Campbell G: Advances in statistical methodology for the evaluation of diagnostic and laboratory tests. Stat Med 13:499, 1994.
6. Campbell MJ: Statistics at Square One. 9th ed. Philadelphia, American College of Physicians, 1995.
7. Carleton RA: Dichotomous disservice. Ann Intern Med 126:589, 1997.
8. Coggon D, Rose G, Barker DJP: Epidemiology for the Uninitiated. 3rd ed. Philadelphia, American College of Physicians, 1993.
9. Coren S: Left-handedness and accident-related injury risk. Am J Public Health 79:1040, 1989.
10. Dawson-Saunders B, Trapp R: Basic and Clinical Biostatistics. 2nd ed. Norwalk, CT, Appleton & Lange, 1994.
11. Day RA: How to Write and Publish a Scientific Paper. 4th ed. Phoenix, Oryx, 1994.
12. Ellis SJ, Ellis PJ, Marshall E: Hand preference in a normal population. Cortex 24:157, 1988.
13. Ellenberg SS: Biostatistics in clinical trials: Part 2. Determining sample sizes for clinical trials. Oncology 3(8):39, 1989.
14. Elster AD: Use of statistical analysis in the AJR and Radiology: Frequency, methods, and subspecialty differences. AJR 163:711, 1994.
15. Emerson JD, Colditz GA: Use of statistical analysis in The New England Journal of Medicine. N Engl J Med 309:709, 1983.
16. Faraone SV, Tsuang MT: Measuring diagnostic accuracy in the absence of a "gold standard" [review]. Am J Psych 151:650, 1994.
17. Friedman GD: Primer of Epidemiology. 4th ed. New York, McGraw-Hill, 1994.
18. Friedman LM, Furberg CD, DeMets DL: Fundamentals of Clinical Trials. 3rd ed. St. Louis, Mosby, 1996.
19. Geronimus AT, Bound J, Waidmann TA, et al: Excess mortality among blacks and whites in the United States. N Engl J Med 335:1552, 1996.
20. Glass GV: Integrating findings: The meta-analysis of research. In Review of Research in Education. Itasca, Peacock, 1977, pp 351–379.

21. Glassman PA, Model KE, Kahan JP, et al: The role of medical necessity and cost-effectiveness in making medical decisions. Ann Intern Med 126:153, 1997.
22. Griner PF, Mayewski RJ, Mushlin AL, Greenland P: Selection and interpretation of diagnostic tests and procedures. Ann Intern Med 94:553, 1981.
23. Joseph L, Gyorkos TW, Coupal L: Bayesian estimation of disease prevalence and the parameters of diagnostic tests in the absence of a gold standard. Am J Epidemiol 141:263, 1995.
24. Haley RW, Kurt TL, Hom J: Is there a Gulf War Syndrome? Searching for syndromes by factor analysis of symptoms. JAMA 277:215, 1997.
25. Huth EJ: How to Write and Publish Papers in the Medical Sciences. 2nd ed. Baltimore, Williams & Wilkins, 1990.
26. Irwig L, Glasziou PP, Berry G, et al: Efficient study designs to assess the accuracy of screening tests. Am J Epidemiol 140:759, 1994 (erratum in Am J Epidemiol 141:697, 1995).
27. Karras DJ: Statistical methodology: II. Reliability and validity assessment in study design, Part A. Acad Emerg Med 47:64, 1997.
28. Kassirer JP: Clinical trials and meta-analysis: What do they do for us? N Engl J Med 327:273, 1992.
29. Kassirer JP, Kopelman RI: Learning Clinical Reasoning. Baltimore, Williams & Wilkins, 1991.
30. L'Abbé KA, Detsky AS, O'Rourke K: Meta-analysis in clinical research. Ann Intern Med 107:224, 1987.
31. Lang TA, Secic M: How to Report Statistics in Medicine. Annotated Guidelines for Authors, Editors, and Reviewers. Philadelphia, American College of Physicians, 1997.
32. Last JM (ed): A Dictionary of Epidemiology. 2nd ed. New York City, Oxford University Press, 1988.
33. Last JM (ed): Maxcy-Rosenau Public Health and Preventive Medicine. 13th ed. Norwalk, CT, Appleton & Lange, 1992.
34. Maher D, Olkin I: Meta-analysis of randomized controlled trials. A concern for standards. JAMA 274:1962, 1995.
35. Marsh GM: Basic occupational epidemiologic measures. Occup Med State Art Rev 11(3):421, 1996.
36. Morton R, Hebel JR, McCarter R: A Study Guide to Epidemiology and Biostatistics. 4th ed. Gaithersburg, MD, Aspen Publications, 1996.
37. O'Brien PC, Shampo MA: Statistics for clinicians. Mayo Clin Proc, 1982.
38. Paulos JA: A Mathematician Reads the Newspaper. New York City, Basic Books, 1995.
39. Paulos JA: Beyond Numeracy. New York City, Vintage Books, 1991.
40. Paulos JA: Innumeracy. New York City, Vintage Books, 1988.
41. Piattelli-Palmarini M: Inevitable Illusions: How Mistakes of Reason Rule Our Minds. New York, Wiley, 1994.
42. Reed JF, Reed JJ: Analyzing the performance of diagnostic tests. Comput Methods Programs Biomed 42:73, 1994.
43. Riegelman RK, Hirsch RP: Studying a Study and Testing a Test. 3rd ed. Boston, Little, Brown & Co., 1996.
44. Saah AJ, Hoover DR: "Sensitivity" and "specificity" reconsidered: The meaning of these terms in analytical and diagnostic settings. Ann Intern Med 126:91, 1997.
45. Sacks HS, Berrier J, Reitman D, et al: Meta-analysis of randomized controlled trials. N Engl J Med 316:450, 1987.
46. Thompson SG, Pocock SJ: Can meta-analysis be trusted? Lancet 338:1127, 1991.
47. Verdonck LF, vanPutten WLJ, Hagenbeek A, et al: Comparison of CHOP chemotherapy with autologous bone marrow transplantation for slowly responding patients with aggressive non-Hodgkin's lymphoma. N Engl J Med 332:1045, 1995.
48. Walker AM: Low power and striking results—a surprise but not a paradox. N Engl J Med 332:1091, 1995.

INDEX

Entries in **boldface type** indicate complete chapters.

Accelerated-voice test, 440
Acoustic reflex decay test, 444
Acoustic reflex thresholds, 443
Adrenocorticotrophic hormone, stress-related increase of, 559
Afferent visual system, evaluative tests for, **449–464**
  Amsler grid, 459–460
  brightness sense tests, 456–457
  color vision tests, 456
  confrontation visual field tests, 457–459
  contrast sensitivity tests, 460–461
  functional visual loss tests, 461–463
  neutral lens density filter, 451, 452
  photostress recovery test, 457
  pinhole occluder tests, 450–451
  pupil testing, 451–456
  Snellen acuity test, 449–450
African Americans, spirometric reference equations for, 497, 498
Ageusia, 466, 474
Agglutination assays, 577
Air pollution, effect on olfactory sensitivity, 472
Airway hyperresponsiveness testing, 491–493, 502
  use in disability assessment, 505–506
Alanine aminotransferase, as liver disease indicator, 565
Albumin, as liver disease indicator, 566
Alcohol use
  effect on gamma-glutamyl transpeptidase levels, 558, 565
  toxicologic testing for, 573
Alcoholism, 423
Aldosterone, stress-related decrease of, 559
Alkaline phosphatase, as liver disease indicator, 565–566
Alzheimer's disease, 423, 471
Amblyopia, 451
American Academy of Otolaryngology, 438
American Board of Clinical Neuropsychology, 415
American Board of Professional Neuropsychology, 415
American Chemical Society, 575
American Medical Association, *Guides to the Evaluation of Permanent Impairment* of, 498, 503, 538, 547
American National Standards Institute, 434
American Optical Hardy-Rand-Rittler pseudoisochromatic plates, 456

American Psychological Association, 414, 415, 417–418
American Standards Association, 434
Americans with Disabilities Act, 489, 540
American Thoracic Society, 487, 496, 497, 498, 506
American Thyroid Association, 568
Ammonia, serum concentrations of, 560
Amsler grid, 459–460
Analysis of variance, 598
Analytic studies, 588–589
Angiography, equilibrium radionuclide, 521
Ankle/brachial pressure indices, 521
Anosmia, 467, 472
Antibody tests, 577–578
Anticonvulsants, as hypocalcemia cause, 558
Anxiety, assessment in independent medical evaluations, 537
Aortic stenosis, 520
Aphakia, 451
Arithmetic mean, 591
Asbestosis, 502–503
Asian Americans, spirometric reference equations for, 497, 498
Asparate aminotransferase
  exercise-related increase of, 558
  as liver disease indicator, 564
Association, statistical, 591
Asthma
  allergic sensitization, 502, 506
  respiratory function tests for, 501–502
    airway hyperresponsiveness tests, 491–493, 505–506
  for disability evaluation, 505–506, 507, 508
  peak flow measurement, 500
Atrial abnormalities, electrocardiographic assessment of, 514
Attention tests, 427–428
Attributable risk, 590
Audiogram, definition of, 433–434
Audiometry, **433–442**
  components of, 436–439
  continuous frequency, 444
  with electrocochleography, 444–445
  evoked-response, 442, 445–446
  for functional hearing loss, 441–442
  high-frequency, 444
  impedance, 444
  medicolegal aspects of, 438–439
  special test applications of, 440
Auditory-Verbal Learning Test (AVLT), 423–424
Autoantibody assays, 579–580

601

Barbiturates, as hypocalcemia cause, 558
Bayes' theorem, 517, 584n
Bayesian analysis, 594, 597
Beck Depression Inventory, 414, 429
Bias, experimental, 590
"Big pumpkin test," 460
Bilirubin. *See also* Hyperbilirubinemia
  fasting-related increase of, 559
  laboratory tests for, 566, 583n
Biostatistics, 591–598
  correlation, 593
  errors, 597
  measures of central tendency and dispersion, 591–593
  measures of spread, 593
  predictive values, 584n, 593–594, 595
  statistical testing, 597–598
Blindness
  bilateral, tests of, 463
  functional, tests of, 461–463
Blood alcohol concentrations, 573
Blood pressure, during exercise, 516
Blood urea nitrogen (BUN), 561–562
Boeing Corporation, workers' compensation claim applications to, 527
Booklet Category Test, 425
Boston Naming Test, 426
Brain cancer, 423
Brain injury. *See also* Head injury
  academic ability evaluation of, 424
  neuropsychological evaluation of, 426, 429–430
Brainstem evoked-response audiometry, 442, 445–446
Brightness sense, assessment of, 456–457
Bronchoprovocation tests, 492–493, 502
Bronchospasm. *See also* Asthma
  exercise-induced, 493, 495
Bruits, 521, 522
Burning mouth syndrome, 475

Caffeine, effect on catecholamine release, 558
California Verbal Learning Test (CVLT), 423, 424
Candidiasis, oral, 477
Carbamate, exposure to, 573
Carboxyhemoglobin, measurement of, 573
Cardiac function, diagnostic testing of, **513–523**
  with ambulatory monitoring, 515–516
  with echocardiography, 519–521
  with electrocardiography, 513–515
  with exercise stress testing, 516–519
  for vascular diagnosis, 521–522
Cardiac output, during exercise, 516
Carotid disease, 522
Case-control studies, 588
Catarrh, 469
Catecholamines
  caffeine-related increase of, 558
  serum concentrations of, 560
  stress-related increase of, 559
Category test, 425–426

Cause-and-effect relationship, 591
Central limit theorem, 593
Chemical color tests, 571
Chemical spot tests, 571
Chemosensory dysfunction, 465–466. *See also* Olfactory disorders; Taste disorders
Chiasmal disease, diagnosis of, 457–459
Chi-square test, 597, 598
Cholinesterase, measurement of, 573–574
Chorda tympani, injury to, as taste disorder cause, 477, 478
Chromatography, use in toxicologic testing, 571
  gas, 572, 584–585n
  with mass spectrometry, 572, 585n
  high performance liquid, 571, 572
Chymopain injections, as back pain treatment, 451
Claudication, intermittent, 521
Clinical laboratory testing, **557–586**
  analytic issues in, 557–558
  automated complete blood counts, 580–581
  automated multichannel chemistry panels, 581–582
  immune functions tests, 576–580
    autoantibody tests, 579–580
    HIV testing, 578–579
    immunoglobulin tests, 576–577
    specific antibody tests, 577–578
  liver function tests, 563–568
  myocardial injury biomarkers, 568–569
  post-analytic issues in, 558
  pre-analytic issues in, 557, 558–560
  quality control in, 585n
  reference ranges in, 558, 560–561
  renal function blood tests, 561–562
  renal function urine tests, 562–563
  thyroid screening, 568
  toxicologic testing, 570–575
Clinical trials, biostatistics use in, 594
Coefficients of variation and determination, 593
Cognitive Behavior Rating Scales (CBRS), 416
Cohort studies, 588
Color anomia, 456
Color vision, 456
Complete blood counts, automated, 580–581
Concentration tests, 427–428
Confidence intervals, 593
Connecticut Chemosensory Clinical Research Center, 466, 468, 475, 476
Contrast sensitivity, assessment of, 460–461
Controlled Oral Word Association Test (COWAT), 426–427
Coronary artery disease, stress testing for, 517
Cortical evoked-response audiometry, 445
Corticosteroids, as hypocalcemia cause, 558
Cranial nerves, of olfactory and gustatory systems, 466–467
Creatine kinase, exercise-related increase of, 558
Creatine phosphokinase, as myocardial injury marker, 568–569

Creatinine, serum concentration of, 561–562
Cross-sectional studies, 588

Decibels, 434
Dementia, 423, 425
Depression, assessment of, in independent medical evaluations, 536–537
Descriptive studies, 588–589
Diabetes insipidus, nephrogenic, 558
Diagnostic and Statistical Manual of Mental Disorders-IV (DSM-IV), 414
Diffusing capacity of the lung for carbon monoxide (DLCO), 501
  use in disability assessment, 505
  use in pneumonioses assessment, 502, 503
Directory of Occupational Titles, 544–545
Disability
  definition of, 538
  rating systems for, 539
  relationship to depression, 536
Distorted-voice test, 440
Distortion product otoacoustic emissions, 446
Diuretics, thiazide, as hypercalcemia cause, 558
Dobutamine echocardiography, 518–519
Doppler echocardiography, 519
Doppler imaging, use with Duplex scanning, 522
Drug abuse
  clinical laboratory tests for, 584n, 585n
  neuropsychological evaluation of, 425
Drugs, effect on laboratory test results, 558
Duplex scanning, 522
Dyschromatopsia, 456
Dysgeusia, 475
Dysosmia, 467–468
  assessment of, 468–469
  etiologies of, 470
  prognosis of, 473–474
Dyspnea, pulmonary function test evaluation of, 506, 508–509

Echocardiography, 518–520
Elderly persons
  functional capacity evaluation of, 548
  olfactory sensitivity decrease in, 471–472
  taste sensitivity decrease in, 478
Electrical injuries, 430
Electrocardiography (ECG), 513–515
  exercise, 516–517
Electrocochleography, 444–445
Electroimmunodiffusion, 577
Electrophoresis
  immunofixation, 576
  "rocket," 577
  zone, 576
Emmetropia, 450
Emotional functioning, evaluative tests of, 428–429
Emphysema, 502
Endemic, definition of, 588
Endocarditis, echocardiographic evaluation of, 520

Enzyme immunoassay (EIA), 577, 578
  use in HIV testing, 578–579
Epidemic, definition of, 588
Epidemiology, 587–591
Equilibrium radionuclide angiography, 521
Errors
  in clinical laboratory test results, 559–560
  statistical, 597
Estrogens, as hypercalcemia cause, 558
Ethylenediamine tetraacetic acid (EDTA), 559–560
Eustachian tube tests, 444
Evoked-response audiometry, 442, 445–446
Exercise, effect on laboratory test results, 558
Exercise electrocardiography, 516–517
Exercise stress testing
  cardiac, 516–519
  pulmonary, 487, 493–495
    for disability assessment, 505
    for pneumonioses evaluation, 502, 503
Experimental studies, 589

Facial nerve test, 444
False-negatives/false-positives, 584n, 593, 594, 596
Farnsworth Dichotomous Test for Color Blindness, 456
Finger Tapping Test, 427
Fistula test, 444
Flame photometry, 575
Forced expiratory volume in one second (FEV_1)
  in airway hyperresponsiveness testing, 492, 493
  in pulmonary exercise testing, 494
  in spirometry, 498, 499, 500
Forced expiratory volume in one second (FEV_1)/forced vital capacity (FVC) ratio, 500, 503
Forced vital capacity (FVC)
  in lung volume measurement, 490, 491
  in pneumonioses, 502–503
  in spirometry, 499, 500
Frank-Starling mechanism, 516
Functional capacity evaluation (FCE), 543–549, 551–556
  medicolegal considerations in, 548
  purpose of, 543–545
  of special populations, 548
  strength assessment in, 546–547
  as work capacity evaluation (WCE), 546, 547–548

Gamma-glutamyl transferase, drug interactions of, 558
Gamma-glutamyl transpeptidase, as liver disease indicator, 565
Gastrin, as hypocalcemia cause, 558
Gaussian curve, 592
Geometric mean, 591
Gilbert syndrome, 559, 566, 583n
Glasgow Coma Scale, 429
Glaucoma, 450

Globulin, as liver disease indicator, 567
Glomerular filtration rate, 561
Glomus tumor, 444
Glucagon, as hypocalcemia cause, 558
Glucocorticoids, stress-related increase of, 559
Gonadotropins
  exercise-related decrease of, 558
  stress-related decrease of, 559
Gustatory system. *See also* Taste disorders
  anatomy of, 466–467

Hair analysis, toxicologic, 572–573
Halstead-Reitan Neuropsychological Battery (HRNB), 419–420, 425, 427
Handicap, definition of, 538
Hardy-Rand-Rittler pseudoisochromatic plates, 456
Head injury
  neuropsychological evaluation of, 425, 429–430
  as olfactory disorder cause, 471, 473
  as taste disorder cause, 477
Hearing, normal, 435
Hearing loss
  functional, tests for, 441–442
  occupational, 433
Heart murmurs, echocardiographic evaluation of, 520
Heart rate, during exercise, 516
Helium dilution method, of lung volume measurement, 490–491, 502
Hematocrit, as automated complete blood count parameter, 580–581
Hemianopia, homonymous, 449
Hemoglobin, as automated complete blood count parameter, 580, 581
Hemolysis, induced, 559
Hepatitis, viral, tests for, 567–568
Histamine challenge test, 492–493
Holter monitoring, 515
Hooper Visual Organization Test (HVOT), 425
Hospitalization, as blood lipid studies contraindication, 559
Human figure drawings, 429
Human immunodeficiency virus (HIV) antibody testing, 578–579
Huntington's disease, neuropsychological evaluation of, 423, 425
Hyperbilirubinemia, 565, 566
Hypercalcemia, drug-induced, 558
Hyperkalemia, artifactual, 560
Hypocalcemia, drug-induced, 558
Hypogeusia, 474
  zinc treatment for, 477–478
Hyposmia, 467, 473–474

Immune function, tests of, 576–580
  autoantibody tests, 579–580
  HIV antibody test, 578–579
  immunoblogulin tests, 576–577
  specific antibody tests, 577–578

Immune tolerance, loss of, 579–580
Immunoassays, use in toxicologic testing, 571
Immunodiffusion, Ouchterlony, 577
Immunoelectrophoresis, 576
  "counter," 577
Immunofluorescence, indirect, 577–578
Immunoglobulins, tests for, 576–577
Impairment, definition of, 538
Incidence, definition of, 587
Independent medical evaluation, **525–542**
  causality determination in, 539
  definition of, 525
  diagnosis formation in, 537–541
  examination in, 530, 533–537
  history taking in, 531–533
  impairment rating in, 538–539
  initial encounter in, 528–531
  legal aspects of, 526, 527, 531, 532
  maximal medical improvement determination in, 540–451
  medical records review in, 527, 528, 529
  report based on, 541–542
  return-to-work prediction based on, 540
  workers' compensation issue of, 532–533, 539
Insulin, as hypocalcemia cause, 558
Intelligence tests, 417, 420–422
Intermittent claudication, 521
International Neuropsychological Society, 415
Interrupted-voice test, 440
Intraocular pressure, 596
Ipsilateral reflex test, 444
Ischemic heart disease, perfusion imaging of, 518
Isokinetic strength assessment, in functional capacity evaluations, 546–547

Jaffé reaction, 560
Jaundice, posthepatic, 566
Job capacity evaluation, 546
Job descriptions, 544–545

Kallman syndrome, 472
Kappa (interobserver agreement measure), 597
Katz Adjustment Scale-Relative's Form (KAS-R), 416–417
Kauffman Test of Academic Achievement (KTEA), 424
Korsakoff's syndrome, 423

Laboratory testing. *See* Clinical laboratory testing
Lacate, serum concentrations of, 560
Lactate dehydrogenase, exercise-related increase of, 558
Language ability, evaluative tests of, 426–427
Lipoprotein
  low-density, 559
  very-low-density, 559
Lithium, 558
Liver function tests, 563–567
Lombard test, 441
Lung, "stiff," 502

INDEX 605

Lung volume, measurement of, 490–491
  in pneumoconioses, 502
Luria-Nebraska Neuropsychological Battery
    (LNNB), 418–419, 420

Magnesium salts, as hypocalcemia cause, 558
Magnetic resonance imaging (MRI), cardiac, 521
Malingering, 537
  brainstem evoked-response audiometry in, 442
  effect on neuropsychological test interpretation,
    418
Mantel-Haenszel test, 597
Manual muscle test (MMT), in independent
    medical evaluations, 533, 535–536
Maximal medical improvement (MMI),
    determination by independent medical
    evaluation, 540–541
Mayo Clinic, 582
Mean cell hemoglobin concentration (MCHC),
    580–581
Mean cell volume of red cells (MCV), 580–581
Mean platelet volume (MPV), 580, 581
Median, 591
Medical records, use in independent medical
    evaluations, 527, 528, 529
Memory tests, 422–423
Mental status examination, 414
Meta-analysis, 590
Metals exposure, toxicologic analysis of, 574–575
Methacholine challenge test, 492–493
Methadone maintenance programs, drug testing
    in, 571
Methemoglobin, measurement of, 574
Methicillin, as hypocalcemia cause, 558
Middle latency responses, 445
Mini Mental State examination, 414
Minnesota Multiphasic Personality Inventory
    (MMPI), 428–429, 532
Mitral valve prolapse, 520
M-mode echocardiography, 519
Mode, statistical, 591
Monell-Jefferson Chemosensory Clinical
    Research Center, 466, 468–469, 471,
    473–474
Motor tests, 427
MUGA (multiple gated acquisition) scans, 521
Multiple sclerosis, 423, 425
Musculoskeletal disorders, independent medical
    evaluation of
  causality determination in, 539
  diagnosis formation in, 537–541
  examination in, 530, 533–537
  history taking in, 531–533
  impairment rating in, 538–539
  initial encounter in, 528–531
  legal aspects of, 526, 527, 531, 532
  medical records review in, 527, 528, 529
  report based on, 541–542
  return-to-work prediction based on, 540
Myocardial infarction
  biochemical markers for, 568–569

Myocardial infarction (*cont.*)
  electrocardiographic assessment of, 514–515
  stress testing after, 517
Myocardial injury, biochemical markers for,
    568–569
Myocardial ischemia, electrocardiographic
    assessment of, 514
Myocardium, perfusion imaging of, 517–518
Myopia, 451

Nasal/sinus disease, as olfactory disorder cause,
    469, 470, 471, 472–473
National Academy of Neuropsychology, 415
National Academy of Sciences, 438
National Institute for Occupational Safety and
    Health (NIOSH), 497
National Research Council, 438
Nephelometry, 577
Neuritis, optic, 450, 460–461
Neurologic evaluation, differentiated from
    neuropsychological evaluation, 414
Neuropsychological evaluation, **413–432**
  definition of, 413
  differentiated from psychiatric and neurologic
    evaluations, 414
  specific tests in, 418–429
Neuropsychological Status Examination, 417
Neuropsychological Symptom Checklist (NSC),
    417
Neuropsychologists
  board certification of, 415
  definition of, 414
  referral sources of, 413, 416
Neurotoxins, occupational, 423
Neutral lens density filter, 451, 452
Nicotine, effect on glucose metabolism, 558
Null hypothesis, 589

Observational studies, 589
Obstructive airway disease, spirometry-based
    diagnosis of, 489
Occupational Safety and Health Act, 433
Occupational Safety and Health Administration
    (OSHA), 434, 488, 497
Odds ratio, 589
Olfactory disorders, 465–474
  aging-related, 471–472
  assessment of, 468–469
  etiologies of, 469–472
  prognosis for, 472–474
Olfactory system, anatomy of, 466–467
Optic nerve disease
  characteristics of, 452
  differentiated from retinal disease, 452–456
Oral contraceptives, effect on thyroid function test
    results, 558
Organophosphate pesticides, exposure to, 573
Otoacoustic emissions, 446
Over-the-counter drugs, effect on laboratory test
    results, 558
Oxygen consumption, maximal, 504–505

Paced Auditory Serial Addition Test (PASAT), 428
Pain assessment
 in functional capacity evaluations, 552
 in independent medical evaluations, 530, 531–532
Pandemic, definition of, 588
Paranasal sinuses, in olfactory dysfunction, 469
Parkinson's disease, 423
Parosmia, 467
Peabody Individual Achievement Test (PIAT), 424
Peak expiratory flow measurements
 of airway function variability, 492
 at worksite, 506
Peak expiratory flow meters, 500
Perfusion imaging, myocardial, 517–518
Peripheral vascular disese, evaluation of, 521–522
Personality tests, 428–429
Phantogeusia, 475, 476–477
Phantosmia, 467–468
 assessment of, 469, 476
 etiologies of, 470
Phenothiazines, effect on thyroid function test results, 558
Photostress recovery test, 457
Physical volume test, 443
Pinhole occluder, 450–451
Platelet count, 580, 581
 relationship to serum and plasma potassium concentration, 560
Plethysmography, 502
 body, 491
Pneumoconioses
 coal workers', 503
 radiographic evaluation of, 502, 503
 respiratory function tests for, 501, 502–504, 508–509
Poisson distribution, 592–593
Postconcussion syndrome, 429
Posture, effect on laboratory test results, 559
Potassium, concentration in serum and plasma, 560
Power analysis, 597
Predictive values, 584n, 593–594, 595
Prevalence, 595
 definition of, 587–588
Problem-solving ability, evaluative tests of, 425–426
Projective tests, 429
Promontory stimulation, 445
Proportional mortality rate (PMR), 588
Prosopagnosia, 456
Prospective studies, 588
Prothrombin times, 566
Pseudocholinesterase, 573–574
Psychiatric evaluation, differentiated from neuropsychological evaluation, 414
Psychological evaluation
 differentiated from neuropsychological evaluation, 414
 in independent medical evaluations, 536–537

Pulmonary function testing. *See* Respiratory function testing
Pupil testing, 451–456

Radial immunodiffusion, 576–577
Radiographic records, use in independent medical evaluations, 527
Radiography, for pneumoconioses diagnosis, 502, 503
Range, statistical, 592
Range-of-motion testing, in independent medical evaluations, 533–535
Rates, epidemiological, 588
Reasoning tests, 425–426
Receiver operating curves, 489, 594, 596
Red blood cell (RBC) count, 580
Red cell distribution width (RDW), 580–581
Reflex sympathetic dystrophy, independent medical examination of, 526
Regression analysis, 598
Relative afferent pupillary defect (RAPD) testing, 452–456
Relative risk, 589
Reliability, statistical, 589–590
Renal function tests, 561–563
 blood tests, 561–562
 urine tests, 562–563
Renin, serum concentrations of, 560
Reproducibility, statistical, 589–590
Respiratory functions, occupational, 487
Respiratory function testing, **485–512**
 algorithms for test selection in, 507–509
 applications of, 501–507
 purposes of, 485–489
 specific test procedures of, 487–488, 490–501
  airway hyperresponsiveness testing, 491–493, 502, 505–506
  diffusing capacity of the lung for carbon monoxide, 501, 502, 503, 505
  exercise testing, 487, 493–495, 502, 503, 505
  lung volume measurement, 490–491, 502
  peak expiratory flow measurements, 492, 500, 506
  spirometry, 487, 489, 495–500, 501–502, 503, 505, 506
 for work ability and disability assessment, 503–506, 508
Respiratory system, components of, 485–486
Retinal diseases, pupil testing for, 455
Retinal nerve dysfunction, characteristics of, 452
Retinitis pigmentosa, 450
Retrochiasmal visual pathway disorders, 450
Retrospective studies, 588–589
Revised Token Test, 427
Rey-Osterrieth Complex Figure Test (ROCFT), 423, 424
Rhinitis, allergic, 465, 466, 469–470
Rorschach test, 429

Scotoma, 449, 458, 459, 460
Seizure disorders, 423

Sensitivity, of tests, 593
  of respiratory function tests, 488–489, 507
Sensory evaluation tests, 427
Sensory-Perceptual Examination, 427
Sex hormones, exercise-related decrease of, 558
Significant Others' Questionnaire, 417
Silicosis, 501
Simultanagnosia, 456
Single photon emission computed tomography (SPECT), for ischemic heart disease evaluation, 518
Smell disorders. *See* Olfactory disorders
Smokers, carboxyhemoglobin levels in, 573
Snellen acuity, qualitative, 449–450
Social Security Disability rating system, 549
Somatoform disorder, 537
Sound localization tests, 440
Specificity, of tests, 593
  of respiratory function tests, 488–489, 507
Spectrophotometry, 571
  atomic absorption, 575
Spectroscopy, inductively coupled plasma atomic emission, 575
Speech reception threshold, 437
Spirometry, 487, 489, 495–500
  for airway function variability assessment, 492–493
  appropriate use of, 496
  for asthma evaluation, 501–502
  BTPS (body temperature, pressure, and water saturation) factor in, 496
  for disability assessment, 505
  equipment and personnel for, 496–497
  for gas exchange assessment, 505
  for pneumoconioses evaluation, 502, 503
  software for, 499–500
  test performance and interpretation in, 497–499
  for ventilatory mechanics assessment, 505
  use at worksite, 506
Standard deviation, 592
Standard error of the mean, 592
Stapedius reflex tests, 440
Static compliance, 443
Stenger test, 441–442
Strength assessment, in functional capacity evaluations, 546–547
Stroke, 423
Sulfhemoglobin, measurement of, 574
Symbol Digit Modalities Test, 425
Symptom Checklist-90-Revised, 429
Symptom magnification, 537

Taste disorders, 465–467, 474–479
  assessment of, 475–476
  etiologies of, 476–478
  prognosis of, 478–479
  terminology of, 474–475
Test results, biostatistical accuracy of, 593
Tetracycline, as hypocalcemia cause, 558
Thematic Apperception Test (TAT), 429
Thyroid function tests, 558, 583n

Thyroid hormones, stress-related decrease of, 559
Thyroid screening, 568
Tinnitus matching, 444
Token Test, Revised, 427
Total lung capacity, 490, 491
Tourniquets, as artifactual hemoconcentration cause, 559
Toxic exposure, neuropsychological evaluation of, 425, 430
Toxicologic testing, 570–575
  specific tests, 573–575
  techniques of, 571–572
Trace metals exposure, toxicologic analysis of, 574–575
Trail Making Test, 424–425, 427
Transesophageal echocardiography, 519–520
Transient event detection, 515–516
Transthoracic echocardiography, 520
Troponin, as myocardial injury marker, 568–569
T testing, 597–598
Tuning fork tests, 436, 437
Tympanometry, 443

Ultrasound, vascular, 522
University of Pennsylvania Smell and Taste Center, 466, 468, 475, 476, 478
Upper respiratory tract infections
  as olfactory disorder cause, 470, 473, 474
  as taste disorder cause, 477
Uric acid, exercise-related increase of, 558
Urinalysis
  for renal function evaluation, 562–563
  six Cs of, 562–563
  use in toxicologic testing, 572
Urine, bilirubin content of, 566

Validity, statistical, 589–590
Variance, 592
Vascular disease, diagnostic techniques for, 521–522
Vasoconstriction, during exercise, 516
Ventricular hypertrophy, electrocardiographic assessment of, 514
Ventricular tachycardia, 515
Verbal Fluency for F-A-S test, 426–427
Visual field testing, confrontation, 457–459
Visual loss. *See* Blindness
Visual perception tests, 424–425
Vitamin A, as hypercalcemia cause, 558
Vitamin D, as hypercalcemia cause, 558
Voice-reflex test, 441

Weber test, 436
Wechsler Adult Intelligence Scale-Revised (WAIS-R), 420, 421–422
Wechsler Intelligence Scales (WIS), 420–423, 427
Wechsler Memory Scale-Revised (WMS-R), 422–423
Wenckebach phenomena, 515
Western blot antibody test, 578, 579
White blood cell (WBC) count, 580, 581

Wide Range Achievement Test (WRAT), 424
Wisconsin Card Sorting Test (WCST), 426
Work capacity evaluation (WCE), 546, 547–548
Workers' compensation
   injury causality determination for, 539
   as independent medical evaluation issue, 532–533, 539
Work sample, 546

Worksite, respiratory function testing at, 506, 508
Work tolerance screen, 546

Xerostomia, as taste disorder cause, 476–477, 478

Zinc supplmentation, as hypogeusia treatment, 477–478
Z transformation, 592